Teaching Deaf and Hard of Hearing Students

Teaching Deaf and Hard of Hearing Students

Content, Strategies, and Curriculum

David A. Stewart

Michigan State University

Thomas N. Kluwin

Gallaudet University

Allyn and Bacon

Boston • London • Toronto • Sydney • Tokyo • Singapore

Executive Editor: *Stephen Dragin*
Editorial Assistant: *Barbara Strickland*
Editorial-Production Administrator: *Joe Sweeney*
Editorial-Production Service: *Walsh & Associates, Inc.*
Composition Buyer: *Linda Cox*
Manufacturing Buyer: *Chris Marson*

Copyright © 2001 by Allyn & Bacon
A Pearson Education Company
160 Gould Street
Needham Heights, MA 02494

www.abacon.com

Library of Congress Cataloging-in-Publication Data

Stewart, David Alan, 1954–
    Teaching deaf and hard of hearing students : content, strategies, and curriculum
      p. cm.
    Includes bibliographical references and index.
    ISBN 0-205-30768-X
    1. Deaf children—Education.   I. Kluwin, Thomas N.   II. Title.
  HV2437 .S74 2000
  371.91'2—dc21   00-063951

Printed in the United States of America
10 9 8 7 6 5 4 3 2 1   05 04 03 02 01

CONTENTS

5 **Teaching Deaf Studies**   **112**

6 **Teaching Mathematics**   **136**

7 **Teaching Physical Education and Extracurriculars**   **157**

PREFACE

We want teachers to form an image of what it is like to teach deaf children. Ideally, this image would be fluid and one that will be shaped and reshaped by the students these teachers have in their classrooms. This fluidity is a reflection of the heterogeneity that deaf children bring to the classroom, the changes in our understanding of the pedagogy of teaching subject matter, and each teacher's growing experiences in the classroom.

The heterogeneity of deaf children is, perhaps, the most complex factor affecting how they learn best and consequently how they are taught. Even in a small class of five students, a range of characteristics may be exhibited in degree of hearing loss; cognition; exposure to experiences that are intellectually stimulating; interactions with others using an effective form of communication; degree, type, and amount of communication experienced at home; ability to learn in a traditional classroom setting; propensity to be distracted; existence of other disabilities; and more.

An image of teaching deaf children that consciously addresses this heterogeneity will help teachers adapt instruction that optimizes each student's opportunity for learning. Thus, one key component of an image of teaching that we are proposing is versatility. This does not mean that every lesson caters to the characteristics of each student—although in some teaching situations, this might be a viable option. More generally, versatility means that teachers use a variety of instructional tools, resources, classroom management techniques, and communication strategies to ensure that the students in their classes have access to meaningful learning experiences.

To help in the formation of a teacher's image of teaching deaf students, we offer this book as a guide about how to teach various subject matter and how to shape instruction that will address the diversity inherent in even a small group of deaf students.

Six chapters of this book cover subject matter teaching in the areas of science, social studies, literacy, mathematics, Deaf Studies, and physical education. Each chapter is a blend of theory and practices, with a heavy emphasis on the pragmatic aspects of teaching each of these subjects. Each chapter addresses the special considerations that teachers face when teaching a particular subject to deaf students. For the most part, these considerations are framed in such a manner that they are applicable across all grade levels. For example, discussion of vocabulary building as a component of effective instruction can benefit teachers at all grade levels as well as across all subject matter. Thus, teachers at the elementary, middle, and high school levels will find the information contained in each chapter to be applicable to teaching their students.

Associated with teaching various subjects are issues that cut across all subject areas. These include issues relating to testing, the use of technology, ethnic and cultural diversity in the classroom, and classroom management. It also includes issues associated with the different types of teaching situations that teachers can find themselves in, such as teaching in a school for the deaf, a separate classroom in a public school, a resource room, or in an itinerant/teacher consultant position. Separate chapters are devoted to each of these issues.

Another important issue is transition. Traditionally viewed as something schools did to help nontraditional students, IDEA '97 (Individuals with Disabilities Education Act of 1997) stipulates that all students with disabilities receive transition planning at 16 years of age and earlier, if necessary. Furthermore, transition is no longer relegated to the placement of students in vocational education programs or sheltered workshops. It entails that schools take a comprehensive view of how to prepare students for post-school activities, including preparation for college and university studies, participating in the community, and using adult services such as those provided by state rehabilitation and interpreting agencies.

Finally, involvement of parents in the learning process is important if deaf children will be given the opportunity to make the best of their school years. Our last chapter describes what teachers can do to help parents understand the challenges that their children face in learning and lays out some strategies that parents can use to help their children overcome these challenges. A foremost responsibility of parents is to engage their children in meaningful learning experiences around the house and in the community that will facilitate the acquisition of language and help build children's knowledge base that is critical to the acquisition of new concepts.

In sum, this book is about what teachers can do to help deaf students achieve success in school. It is a book that is mostly about the practice of teaching. In the science chapter, for example, we make the assumption that what teachers know about teaching science to hearing children in general can be applied to deaf children. Thus, our focus was to examine specific challenges associated with teaching science to deaf students and then describe how lesson plans can be developed that address these challenges.

Another key aspect of the book is that it contains a range of teaching practices that are applicable across all subject matter teaching. However, we do not repeat discussions of these practices in each of our subject matter chapters because the principle for applying the practice in one area can be transferred to another area. Thus, the reader is encouraged to read all of the chapters to glean ideas for teaching any subject to deaf students.

This book was a major undertaking and the content reflects our total of over fifty years of involvement in the teaching of deaf children in a variety of capacities. These experiences include teaching deaf children in a self-contained classroom at a school for the deaf, researching how other teachers teach deaf children, examination of the communication strategies used by teachers, surveying over a thousand teachers of the deaf in public schools, working with parents of deaf children, and preparing teachers of the deaf at the university level. We alone, however, could not have put together this book without the invaluable directions and feedback of our colleagues in the field, both at the school and university levels of teaching. To these people we give our profound thanks: Glenn Anderson, Stephen Butterfield, Susan Dickinson, Vincent Daniels, Kathleen Ellis, Michael Karchmer, Harry Lang, Carol LaSasso, Diane Little, Donald F. Moores, Martin Noretsky, and Alison Sandberg. We would also like to thank the reviewers of this book, James C. Blair of Utah State University and Jack Foreman of The University of Tulsa, for their time and effort.

1 Teaching Deaf Children: Characteristics and Themes

CHAPTER OUTCOMES

After reading this chapter, you should be able to:

1. Describe how characteristics of deaf students can affect their learning.
2. Describe the different types of teaching situations for teachers of the deaf.
3. Describe the relationship of the four recurring themes of this book to teaching deaf students.

Here is one way some deaf high school students learn about frogs: In a laboratory they dissect a frog, identify parts of the body and internal organs, study the function of various parts of the body, and take a written test to see how well they have memorized information about parts of a frog and their respective functions. The teacher will lecture, and the students will use their science textbooks to gather information pertaining to the science experiment. The lesson is very much a routine for the students. They might talk to one another during the dissection but in general each student works independently.

Let's redesign the above lesson, but this time incorporate a student-centered approach to teaching science; one that empowers the students in the learning process. In this new lesson, a class is divided into small groups of two to three students. A list of instructional objectives related to dissecting a frog and learning about the functions of various parts of its body is given to each student. Two examples of objectives are "the student will demonstrate how to make a clean dissection of a frog that will reveal the leg muscles," and "the student will describe how muscle mass is related to the leaping ability of frogs." With assistance from the teacher, each group decides upon a strategy for meeting the objectives. The students can use any resources to help them gather information pertaining to the experiment. Rather than a written test, an alternative assessment strategy is used whereby the students are required to demonstrate mastery of the instructional objectives by putting together a presentation about frogs. Criteria for evaluating this presentation are shared with the students.

The redesigned lesson aims to facilitate learning by incorporating the following concepts:

1. *Awareness.* Students are informed at the beginning of the experiment what they are expected to do (i.e., the list of objectives that is passed out) and the criteria for success (e.g., a presentation about frogs that can be understood by peers).
2. *Cooperative learning.* Students work with each other to plan how they are going to meet the objectives of the lesson.
3. *Science talk.* Each student is given an opportunity to talk about science—what they are doing, what they are observing—to their group partners.
4. *Language experiences.* By engaging in science talk, the students should be better prepared to write about the science experiment.
5. *Empowerment.* Each group develops a strategy for dissecting the frog, identifying parts, and gathering information about the functions of different parts of the body.
6. *Engagement.* Students can use a variety of resources to gather information, including any type of reading material (e.g., books about frogs, textbooks, magazine articles, encyclopedias, and web sites). The key is that the students make the decision about what they think would serve as the best source(s) of information for them to use.
7. *Socialization.* Students have opportunities to interact in a socially acceptable manner that is conducive to the group completing the task on hand.
8. *Portfolio assessment.* By creating a presentation, the students are able to select the manner of presentation in which they feel most comfortable. Included in this selection process are the format of the presentation and the mode of communication (e.g., one student might feel most comfortable with a presentation that is essentially written while another student might prefer to make a presentation in American Sign Language).

The redesigned lesson encourages **deaf students** to learn in a multitude of ways while they also attend to and direct the learning process. For deaf students this type of lesson helps them in a number of ways, for example, development of language skills through the use of cooperative learning strategies—students must use vocabulary and sentence structures that will be understood by others; students demonstrate their knowledge according to their strengths in using various forms of communication; and students have a chance to listen to others talk about science in a small group and in so doing refine their own thoughts about the concepts they are learning.

In a sense, what the redesigned lesson does is help deaf students access science-related content and concepts through greater involvement in the learning process. This book is about designing instructional activities that are appropriate for teaching deaf students. It is not, however, a textbook about the theoretical underpinnings of best practices. Nor is it a listing of good teaching principles gleaned from an extensive review of the literature. This information is extensively covered in the literature (see the box titled "Principles of Effective Teaching"). What we have done is to use our understanding of the literature on research and teaching, our experiences as teachers, and our years of observations of teaching practices to put together this pragmatic book about how to teach deaf students.

What Is a Deaf Student Like?

When we talk about deaf students, we are talking about any student who has a degree of hearing loss severe enough to adversely affect his or her learning. In this group we include those students who are referred to in the literature as being **hard of hearing, deaf, hearing impaired**, and **Deaf** (i.e., those students who use sign language as their primary means of communication and have some affiliation with the Deaf community). This book is not geared to any particular type of method of communication; the information provided herein can be applied to the teaching of all deaf children irrespective of the mode and language of communication they use.

Kluwin and Stinson (1993) described several different types of deaf students based on their longitudinal study of deaf students in local public school programs:

1. Students with moderate hearing loss, intelligible speech, above average achievement, and placed in a general classroom without an interpreter.
2. Students reading on grade level with a more severe hearing loss but have intelligible speech and use assistive listening devices and an interpreter.
3. Profoundly deaf student who are reading below grade level who have a mix of placements. These students prefer signs but will use speech as appropriate.
4. Less able students with severe hearing loss whose family has never adjusted or responded to the diagnosis of the hearing loss. These students read considerably below grade level.

Students in each of these categories can also be found in schools for deaf children.

Variation occurs when we include the student's race or the family's educational level or economic situation. In addition, further delineation can be made based on whether a student has deaf or hearing parents. Deaf children will also experience different communication philosophies, friendship patterns, and history of placement situations. These differences, along with the age at onset of deafness, the age of the diagnosis of the child's hearing loss, the availability of early services, and the family's response to those services, influence how the child performs in school.

Family Traits and School Success

Families are an integral part of the education of any child, but because deaf education is built on a model of early intervention with the family, the family and its response to the diagnosis take on special significance. The family directly influences the child's eventual success in a number of ways, including by its physical and economic resources, overall emotional support, emotional climate, life and career expectations, and values toward education (Kluwin & Gaustad, 1992).

Of critical importance is primarily the mother's role in the education of the deaf child. That influence includes the quality of the physical care of the child; the handling of communication issues, such as involvement in auditory training and learning to sign; and leading the rest of the family in communicating with the deaf child (Kluwin & Gaustad, 1991). Families that have two parents who share values about the education of the deaf child tend to be more effective in producing academically successful deaf children than other types of families.

A combination of high parental expectations for success and specific parental behavior, such as checking homework and taking children to appointments as well as to cultural events, factors into the equation for producing successful children. The extent to which parents support achievement as well as their expectations of academic success predict much of a deaf child's success in school (Bodner-Johnson, 1986; Kluwin & Gaustad, 1992). Parents who adapt their behavior to the child's deafness bolster this support. For profoundly deaf children, this could mean learning sign language and exposing the child and the other members of the family to contact with the Deaf community. For many deaf children, it means that the parents make use of technology such as assistive listening devices, captioned TV, home computers, and captioned videos.

Social Class, Income, and Education.   Social class, which is often confounded with race or language in the United States and Canada, can mitigate or exacerbate the effects of deafness on the education of a child. Affluent families, because of access to health insurance and better health care, can reduce the incidence of some etiologies of deafness, for example, otitis media infections. Or they can reduce the severity of the condition through better access to assistive devices or prosthetics such as cochlear implants. Access to maintenance antibiotics or surgery to drain fluids in the middle ear can eliminate mild degenerative hearing losses. Greater access to medical care and medical services also can lead to earlier diagnosis and the start of medical therapy, if applicable, and educational programming.

Family income is systematically related to social class, and we mentioned above how income and social class together can impact deafness primarily because of access to health care. Family income and social class are also related to the parent's educational level because as the parental education level rises, so does income and social class. Parents who not only espouse high educational expectations but also act on those expectations produce children who do better in school. Across cultures and time periods, the mother's educational level is the most consistent predictor of a deaf child's success in school; this is true for both deaf and hearing mothers (Bodner-Johnson, 1986; Kluwin & Gaustad, 1992).

Communication Practices Within the Family.   Communication options for families of deaf children are varied. Some of the more common options include one or more of the following: speech (English or a second language commonly spoken in the home such as Spanish), audition, sign communication (American Sign Language, contact signing, or various formal types of English signing), fingerspelling, or cued speech. Moores, Kluwin, and Mertens (1985) studied communication practices among 176 deaf adolescents in local public schools from three cities across the United States and reported 175 unique family communication patterns. Combinations included mother, father, and hearing siblings who spoke to the deaf child who in turn spoke to them; single and married mothers who used signs; and various combinations of sibling communication patterns. Kluwin and Gaustad (1992) conducted a follow-up study but used a different set of definitions to classify family patterns. They found two dozen combinations of communication behavior in over 200 families.

Beyond the issue of varied communication modes and language in the home, there is the question of the impact of various communication decisions on the deaf child and on other family members. Vernon and Andrews (1990) described a tendency for hearing siblings to turn outward from the family or relationships with some member of the family when the family's choice of communication makes it difficult, if not impossible, for these siblings to interact with the deaf child in a meaningful way. This can occur when a family that decides to use speech makes it difficult for the deaf child to communicate with other members of the family. Conversely, a family that decides to focus on sign communication may make it difficult for a hearing parent or sibling who does not acquire proficient signing skills. Another unfortunate outcome occurs when the mother acquires the role as the family interpreter for the deaf child. This role compounds the stress on her role as a mother to the deaf child and to the hearing children in the family.

The role of the mother in developing a functional family communication system cannot be emphasized enough. The mother's choices, however, are impacted by several factors, including the degree of the child's hearing loss and the mother's educational level. This means that these factors enter into the prediction of the academic success of a deaf child at more than one point. For example, the greatest influence on the decision of the father and sibling to learn to sign is the mother's use of signs (Kluwin & Gaustad, 1992).

Educational Experiences. In the next section of this chapter, we describe the different teaching options you will have as a teacher of the deaf. These options translate into a variety of educational experiences for a deaf child. Educational placement is a key option, and there have been changes over time for a variety of reasons (Moores, 1992). In general, about one in four or five deaf children will be in a school for the deaf; however, only half of those will be living at the school. This number typically does not include those children who have a mild or moderate hearing loss. These children are essentially hard of hearing and are placed in the general education classroom. The rest of the children will be in local public schools, but only about half of those children will have had any significant contact with hearing children (Kluwin & Stinson, 1993). The other half will be in self-contained or separate special education classes where the students are all deaf or there may be a few hearing students with other special education labels.

Children's abilities and parents' changing understanding of the effect of deafness on learning combine to produce complex combinations of educational experiences. There has never been a time during which all deaf children attended one type of program (Moores, 1992), and many children have experienced more than one program. Therefore, teachers can expect to encounter children who have been through a number of placement situations and communication philosophies. According to Kluwin and Stinson (1993), they can range from students who spend all of their years of education in a school for the deaf to children entering high school who have been in eight different educational settings in eight years.

What Is It Like Being a Teacher of the Deaf?

The education of deaf children in the United States and Canada is every bit as diverse as the general education systems. There are public, private, or parochial schools. In addition, teachers of the deaf could find themselves in a school for the deaf, in either a residential or a day program. It is possible that as a teacher you could spend your entire career in one school in a small town or ride the subway in a big city from one school to another. The common view is the teacher who teaches in a school for the deaf where all of the students have a severe to profound degree of hearing loss. Indeed, this has been the case for much of the past two centuries.

However, before the establishment of the American School for the Deaf in Hartford in 1817—a landmark recognized as the starting point for the formal education of deaf students in the United States—the education of deaf students was a sporadic affair marked by isolated tutorial situations such as the plantation school that was the predecessor to the Virginia School for the Deaf and Blind in Staunton, Virginia. But even as the education of deaf children moved toward the establishment of residential schools state by state, there were early experiments with other approaches. For example, in 1848, in parallel with the rise in education of German immigrants and native-born Americans in German language schools, there appeared in Baltimore a "mainstream" program for deaf children.

During the second half of the nineteenth century until about World War I, the education of deaf children was divided between rural residential schools for the deaf and urban day schools for the deaf. Wisconsin was a leader in the day school movement, with a string of day programs dotting the shores of Lake Michigan.

The golden years of the residential schools were from about 1910 around 1950. One factor that capped their growth was the considerable cost of establishing a new school. The high water mark in enrollments was during the Great Depression, when any poor child with a hearing loss was likely to be sent to the state residential school to ensure the child ate regularly.

After World War II America changed, and as a result the landscape of educating deaf children changed also. Families became smaller, and people moved to the suburbs. At the same time, new road systems were built, and school districts got larger. The population density of America increased. Along with these demographic changes, values changed as well, with education becoming increasingly important (Moores, 1992).

During this period, families became more able and more likely to support a child with a disability at home, while at the same time facilities for the education of children with disabilities began to appear within local school systems. New ideas about teaching children with disabilities started appearing too. The first change was a small increase in the number of deaf children in local public schools during the 1960s. Then two events occurred that impacted the number of deaf students and their placement especially in public schools. First, a rubella epidemic in the 1960s led to a significant increase in the number of deaf children that were born. Many of these children ended up in schools for the deaf, causing these schools to swell to capacity. Local public school programs started to take up the excess population and mainstreaming was on its way to becoming the educational placement containing the largest number of deaf students.

The second event was the passage of Public Law 94-142, the Education of All Handicapped Children Act, in 1975. Later renamed the Individuals with Disabilities Education Act (IDEA), this federal law mandated that every child with a disability had the right to a free and appropriate education alongside peers without disabilities. It also required that children with disabilities be placed in the least restrictive environment. This federal law led to a net growth in the number of deaf students being educated in public schools either in a **self-contained** program or in a general education classroom with support services. By the 1980s most schools for the deaf began to experience a steady decline in enrollment.

Today, about four out of every five children with a hearing loss are in local public school programs; meanwhile, about half of the students in schools for the deaf commute to and from home everyday. This is a considerable departure from the days when almost all students at a school for the deaf were residential. We can expect further decline in the number of students attending schools for the deaf as the ability of programs to help deaf students achieve comes under closer scrutiny by parents who have a greater understanding of laws such as IDEA and are prepared to search for the best program possible for their deaf children within their local school districts. In addition, the number of children with cochlear implants is growing, which may result in changes in the landscape of deaf education in the years to come. Although predicting the direction of these changes is difficult, it is reasonable to say that children with cochlear implants will likely be in local school programs, as opposed to schools for the deaf, because integration with hearing peers is a major reason for getting an implant for a profoundly deaf child.

Career Options for Teachers of the Deaf

Currently, there are four basic types of teaching situations for teachers of the deaf:

- Teaching in a traditional or self-contained classroom
- Teaching in a resource room
- Teaching as an itinerant teacher or teacher consultant
- Teaching in a team teaching classroom

Teaching in a Traditional or Self-Contained Classroom. The traditional or self-contained classroom is a place where you teach a group of relatively homogeneous deaf students in a single classroom. This is probably the most common image carried by prospective teachers of the deaf. These tend to be small classes of four to seven students. If the class is in a school for the deaf or in a large public school program, the students will likely be grouped by age. However, if the class is in a local public school classroom, students might vary in age by several years, and you might find yourself teaching three or four different grade levels of the same subject matter.

Teaching in a Resource Room. Kluwin, Stewart, and Sammons (1994) described **resource room** teaching as varying widely from larger groups of children down to single students in a closet that had been converted to a classroom. As a resource room teacher, you will not necessarily have a specific class of students, although you may have several students at one time for a particular subject, such as a language arts enrichment class. More generally, teaching in a resource room will involve instructional activities ranging from one-on-one tutorials to several students learning different topics at the same time. At most you may see five or six students at one time, but more commonly only one or two students will be in a resource room at a time. Resource room teachers work at all levels of schooling but a greater percentage of resource room classes exist at the high school levels.

Teaching as an Itinerant Teacher or Teacher Consultant. Luckner and Miller (1994) created a picture of the life of an **itinerant teacher** of the deaf (or as is the preferred nomenclature in some states, the teacher consultant). Most itinerant teachers directly instruct between eight and twelve students and consult on six to eighteen additional students spread across five to nine different schools. To accomplish this, these teachers will drive between five and nine hours per week and will only provide fourteen to twenty hours of direct services to students weekly. The itinerants spend twice as much time in their cars as they do consulting with general education teachers.

Teaching in a Team Teaching Classroom.   **Team teaching** or co-teaching involves a general education teacher and a teacher of the deaf teaching a group of hearing and deaf children. In co-teaching situations, smaller classes of about twenty-five students are created. Five or six deaf students are combined in a classroom with fifteen or more hearing students. Although the class is planned jointly by a teacher of the deaf and a general education teacher (Kluwin & Gonsher, 1994), the teacher of the deaf tends to take on the responsibility of implementing the deaf students' Individualized Educational Plans (IEPs).

How Do Teachers of the Deaf Think About Themselves?

Luckner (1991) looked at itinerant teachers, teachers in integrated settings (i.e., public schools), and special school teachers (i.e., schools for the deaf) and noted many similarities and differences in their skills. The integrated teachers were those who had self-contained classrooms or resource rooms. The teachers who worked in special schools were in schools for the deaf, either residential or day. A major difference was revealed between the itinerant teacher and the other two types of teachers: Itinerant teachers taught only single students who are, for the most part, hard of hearing. In addition to providing supplementary teaching to these students, the itinerant teacher performed tasks related to helping hard of hearing students function in the hearing and speaking environment of the general education classroom. Thus, they are involved in the assessment of residual hearing and speech and provide information to parents on the importance of amplification. Teachers in an integrated setting also found themselves assessing hearing and speech.

Teachers in self-contained classrooms in public schools shared a critical responsibility with itinerant teachers in that both of these teachers are often called upon not only to teach but to be consultants for the general education teachers and other school personnel who have contact with deaf students.

There is also an overlap between teachers in public school settings and those in schools for the deaf. Both focused on small classes of diverse deaf students. They both have the responsibility for implementing IEPs and handling curriculum matters.

Obviously, there are differences in the way teachers of the deaf work. Moreover, each of these teaching situations calls for different skills and approaches to teaching.

Repeating Themes in This Book

This book is divided into four sections: Introduction, Subject Matter Teaching, Issues in Cross-Curricular Teaching, and Other Teaching Issues. In addition, this book has four general themes that are repeated throughout the section on Subject Matter Teaching. These are not principles per se, although they often draw from the disciplines of cognitive psychology and learning theory. Instead, these are four ideas that are crucial to the teaching of deaf students. As such, they need to be considered when planning instructional activities.

To understand the rationale for our four themes, it helps to look at the experiences of a deaf child. Statistically, a deaf child is most likely to be born into a hearing family—often a family that has had no experience with a deaf individual. Further, that child on average is not likely to be diagnosed as having a hearing loss until almost eighteen months of age when other children are babbling along through the one-word phase of language development or beyond.

In the hearing world, a lot of information is transmitted incidentally. Parents talk about how to handle day-to-day problems within earshot of their children. Active communication takes place when curious children who see anomalies in their world have these anomalies explained to them. In addition to access to this kind of vicarious experience, hearing children accompany parents on outings and to events that are open to the children because of their hearing. These include the theater, movies, guided tours of museums, and art galleries. Also included are the mundane activities such as shopping, talking to a neighbor, and listening to someone talking on the telephone. Direct experience for the hearing child is not difficult to come by because it is omnidirectional.

Deaf children with hearing parents are cut off from vicarious and direct experience in a number of ways. During their critical years of learning language, their parents are often struggling to cope with the implications of the diagnosis and are struggling to seek a solution. Even if the parents opt for a form of sign communication early on, their development of signing skills cannot match the rate at which their child would be developing language if the child could hear. It is hardly surprising that deaf children bring to school a rather meager volume of meaningful experiential background.

Thus, deafness is a communication problem not just in the immediate sense of making conversation difficult, but in the long-term sense of depriving many deaf children of access to necessary experiences and information. In addition, most deaf children are the only individuals with a hearing loss in their family and neighborhood and among their parents' friends and acquaintances. More to the point, outside of the school environment they are not likely to come in contact with other deaf people who can serve as role models in a variety of life experiences such as community involvement, working, and marriage. Hence, these children either do not or rarely come in contact with people who share their visual connection to the world.

As a result of the lack of experiences and the absence of adequate opportunities for communication that most deaf children have in their home environment, we want to stress four themes throughout the book that help provide a more comprehensive approach to tackling the learning needs of deaf students. These four themes are the following:

- Creating authentic experiences
- Integrating vocabulary development
- Creating opportunities for self-expression
- Providing deaf role models

Creating Authentic Experiences

Language and knowledge will be acquired when the context in which they are presented is meaningful to deaf children. Clarke (1983) made the point that the benefits of many traditional language programs used with deaf children are limited because of the lack of connections to real-world or **authentic experiences**. A series of disconnected sentences in a language book is only as relevant as a child's linguistic and experiential background will make it. In the absence of much real-life experiences, deaf children become restricted in their ability to acquire new vocabulary and formulate new sentences.

Reflecting on their years of studying conversations, Clarke and Stewart (1986) observed that they "have yet to hear 'Today is Tuesday, yesterday was Monday, tomorrow will be Wednesday; it is sunny and cold' " (p. 162). Yet, the day and weather charts are a ubiquitous feature in many classrooms for young deaf children. Teachers need to question everything they do in the classroom. They might ask themselves, for example, what is the importance of looking out of the window then placing a picture of a cloud on a chart below the word "Monday"? Indeed, the challenge for all teachers of the deaf is to optimize the learning environment of their deaf children, which they can do by ensuring

> that conversation, facilitative activities, and specific systematic experiences which involve authentic real-world language transactions become an integral part of education programs. (Clarke & Stewart, 1986, p. 163)

Authentic experiences are especially important for deaf children because they may not have had the same experiences as hearing children have had. Because of gaps in experiential background, deaf children may lack the scripts or schema for performing specific actions.

Scripts, schemas, plans, and goals are terms that cognitive psychologists have applied to the routines we have internalized that permit us to carry out multistep tasks like ordering food in a restaurant or getting dressed in the morning. Schema theory proposes that "what is comprehended during reading or communication integrates in some conceptual way with what already exists in the mind of a person" (Luetke-Stahlman & Luckner, 1991, p. 240). Luetke-Stahlman and Luckner (1991) described the role of schema theory in learning in the following passage:

> A fundamental tenet of schema theory is that messages do not, in themselves, carry meaning. On the contrary, the message provides cues and directives for individuals as to how they should, using their own previously acquired knowledge, construct meaning. This previously acquired knowledge is stored in memory in the form of abstract cognitive structures called *schema.* The purpose of schema is to serve as a cognitive template against which incoming data can be matched. (p. 240)

Scripts or schemas are learned incidentally as well as taught directly. Take the following announcement that a mother might give to her 6-year old son:

> First, we are going to the ATM because I need cash before going to the grocery store. If you behave in the grocery store, there will be a stop at the ice cream stand on the way home.

By saying this, the mother is teaching the component parts of a sequence with outcomes and alternatives. Similarly, many parents go through a series of questions such as the following when putting their children to bed:

> Did you brush your teeth?
>
> Did you wash your face?
>
> Are your toys off the floor?

Are your dirty clothes in the hamper?

Where did you put your wet washcloth?

By asking these questions, the parents are teaching their children a schema.

Schema are important because they expose children to patterns and sequences in life. Most deaf children receive far fewer opportunities than their hearing peers to experience new schema or to ingrain old ones because parents may take them directly through the sequence without verbalizing it or without giving the child the opportunity to experiment with sequencing. In general, the child fails to learn the concept of sequencing and fails also to learn specific sequences.

Clearly, the first reason for using authentic experiences is to provide the deaf child with the opportunity to construct and verbalize sequences. The process of acquiring schema or scripts is a lifelong process that requires different scripts at different points in time. No individual ever learns all of the necessary scripts at one point, and for this reason the teacher of the deaf constantly needs to be providing new opportunities for learning them.

What differentiates an authentic experience? Authentic experiences are immediate and universal. They are immediate in the sense that they will happen now or if not this minute at least tomorrow. A mock United Nations theme for 10-year-olds can be an example of experiential learning. However, this type of learning is further accentuated if the teacher brings in a picture of a 10-year-old child starving in Angola or of one murdered in the Balkans. The visual images heighten a student's attention to the theme. Often teachers have to struggle trying to make a school experience authentic for children because the experience is not immediate. The immediate experience of colonial life is the field trip to the living history museum where pigs are fed, corn is ground, and the scale used to depict objects is very human. An example of an immediate experience in science is taking care of a living thing or walking out in the woods to collect pond scum or different kinds of leaves.

The universal aspect of an authentic experience is that it is the same wherever it occurs. Measurements of a student's body or measurements for a club house can occur anywhere. They are not tied to the confines of the classroom or the school. How much of you is one inch? Or one foot? Or one yard? Whatever your answer is, it will remain the same anywhere you are.

The authentic experience is credible. If you are teaching a language arts class, for example, you create credibility by having the students write their own children's books or compose a classroom newsletter to inform their parents about an event that they are sponsoring in their classroom. In science, credibility is evidenced when the students learn about the development of life by tracking the growth of a single plant or animal through the course of a year.

Integrating Vocabulary Development

The process of vocabulary development is integrated in at least three ways:

- Words are parts of related concepts.
- Words are presented in contexts.
- Words are everywhere.

Words occur in bunches. In science, *fossils* are found in *sedimentary rocks,* which are found in *quarries.* In language arts, *stories* or *narratives* have *characters* who are involved in the action of the *plot.* In social studies, *voting* is a *right* and a *responsibility* of a *citizen* in a *democracy.* In Deaf studies, *access* to *visual information* is a key issue in the *Deaf community.* Since the meanings of words are parts of related systems, they need to be taught as related collections. It is not enough to provide a list of words. Instead, the words on the list must be related to each other, and the relationships among the words must be explained and clarified.

Words do not occur in isolation. They appear in contexts. The contexts define and refine the meanings. A spring is a season of the year, a coiled bit of metal, a leap or jump, a small body of water, and many other fairly unique items in reality. The word *spring* should not be taught alone but the place where the word occurs physically and conceptually should be presented as well. In other words, this spring shows up in a mattress ad. Is it the same spring that shows up on a calendar?

Words are everywhere! There is writing on cereal boxes, on the handles of tools, and on parts of a car that you can't even get at. Why shouldn't words be everywhere in the classroom for the deaf child too? In an integrated approach to vocabulary development, words appear on charts, on bulletin boards, and on objects in the room. The classroom must be a place where a deaf child cannot look without seeing a word. It must also be a place where vocabulary is provided to help deaf children grapple with new concepts.

Words are in conversation also. Students are better able to expand their vocabulary when they see how words are used in daily discourse and when they are given opportunities to incorporate new words into their own dialogue.

In our discussion of subject matter teaching, we will suggest specific ways to introduce vocabulary, but one general way is to situate the words in both their physical and linguistic contexts. For example, teachers can put the back of a cereal box, a set of instructions on how to assemble a barbecue, or the newspaper comics on the bulletin board or on a bare wall with target words marked. They can create charts that convey the word in the context in which it occurs. Doing things like this becomes second nature for effective teachers, all of whom can benefit from a healthy dose of creativity.

The old Jericho Hill School for the Deaf in Vancouver, British Columbia, was on a hill overlooking the bay. If one of the authors had been a student there he'd have spent half of his time on sunny days staring out the windows—like he did in a Catholic elementary school in Wisconsin. But the astute teacher would outfox him because every time he looked up and out that window a new word related to a familiar concept would have greeted him. In the first grade, it might have been *blue* or *ocean* or *ship*. By the eighth grade it would be *vessel* or *circumnavigate* or *tempest* or *becalmed*. The important point is that teachers need to make words visible.

Creating Opportunities for Self-Expression

The flip side of the schema issue is the practice of complex verbal routines and, in particular, self-expression. This takes a multitude of formats. When you are in preschool learning about the bunny running around the tree and into the hole, this helps you learn to tie your shoes. When you are in high school preparing to move into a world where you will earn a living, become a registered voter, and make major life decisions, you have to become engaged in self-expression to control far more complex processes. Basically, then, self-expression is the following:

- An opportunity to practice elaborate verbal skills.
- An opportunity for definition and refinement of ideas.

Adolescents with their in-groups and out-groups and constant interaction are the clearest example of school-aged children defining themselves through self-expression. But they are not the only ones. Self-expression is very much a part of the learning process that takes place in the classroom. An 11-year-old boy checking an understanding of the scientific method and a 14-year-old girl making sure that she understands the steps for structuring the algebraic solution to a word problem benefit from expressing in their own words the processes that they are using.

Self-expression is also important in testing. Testing is usually a one-way street in that the teacher creates all of the conditions for expression. However, testing in this manner also raises the possibility that the teacher might get the appropriate response to a question for inappropriate reasons. If you ask a student to read a passage and give the student four multiple choice questions to "test comprehension," the student will get at least one right by chance. He or she could also arrive at the correct answer by eliminating options. As a result, what does the student know? More importantly for you as the teacher, what do you know about what the student knows?

Now, let's suppose the student has to convert the information inside his or her head into another form and express it to you. In this way, you will get a fuller and more accurate image of what has been learned. For example, you have the students read: "My love is like a red, red rose." You ask them to write the next line of this poem. They might write:

> My love smells like a flower.
> My love is like a blue balloon.
> My love is like a glowing sunset.

Which child has grasped the idea of the line? The first child has stayed in the concrete idea of a flower and missed the nature of a metaphor. The second child has understood the metaphor but missed the underlying passion of the image. The third child has grasped the notion of the implied metaphor, a visual image, and beauty. Self-expression can reveal much about the depth and direction in which information has been processed.

Providing Deaf Role Models

Have you ever asked: Who am I? Children ask that question and then they go looking for answers. Will deaf children have the information they need to answer this question in the absence of positive contact with deaf adults? Possibly. But more realistically, every deaf child should have the opportunity to meet and interact with deaf adults from all walks of life.

There is the possibly apocryphal story about a fairly new teacher of the deaf at a residential school for the deaf in the American South during the 1950s. This teacher comes upon a deaf child in the school who is crying. The new teacher asks the child why he is crying. The child responds that he is going to die when he is 18 years old. The teacher is appalled at such nonsense and asks:

Why do you think you'll die when you turn 18?

The child responds,

I have never seen a deaf person older than 18.

A role model does several things for a child. A role model should be a positive image of adult behavior. A role model should be a benchmark or reality check not for the limits of success but for the means to achieve success. The role model does not say, "I did it" but rather "This is what you need to do to succeed." As we will indicate in various parts of this book, schools provide many opportunities for exposing deaf children to deaf role models.

Conclusion

Deaf students arguably present the most complex challenge for teachers of any group of students in both the general and special education populations. Every corner of their educational process is multidimensional and each dimension has the potential to significantly impact their academic achievement. These dimensions include:

- The status of the parents in areas such as the presence of deafness among the parents, economic situation, educational levels, ethnic affiliations, and ability to communicate with the deaf child in a particular form of communication.
- Educational placement options available to the students.
- Individual characteristics, such as the degree of hearing loss, the age at onset of deafness, exposure to early childhood education, learning characteristics, and proficiency in communication.

These dimensions are not exclusive and their interactions lead to compounding effects that either enhance or disadvantage a deaf student's education.

Teachers of deaf students must therefore be prepared for a host of teaching situations, few of which will remain constant through the year. As student characteristics change, so too will the teaching demands. Thus, teachers must bring to the classroom a strong belief in meeting the individual learning needs of each student.

Finally, to meet the diverse demands of their students, teachers should integrate, across all teaching situations and instruction, central themes in their planning that will help deaf students gain the language and experiential background that they need for accessing and learning the curriculum. Four such themes are:

- Creating authentic experiences
- Integrating vocabulary development

- Creating opportunities for self-expression
- Providing deaf role models

These themes are highlighted in our discussions of subject matter teaching.

KEY WORDS AND CONCEPTS

authentic experiences: Experiences that have real-life meaning to children, such as experiences in which children can directly engage (e.g., hands-on learning, field trips, writing a letter to an editor) or to which they can relate (e.g., discussion about how children their age attend school in other countries).

deaf student: Any student who has a degree of hearing loss severe enough to adversely affect his or her learning. Under this generic term we include those students who are referred to as being hard of hearing, deaf, hearing impaired, and Deaf.

deaf: A term that refers to any person with a hearing loss that is serious enough to impede educational progress.

Deaf: A term used by various authors to refer to people who have some degree of hearing loss, use sign language as their primary means of communication, and are in some manner affiliated with the Deaf community.

hearing impaired: A term used by some authors to refer to any person with some degree of hearing loss.

hard of hearing: A term referring to a person who has some degree of hearing loss but is able to function in the hearing and speech modalities either with or without the use of assistive listening devices such as hearing aids.

itinerant: Instruction by a teacher who teaches several students in a pull-out setting in different schools. The itinerant teacher typically travels from school to school on a daily basis, and the instruction is direct. A single itinerant teacher of the deaf may be responsible for a wide range of students with varying academic levels or for all deaf students in a particular geographic part of a large city. Another term for itinerant teacher is **teacher consultant**, reflecting increased contact with other teachers.

resource room: Classroom instruction in which the student leaves the general education classroom for assistance in a particular subject area. This type of arrangement is also referred to as a pull-out instructional setting. The resource room teacher collaborates and consults with the general classroom teacher

self-contained: Classroom instruction in which a small group of students who have similar disability labels or academic performance ability are taught in a single classroom, separated from the general education classroom. Included in self-contained classrooms are teachers who teach in a school for the deaf.

team teaching: Also referred to as **co-teaching**. In a team teaching situation, two teachers in the same classroom provide instruction. Usually one of the teachers is the main leader. Both can teach the same lesson or teach alternately. How a classroom is set up is dependent upon the characteristics of the team teachers, including their preferred instructional styles.

QUESTIONS

1. What factors caused the population of schools for the deaf to decline in the latter part of the twentieth century?

2. What parental factors are related to enhancing the overall education of a deaf child?

3. How does the communication behavior of the mother of a deaf child influence the communication behavior of other members of the family?

4. Of the four types of teaching options (teaching in a traditional or self-contained classroom, teaching in a resource room, teaching as an itinerant teacher or teacher consultant, teaching in a team teaching classroom), which would you prefer as your career choice? Explain your answer.

5. Why is it important to integrate vocabulary development when designing lessons for deaf students?

6. Why should teachers expose their deaf students to deaf role models?

7. Explain why deaf students need opportunities for self-expression at school.

8. Describe what you think an authentic experience entails for a deaf child.

ACTIVITIES

1. Develop a list of questions that you would like to ask an itinerant teacher, a resource room teacher, or a teacher working in a self-contained classroom. These questions should attempt to create a picture of a typical day of instruction in the activities of a teacher of the deaf. Then contact one of each of these types of teachers and conduct a brief interview.

2. Create a list of questions that you would want to ask a parent of a deaf child. These questions should be centered around such themes as communication, involvement in community activities, educational and career expectations, and so forth. Use this list to interview a parent of a deaf child.

3. Describe an idealized day in the life of a deaf child one Saturday in the summer. In this description ensure that the child has opportunities to engage in authentic experiences that will translate into better preparedness for learning in the classroom.

Principles of Effective Teaching

Jere Brophy is a leading researcher in the field of education. His work is extensively published in academic journals and books. Through years of research he has pieced together those principles of teaching that define an effective teacher. These principles address generic aspects of curriculum, instruction, and assessment as well as classroom organization and management practices that support effective instruction. He focuses on learning outcomes but with recognition of the need for a supportive classroom climate and positive student attitudes toward schooling, teachers, and classmates.

These principles are the following:

1. Students learn best within cohesive and caring learning communities.
2. Students learn more when most of the available time is allocated to curriculum-related activities and the classroom management system emphasizes maintaining their engagement in those activities.
3. All components of the curriculum are aligned to create a cohesive program for accomplishing instructional purposes and goals.
4. Teachers can prepare students for learning by providing an initial structure to clarify intended outcomes and cue desired learning strategies.
5. To facilitate meaningful learning and retention, content is explained clearly and developed with emphasis on its structure and connections.
6. Questions are planned to engage students in sustained discourse structured around powerful ideas.
7. Students need sufficient opportunities to practise and apply what they are learning and to receive improvement-oriented feedback.
8. The teacher provides whatever assistance students need to enable them to engage in learning activities productively (i.e., scaffolding).
9. The teacher models and instructs students in learning and self-regulation strategies.
10. Students often benefit from working in pairs or small groups to construct understandings or to help one another master skills.
11. The teacher uses a variety of formal and informal assessment methods to monitor progress toward learning goals.
12. The teacher establishes and follows through on appropriate expectations for learning outcomes.

As you go through this book, you will recognize that many of the instructional strategies that we have presented are based on the principles above.

(Taken from *Teaching* by Jere Brophy. Available on the Web site www.ibe.unesco.org)

2 Teaching Science

CHAPTER OUTCOMES

After reading this chapter, you should be able to:

1. Explain why science appeals to deaf students.
2. Describe four main challenges that teachers of the deaf face when teaching science to deaf students and address these challenges when preparing a unit or lesson plan.
3. Incorporate strategies related to effective preparation and teaching when designing a science unit.
4. Use a variety of strategies to engage deaf students in talking about science.
5. Use science lessons, including hands-on activities, as a way of teaching reading and writing to deaf students.
6. Use portfolio or performance-based assessment that relies on a variety of indicators of success to evaluate student performance.
7. Use mapping strategies to help students think about a science concept that can also be part of a student's science portfolio.

If you had to select a subject that both appealed to and contrasted with the learning style of most deaf children, you would probably pick science. The media is soaked with current events that revolve around science. There are the proverbial science topics that include reports about global warming, the shrinking ice cap, hurricane patterns, chronic back problems, diet plans, another link to the evolution of humans, the age of the universe, the good and bad news about cholesterol, and the effects of noise on hearing. There are the customary battles involving the tobacco industry and legislators; prescription drugs and health management organizations (HMOs); and salmon fishermen and loggers. You cannot pick up a newspaper or a magazine (Yes, even teen magazines can't avoid science: "Facial care for your big date!") or turn on the TV without encountering something that children can and do study in their science classes. Unquestionably, there is a lot of help for teachers keen on motivating their students to learn about science.

Then there is the reality of how this subject can best be learned. Reading helps as does a large vocabulary. The ability to learn from observations is central to learning science. Also important is the capacity to describe and analyze one's thoughts about science concepts using print, signs, or speech or all three. As teachers, you will need to give deaf children the tools necessary to access the world of science.

What Is Science?

Science is about making sense of the world around us. The more we understand about biology, chemistry, geology, astronomy, physics, and other sciences the better equipped we are to understand who we are and why things are the way they are. Science is also about discovery. Few disciplines challenge our intelligence in the way science does.

In children's discovery of science, they learn about Copernicus in the sixteenth century, discovering the theory that the sun, not the earth, was the center of the universe. They study about Newton discovering the theory of gravitation, Dalton the theory of atoms, and Einstein the theory of relativity. They trace the means by which Gutenberg invented the printing press, Watt the steam engine, Edison the phonograph, Fleming the medicine penicillin, and Weitbrecht the teletypewriter (TTY) modem used by deaf people.

But discovery need not always be associated with the great names in science. Somewhere along their road to great discoveries, scientists were content to make small discoveries. They learned that a hot sun made blacktop too hot to walk on barefoot; that blowing on a window on a cold winter day caused water to appear on the pane; that some leaves were smooth and silky to the touch while others were soft and velvety; that no matter how much you shook, oil and water wouldn't mix; and that tadpoles eventually grew legs and jumped out of the water—discoveries that allow all children to be scientists.

This is the premise for the chapter. We assume that all children are natural discoverers and that our job as science teachers is to provide a platform to allow children to make sense of their discoveries. We teach science because all children are budding scientists. And for deaf children, we add the further task of using science as a springboard for language development.

Science and the Deaf Student

In line with society's march through the technological age, there is a Web site (and possibly more than one site is available) devoted to expanding our understanding of how best to teach science to deaf students (see section "A Sampling from the Internet" in this chapter). This is one indication of the appeal of science to deaf students. Evidence in support of this appeal is offered by Lang and Meath-Lang (1985) who found that more than 80 percent of the 329 students they studied from nine schools for the deaf enjoyed science.

Deaf students should not only be given the opportunity to study science at all levels but encouraged to do so. There is so much in life that they and the rest of us use and enjoy, and for these things we all owe thanks to the legions of scientists who are constantly striving to improve the quality of life. Scientists gave us coconut flavor lip balm, low-calorie blue cheese dressing, spandex, tanning salons, DVD movies, captioned TV, and national forests for trekking. They are helping us to live a longer, healthier life, to have smooth skin and children without ear infections, and to travel to faraway exotic places in shorter periods of time. They gave deaf children auditory trainers, alerting devices that flash lights in place of school bells and fire alarms, and video technology that allows signers to record their stories in American Sign Language.

Deaf and hard of hearing scientists have also made important contributions to the world of science. They discovered scientific principles and chemical elements, founded fields of science, pioneered in rocketry, and received Nobel Prizes for their work (Lang, 1994; Lang & Meath-Lang, 1995).

In short, we cannot avoid being influenced by the work of scientists, and we must explore this influence with the deaf children we teach. *To do so we must focus on teaching the language of science to give deaf children the linguistic tools for internalizing science concepts.* This means teaching all relevant science terminology such as those associated with the growth of *epiphytes* in a rainforest, *refraction* of light waves, *repelling* of magnetic fields, *reproductive* cycle of fish, and *thermonuclear reactions* of the stars to children who are identified as being delayed in their acquisition of language; terminology, by the way, that is found in most elementary science curricula.

Interestingly, science lends itself to **visual learning** and **hands-on activities**—two elements of teaching suited to the learning needs of many deaf children. In fact, in this chapter, one of the premises for teaching science is that teachers need to go beyond the science objectives of their lessons and seek ways to use science as a means of teaching language. Lang and Albertini (2000) found that teachers felt that deaf students' writing samples associated with hands-on activities aided teachers in evaluating students' comprehension. The teachers saw the benefits of incorporating writing into their science teaching. Using four different writing strategies to evaluate how well students could construct meaning in science from their hands-on activities, teachers revealed that writing helped in the construction of meaning, in identifying possible misconceptions, and in areas on which to focus in subsequent lessons.

The notion of integrating language with science is one way of helping deaf students grapple with the many language variables associated with learning science. These variables include vocabulary, textbook reading levels, and the ability to write down meaningful observations and scientific reports. Teachers of the deaf need to be cognizant of the role of language in learning science and need to address language instruction in their science lessons. This does not mean, however, that teachers need to focus on simple science concepts and easy-to-learn science terminology in an effort to help deaf children learn. By doing this they might unconsciously create a science curriculum that has a built-in inertia to language acquisition.

Thus, learning language should be an expected outcome of good science teaching. Indeed, some bilingual education proponents believe that science provides an ideal school platform for students to learn a second language because of the connections to hands-on learning—a connection that helps students visualize the meaning of words and phrases (Stewart, 1992).

What TIMSS Has to Say About Science Education in America

The most extensive study of science achievement in the United States was conducted by researchers associated with the Third International Mathematics and Science Study (TIMSS). Depending on the variable being studied, TIMSS compared the science achievements of students in up to fifty countries and then attempted to explain discrepancies by comparison of curricula, textbooks, and teaching practices (Schmidt, McKnight, & Raizen, 1997; Schmidt et al., 1999).

Although the TIMSS study did not look at the achievement of deaf students, if deaf students are going to be integrated with hearing peers then it would be beneficial to them to be in a class where students in general are performing well. This is not to say that the deaf students are achieving at the same level as their hearing classmates when they are in such classes. To achieve well, deaf students must be able to do the work and to maintain pace with the proceedings of the classes. This may be a difficult task for some to do because the TIMSS researchers discovered that the science curriculum in the United States demands that teachers cover a lot more topics in a given period of time than do the science curricula in other countries. In other words, students are given a shorter period of time in which to absorb and understand science concepts. This has serious implications for deaf students whose language skills are weak. These students have the dual challenge of having to master the science concepts and the language associated with the science all within a timeframe that other countries consider inadequate for their general education students.

Four Challenges for Science Teachers of Deaf Students

To know how to teach science to deaf students we have to examine how well equipped they are for learning science. Consider first what the National Science Education Standards (National Academy of Science-National Research Council, 1996) have to say about the importance of learning science:

> [E]veryone needs to use scientific information to make choices that arise every day. Everyone needs to be able to engage intelligently in public discourse and debate about important issues of science and technology. And everyone deserves to share in the excitement and personal fulfillment that can come from understanding and learning about the natural world. (p. 23)

This passage brings forth several implications. To acquire scientific knowledge implies that students must

- Learn about science-related concepts and retain this information.
- Be able to speak intelligently about this knowledge, implying that they have a command of the language of science and discourse skills.

- Engage in critical thinking to recognize important issues relating to science, which calls for an access to literature, discussions, and experiences that accentuate this importance.
- Gain an appreciation for the value of science, implying that their experiences involve them in activities that reveal the thrill and satisfaction that science brings to their lives.

Teaching science means interrelating many different facets of children's lives and ways of thinking. This is true for all children. But ensuring that it happens for deaf children requires that we plan meaningful learning experiences and make accommodations for the learning needs they bring to the classroom that are often different from those of their general education peers. Following are four challenges that deaf students pose to their science teachers:

1. *Deaf students need greater access to **authentic learning experiences**.* Encounters with events help children form new understandings or concepts. Experimentation in the classroom, laboratory, or field provides new information that challenges these understandings. It is these challenges that enable children to learn. It follows that the more experiential knowledge that children bring to these experimentations the better positioned they are to further their understanding. All children gain experiences by going places with their parents and others and talking about things. Deaf children may well go to the same places that other children go but the experiences they gain from such visits will likely be markedly different because they often do not have effective communication with their parents and significant others.

We cannot overstate the importance of authentic learning experiences in building up knowledge or the extent to which deaf children miss out on opportunities to gain experiences. Let's do a snapshot analysis of the wealth of knowledge associated with a seemingly simple experience of one of the authors, who was driving in the country with two of his children when he spotted Venus and Jupiter perched above the Western horizon shortly after sunset. While driving he pointed this out to his children and a discussion about planets ensued. Their short discussion touched upon many facts including the following:

- Venus and Jupiter appear in the sky before the stars do.
- Venus and Jupiter change positions in the sky.
- These two planets are not always aligned so that they look close to each other.
- Venus always appears in the Western sky.
- Venus is always the brightest object in the sky other than the moon.
- Venus is smaller than Jupiter but it looks bigger and brighter to us because it is closer to Earth than Jupiter.
- Planets look just like stars in the sky.
- Stars give off their own light but planets reflect light from the sun.

This discussion lasted about four minutes and the hearing children were 6 years and 9 years of age. Did the children retain all of this information? Perhaps not, but what they did gain was the experience of an observation that was enhanced with intellectual discussion. Imagine a deaf child sitting in the back seat of a car while his or her parent is driving along the same road in the dark. What do you think the parent would have said given a perfect viewing of Venus and Jupiter? Would the parent think to talk about these planets once out of the car? What would you have said if you were the driver?

2. *Deaf children need vocabulary that is conducive to the acquisition of science concepts.* This vocabulary needs to be in English but for those deaf children who rely on signing for communication then they also need exposure to the vocabulary of American Sign Language and/or other sign communication systems. We use language to help internalize our experiences. Language enables us to share our thoughts, ask questions, formulate opinions, and pursue arguments with others. The more language children know and the larger vocabulary they possess the greater "flexibility and ability to construct and reconstruct meanings" they will have (Scott, 1992, p. iv). In other words, children are active in their learning process and require the linguistic tools that will facilitate this process.

Take a unit about fossils. A dictionary defines a fossil as "a remnant, impression, or trace of an animal or plant of past geologic ages that has been preserved in the earth's crust." Suppose you had deaf students studying a butterfly fossil from the Pleistocene era, what language might they encounter? The students might study the *location* in which the *fossil* was found such as a *quarry* dug deep into *sedimentary* rocks. They might connect the *well-preserved nature* of the fossil with the fact that the quarry was in an *arid* area that had experienced little *erosion* over time. They might learn that this particular *specimen* is *related* to the *Monarch* butterfly and was present in *abundance* during the *Pleistocene era.* Learning these words and the concepts associated with them is critical to students learning and appreciating science. Teachers must not use a deaf student's language level as a reason not to teach relevant science terminology.

3. *Deaf children need opportunities to talk about science-related matters with others.* We are talking about in-depth discussions of something of interest at an opportune time. Adult-mediated and peer-mediated interactions are critical to the development of a deaf child's language and social skills. Children engaged in a hands-on science activity should be encouraged to verbalize throughout the activity to help them structure their thinking about a science concept. Hearing children do this naturally, partly because they can hear and speak to others while looking at something and also because given the typical size of public school classes they are usually assured of an audience. For deaf children, eye contact is critical, and hence they must often divert their attention from an experiment in order to talk to someone.

Hand in hand with the need to talk about science while an experiment or observation is occurring is the need for discussions that are intellectually stimulating and challenge children's thoughts about something. Opportunities to do this are everywhere, but teachers need to recognize them. Let's take a simple discussion about how a rock feels or looks. Is the surface of a rock rough, jagged, ragged, craggy, uneven, or sharp? Which word do you think a deaf child might use? Which word might you use? You would probably select a word based on the feature of the rock that most caught your attention, and it might depend on the context in which the rock is being examined as, for example, a rock held in the hand, a picture of a rock, a rock being observed in the distance, or a rock that was just passed through a rock crusher. Would you then use this word with your deaf students? If a deaf student said the rock felt rough, would you be content with that description or would you pursue an elaboration including an explanation of why the rock felt rough along with a suggestion for other words that can be used to describe the rock? Creating opportunities to talk helps expand a student's vocabulary, which in turn helps expand the student's opportunities to talk about science.

4. *Deaf children need science role models.* Can you name three people involved in science? Are any of these three people deaf and if none are, can you name a deaf person who is involved in science? If you are having difficulty identifying deaf people in the field of science, it may be because your focus on science is too narrow. Consider these science-related careers: horticulturist, landscaper, farmer, swimming pool maintenance worker (measuring the chlorine level of a pool and adding chemicals to the water are science-based tasks), dental assistant, and hair stylist (a person who must have an understanding of chemicals and their effects on the scalp and hair). Chances are that you do know a deaf person whose knowledge of science is an advantage in, or even essential to, his or her career.

All children benefit from contact with role models, and one of the challenges for science teachers is to introduce deaf children to deaf role models in the field of science. This does not downplay the value of scientists who are hearing because they have been adequately covered in textbooks. What textbooks do not show, is that a hearing loss, a different method of communicating, and even a different type of social group do not prevent success in any area of endeavor, scientific or otherwise.

The American inventor, Thomas Edison, declared that his deafness was an asset; that not being able to hear insulated, rather than isolated him, from society (Lang & Meath-Lang, 1995). He began losing his hearing when he was twelve years old, and by the time he was a young adult communicating by pen and paper was a necessity. Given he was the inventor of such products as the phonograph and wireless telegraphy machine, it is not surprising to note his ingenuity in communicating with others. At theaters, "his wife 'interpreted' for him by tapping out on his knee the code for words spoken on the stage" (Lang & Meath-Lang, 1995, p. 109). Edison even proposed to his wife using the Morse Code. Stories like these tie in the human qualities of being a deaf person with the work and accomplishments of this person. They are a source of inspiration and hope for deaf children who are exploring education and career options.

Human speech was first transmitted over radio waves by the American scientist R.A. Fessenden in 1900—a significant event because it stressed a most essential form of communication, speech. But, like Alexander Graham Bell's telephone, Fessenden's pioneering work with radios isolated deaf people in a hearing- and speech-driven society. We are now witnessing the first pioneering efforts of the twenty-first century—and one that many deaf people eagerly anticipate—the improvement of the capacity of home computers to allow people to communicate in signs, speechreading, print, or sound with whomever they please. To deaf people, this new technology is the antithesis of Fessenden's invention and one that serves to integrate rather than isolate deaf people into society. The elements of this technology are already in place in the form of videophones and cellular communication. Advancement of this technology will give deaf people access to a greater part of society. A deaf man, Robert Weitbrecht, did this with his invention of the TTY modem in the 1960s. This invention allowed deaf people to use the telephone to communicate with others.

Helping Deaf Children Learn Science

Learning is an interactive process that encompasses many elements of the environment and the learner. Students learn science by making sense of what they know about things, and how they do this is influenced by the people with whom they interact. Furthermore, all people are influenced in their thinking by the culture or cultures in which they are in contact. In essence, a person's knowledge of science is constructed within the context of social and cultural forces. This is how a constructivist would define science learning. Thus, learning "is not simply the act of an individual learner, but a product of social interactions between groups of learners" (Barba, 1995, p. 100). It is with a social constructivist's mindset that we now explore how teachers can best help deaf children learn science.

We select as our vehicle for talking about teaching techniques the theme "How Plants Grow." We will explore this theme using the following six elements of a **unit plan**: preparing the unit or lessons, designing the lessons, introducing students to the language of the experiment, engaging students in science talk, planning authentic experiences, and creating a reading center. A seventh element is evaluation or helping students demonstrate their knowledge; this will be discussed later in the chapter. These elements are in no way restricted to the delivery of a unit plan on science; they can be applied across a variety of instructions and subject matter.

Preparing for the Unit or Lessons

Preparation is essential. Experience as a teacher and with a particular science theme may make a teacher better able to prepare a lesson but it does not lessen the need to prepare. Preparation involves a number of actions that need to be thought out, written down, researched, or collected. Setting up for an experiment is an example of preparing for an experiment, but if that's all you do then you may be neglecting the four challenges to teaching science to deaf children described earlier in this chapter.

The first step is to consider the **curricular goals** and **instructional objectives** (learning outcomes) that will guide your teaching. Here the school's curriculum should be consulted. This is a critical part of the overall success of a science program for deaf students. Teachers of deaf students have been known to teach from science textbooks that their students are capable of reading; such as using a third-grade science book with tenth-grade deaf students. Language should not dictate the level of science that a deaf student is studying. Language must not be a barrier for teaching age-appropriate science concepts to deaf students. Deaf students must learn the concepts that their same-age peers are learning.

There are several ways in which a curriculum can be shaped. These ways include using curricular-based textbooks, personally pulling together and designing one's own set of science units that cover curricular goals, and designing science units that are a part of thematic teaching across several subject areas. Whichever route you decide to pursue, you should think about incorporating the suggestions in this chapter to enhance science learning for deaf students.

For our theme about how plants grow, we have selected the following content standard designed for the elementary grades:

> Describe life cycles of familiar organisms. (Key concepts: Life cycle stages—egg, young, adult, seed, flower, fruit. Real-world contexts: Common plants and animals such as beans, apples, butterflies, grasshoppers, frogs, birds). (Michigan Curriculum Framework, Michigan Department of Education, 1996, p. 73).

Note the language processes embedded in this science standard. You could have students draw and label the life cycle of a plant or animal. The only language process you would be emphasizing is vocabulary. It would be a much richer linguistic experience for the students if you have them also describe verbally or in print the life cycle. Therefore, define the activity "describe" to include the ability to use language to identify and connect the different forms of a plant or an animal cycle.

Content standards as shown above tell us what it is that a student will learn, are often broadly defined, and often involve learning a number of concepts. A content standard can be broken down to specific goals that you are going to teach. Two specific curricular goals at the fifth-grade level that are associated with this content standard are the following:

a. The student will be able to use observation skills to analyze a plant's structure and function.

b. The student will be able to analyze the relationship between function and structure using observation techniques.

These goals are also broadly defined but they suggest that teachers select a particular aspect of the life cycle, which we can do by creating specific instructional objectives that will help us accomplish the goals stated.

Whereas content standards and curricular goals can be found in a curriculum, instructional objectives are created by you, the teacher. It is with instructional objectives that you take into account the various learning levels of your students. You use your instructional objectives and not the science experiment per se to separate the students in the event that they are working at different levels. Many science experiments can be conducted by a wide range of students; the key for the teacher is to assign different instructional objectives that match each student's learning level. Instructional objectives should be stated in terms of outcomes, noting what it is that a student will be able to do after a lesson is completed. Some possible instructional objectives are the following:

a.1 The student will be able to describe in writing two functions of a plant seed based on two weeks of observing a corn seed growing inside a glass jar.

a.2 The student will be able to draw and label the parts of a corn plant.

b.1 The student will be able to identify the structure of a plant that corresponds to a particular function associated with the growth of a plant. The learner will be able to describe the function to the class using whole sentences (in signs and/or speech).

b.2 The student will be able to write a prediction about what would happen to a growing plant if the function of the roots was stopped.

Note how each of these objectives provide clear and specific directions for a student to perform. For example, in a.1, the student is expected to describe *two* functions of a plant. This specificity provides a focal point for what is going to be taught.

This is a good time for the teacher to consider integrating the science unit with other subject matter. As an example, we will do this with language arts. Once again, the curriculum is consulted. In a fifth-grade language arts curriculum, there is a section called "Study and Research Skills" that contains the following goal:

> The learner will be able to work in a group, as an actively participating member, to decide on a research topic, plan the project, set goals, make timelines for completing the project on time, develop a thesis statement, collect, compile, and synthesize information from a variety of sources, prepare a group presentation to inform others on the topic, and participate in the presentation using visual/audio aids.

We now have all of the elements necessary to plan one or more lessons relating to the growth of plants.

Designing the Lessons

We use the instructional objectives to design a science experiment that may be stretched over more than one lesson. As it happens, all of the above objectives can be covered in a single science experiment:

The Experiment.   Four to six corn seeds (or bean seeds) are first soaked overnight and are then placed in a tall, wide-mouthed jar with a moistened paper towel pressing them against the glass. The paper towel is held in place with crumpled squares of wax paper. The jar is placed in sunlight, and the paper towel is moistened daily with a spray bottle. The seed will sprout in a couple of days. Over a two-week period the children will observe and measure the growth of the roots, stem, and the leaf. Cutting off the roots of one of the plants midway through the experiment will halt further growth of the plant. This experiment can occur at anytime during the school year, but early spring is a preferable time because of the blooming plants outdoors.

Once the experiment is selected, you need to decide how you will keep the students informed of their progress through various aspects of the experiment. You have many options, and a combination of several is probably the best:

■ Draw a chart that contains labels and descriptions of all of the relevant parts of the experiment.

- Describe the experiment to the students verbally and have them describe back to you the key elements of the experiment. This is a good strategy for testing your students' understanding of vocabulary and language structures.
- Write out the steps in the experiment and have the students describe to one another what they think the experiment is about.
- Demonstrate and describe the steps in the experiment and have the students write the experiment out.

Whatever you decide, keep in mind the language challenges associated with teaching science. Deaf students may have difficulty following directions (see, for example, Chapter 1 for a discussion of schema and how children acquire them). Descriptions of a science experiment can be used to help students overcome this difficulty. Make your descriptions progressively more difficult throughout the school year.

Introducing Students to the Language of the Experiment

Make a list of words associated with the experiment:

plant	seed	grow	germinate	sprout
sunlight	leaf	stalk	photosynthesis	root
root hairs	nutrients	procedure	length	measure
moist	moisten	damp	jar	shade
predict	rotate	oxygen	chlorophyll	etc.

The list contained in this chart is a teacher list of key vocabulary words that may be different from what might be shown to the students. Indeed, there are different ways in which vocabulary words can be presented to deaf students. One such way would be to have the students label their own illustration of a plant and associated processes such as photosynthesis. Figure 2.1 shows an example of such an illustration.

Make few assumptions about what words you think your deaf students will understand. If the words are important to your experiment then put them in your vocabulary list. If you use signs, go through the list and place an asterisk next to the words for which you know the signs. Use a reference text to look up signs for words that you do not know. A particularly useful reference is *Signs for Science and Mathematics* (Caccamise & Lang, 1995). You might also wish to contact someone for help if there are too many words for which you do not know the signs. Now place a large dot next to these words, which you are going to express through fingerspelling.

Include in this list those words that have a sign but for which you are going to fingerspell most of the time in order to help expand the student's written vocabulary. For example, you might use the same sign for *damp, moist,* and *moisten,* which the students might identify more readily with the word *wet.* If you are signing something and you mean the word *damp* then also fingerspell it to help students make the association of the sign with

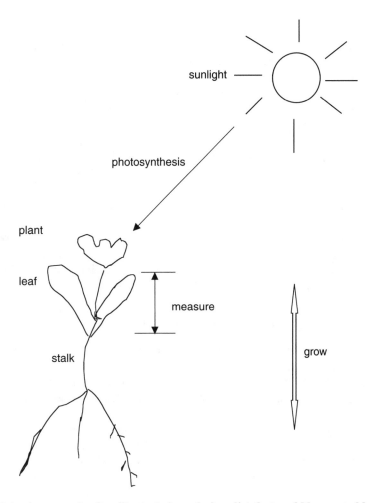

FIGURE 2.1   An example of an illustrated vocabulary list that could be created by a deaf student.

its different printed forms and the different ways in which each of these words are used to describe things in English.

Think about how you are going to work these words into your lessons. You can use them in your chart that describes the experiment; you can have the students create a mapping of words they associate with the experiment; you can use them in your verbal descriptions of the experiment; and so forth. Write the words down on cards that you will use to reinforce students' learning of them. Have the students write some of the words on cards and provide definitions for them. Do note, however, that working with new vocabulary can be a labor-intensive activity for some deaf students and can be fruitless without reinforcement through other activities.

Now, think about how you can use the words incidentally throughout the day. There are not enough hours in a day to "teach" English to deaf children. Hearing children may hear words hundreds of times before they absorb them into their vocabulary. It is important for teachers to use words repeatedly and in different contexts, and this should be planned. For the present lesson, you might do this by:

- Looking out the window and observing the growth of plants.
- Taking the students for a walk around the school and having them point out the many different plants that are coming to life again in the spring.
- Having the students suggest ideas for a science experiment about seeds growing to become plants.
- Talking about the length of hair and discussing how the growth of hair might be measured.
- Standing in the shade and asking the students why they feel cool.

If you do activities such as these on a regular basis it becomes a habit, and you are helping your students acquire new vocabulary more rapidly.

Engaging Students in Science Talk

Let your students know that they are scientists. All children are naturally curious, and in science we need to teach them the language of a scientist. A part of this involves exposing children to the terminology of science as described earlier. Another part is helping students frame their curiosity in the form of questions. And from these questions, help your students develop a sense of how to answer questions in a way that others can understand. To do these activities, it will help if you model how questions are asked and answered.

Develop a list of questions for the different parts of the seed experiment—for example, consider what questions you might ask in preparation for the experiment, as an introduction to the experiment, to draw analogies with real-life experiences relating to growth, to relate to the growth of other plants, to satiate your students' inner curiosity of "what makes it all happen," and so forth. Following are some questions about the growth of seeds and related matters:

1. How do seeds open up?
2. Where does the food come from to make a plant grow?
3. Why do plants produce seeds?
4. What would happen if a plant never produced any seeds?
5. How many different kinds of seeds can you eat?
6. What does the word *edible* mean?
7. What makes some seeds taste good?
8. How long can a seed live before it won't grow anymore?
9. Why is sunlight important for helping plants grow?
10. What happens to seeds that are always in the shade?
11. Can a seed grow without water?
12. Can a corn seed germinate without dirt?
13. How do seeds move from one place to another?

14. What animals eat seeds?
15. Why does corn grow faster than you do?
16. What will happen if we leave one side of the jar toward the sunlight all of the time?
17. What will happen if the paper towel is not kept moist at all times?
18. How can you measure the growth of the corn?
19. How can you show the growth of the corn over a period of two weeks?
20. Why do corn seeds always grow to become corn plants?
21. What kind of soil will corn grow best in?
22. What is a cob and why do we say "corn on the cob"?
23. What is a stalk of corn and why do we say, "the man was stalking the deer"?
24. What do roots do?
25. How does water get into the root and up through the plant?
26. How fast will the corn grow?
27. Can popcorn be planted so that it will grow?
28. What makes a popcorn pop? (Hint: the same thing that helps a seed germinate)
29. Can the corn plant be moved from the jar and planted in soil?
30. What other experiments can you do with seeds?

These questions may appear obvious, and you might even think that it is not necessary to write them down. Our numerous observations of teachers teaching science, however, indicate otherwise. Teachers tend to do most of the talking and ask very few questions. The questions appear to be limited by the instructional moment in that teachers feel the need to "get on with the lesson." Questions also seem limited by the fact that some teachers may not have the requisite skills to sign them or to get the meaning of the question across in whatever modality and language they are using. They may feel limited by the language of their students. Or they may feel intimidated by their lack of fluency in signing. Both of these excuses are poor and heighten rather than weaken the need to write questions down. Therefore, do make a habit of writing a list of questions relating to your science lesson. Practice signing and/or saying these questions. Think of prompts that you might use to help clarify the meaning of a question or to help a student answer the questions. In class, ask these questions over and over and encourage your students to put forth any answer they can think of. Hazarding a wrong answer is a part of being a scientist.

You too should assume the role of a scientist and answer some of the questions. This allows you to model the language related to responding to questions. As with the students, if you do not know an answer you should allow yourself to make an intelligent guess, explaining to the students the reason for your answer.

This leads us to another strategy for engaging students in science talk. When a question is asked for which a student does not know the answer, teach the student a strategy for finding the answer. The following five steps to answering a question may be of help to some students:

Step 1: What is the question? Do I understand what is being asked? Can I repeat the question in a different way?

Step 2: What do I need to know to answer the question? Do I understand the question well enough to know what to look for? Who can help me understand the question?

Step 3:   How can I go about finding the answer? What can I do to get the information needed to answer the question?

Step 4:   Where do I go to get the information that I need to answer the question? Is this a question that I can answer by reading, by conducting an experiment, or by asking someone for help?

Step 5:   Am I ready to answer the question? If yes, then answer it. If no, then go back to step 1.

Place these five steps on a chart on a wall. Write the steps on a laminated, colored bristol board that the students can keep in their desks or take home with them to refer to when necessary.

When practical, make a point of writing down questions that your students have asked before, during, and after an experiment. This reinforces the importance of language as a means of expressing one's knowledge of science. It is also a good opportunity to demonstrate examples of how questions are written. Display these questions above your science **reading center** on a chart and encourage your students to add to the chart. You and your students might not be able to answer all of these questions but that is the way of a scientist.

Finally, science talk should be encouraged throughout an activity because it helps students structure their thinking about a science concept. During an experiment have your students describe what they are doing or observing and help them attach words and signs to their descriptions. You could also have students take turns conducting an experiment while another student describes what is happening. The point is to engage students in talking about science often.

Planning Authentic Experiences

Not every teacher has the pleasure of being able to go on weekly field trips. But field trips are essential to deaf children's acquisition of science knowledge because deaf children miss out on too many incidental learning opportunities through their diminished access to the language of their home environment. Attack this problem by planning authentic language and learning experiences for the students. Consider the present experiment. We have already talked about a walk around the school to identify growing plants. This activity is simple and cheap, plus if the students engage in a lot of discussions it can become a beneficial language learning experience.

A field trip to a horticultural garden or a plant nursery would be a suitable experience. If you know of one that employs a deaf person, that would enhance the value of the experience. As described in greater detail in Chapter 3, the field trip needs to be planned carefully, accounting for the many language learning opportunities associated with the trip. In conjunction with a trip to a horticultural garden the students might do any or all of the following activities:

- Write a letter to the director of the garden to ask for permission to visit.
- Search on the Internet to see if the garden has a Web site.
- Use a map to describe the directions the school transportation will take to get to the garden.

- Prepare a list of questions to ask someone who works at the garden. Arrange for a time so that the students can write the responses to the questions during the field trip.
- Assign one or two students the responsibility of being field-trip reporters.
- Take Polaroid or digital pictures during the trip and write a caption for each picture taken.
- Write a report on the field trip using information from the questions that were asked, the pictures taken, and the reporters' notes.
- Write a thank you note to the person who gave the class the tour of the garden.

Another authentic learning experience is to have the students bring the materials needed for an experiment to class. In the present experiment, they need four to six corn seeds, a tall wide-mouthed jar, waxed paper, a spray bottle, and two to four sheets of paper towels. Have the students write this out and take it home to show their parents. Write a letter to the parents containing a checklist of things that their child has to do when gathering the materials. The child might, for example, have to explain why each material is needed, name or spell the item being collected, and if the items are not in the house, then the child should have to discuss with his or her parents where to find or buy the items. The students can top this off by writing a brief paragraph describing how they gathered the materials.

Creating a Reading Center

All classrooms should have a reading center that is related to the science unit being taught. You do not need books relating to each experiment that you will teach, but you do need a collection of reading materials associated with the theme of your unit. You might try to make the reading center a place that the students want to visit by allowing them to participate in the design and building of it. It should be visually appealing with posters. Most importantly, it should be accessible and practical by providing a range of reading materials at levels that will appeal to your students. Magazines, storybooks, resource books, and picture books have a place in all reading centers. So too does access to the Internet.

Stock the reading center with some of the more obvious choices such as the *National Geographic* and *Discovery* magazines. Also include gardening catalogs, which are wonderful sources of pictures for collages and other artwork. For younger children, include different versions of "Jack and the Beanstalk" and books such as *The Giving Tree* that can generate discussions about our dependency on the food chain and our responsibility for caring about nature. Be creative in the books you select. If you can find a teen magazine that has a feature on a teen movie star who lists gardening as a hobby then you have probably set a new standard for making literature interesting to your students. Many public libraries have collections of used books that they sell for less than a dollar. Bazaars and rummage sales are also excellent sources for stocking up on magazines and books on gardening and nature.

Have an adult, deaf or hearing, come to your class to read a book or talk about a book about plants that he or she enjoyed reading. Last, you read, too—not just to the students but also to yourself. Talk about what you have read and what you have learned. Show your excitement when talking about reading. Share with your students some of the things that you would like to read about and how you plan to go about reading them.

. . . and Don't Forget the Role Models

Although including role models is not a critical element in all lesson plans, it should be an important consideration in the design of a unit plan. As discussed earlier, role models are a source of inspiration for children to learn about things. They also can help children begin to think about possible career choices that are of interest to them. In the unit plan on plants, one person that immediately comes to mind is George Washington Carver, an African American agricultural scientist. Working in a laboratory, he invented some 300 synthetic products from peanuts including butter, milk, cheese, flour, wood stain, dyes, and soap. From the sweet potato, he developed over 100 products including tapioca, starch, vinegar, molasses, paste, and rubber.

Then there is Charles Bonnet, a deaf naturalist. Born in Geneva, Switzerland, in 1720, Bonnet was educated by private tutors because his parents wanted to remove him from his peers who teased him about his deafness (Lang & Meath-Lang, 1995). He spoke of his deafness in terms of the hardships it caused him:

> It was my deafness, which had already begun to manifest itself, that frequently made me the object of scorn in the lessons and lectures and exposed me without stop to ridicule. (Lang & Meath-Lang, 1995, p. 43).

He did not succumb to teasing and ridicule but became well educated. His perseverance led to a life of dedicated work in the area of science, and he was recognized for his study of plants and animals. In the area of botany, he was one of the first scientists ever to study the process of photosynthesis. At 20 years of age, the French Academy of Sciences appointed him as a corresponding member (Lang & Meath-Lang, 1995).

Other Ways to Help Deaf Children Learn Science

What we have been describing are ways to shape your science teaching in order to enhance your deaf students' acquisition of science knowledge and skills. The methods described emphasize the need to focus on the language aspect of learning science. But there are many ways to teach science, and we encourage you to explore their benefits while incorporating the four challenges of teaching science to deaf students into the application of these various science teaching methods in your classroom.

Burton and Campbell (1997), for example, espouse the "Seven E" teaching model that relies on seven steps to effectively teach science. These seven steps all have to do with sound teaching practices and involve the following self-explanatory instructional goals: expectation, enticement, engagement, explanation, exploration, extension, and evidence. For deaf students, you could have more "E" goals. In particular, consider incorporating evolving language experiences that begin with the expectation of what the science lesson is all about and end with your evaluation of the success of the instructional unit in teaching certain science concepts.

The National Science Resource Center (1997) has published a list of questions that teachers should ask when selecting inquiry-centered science curricular materials. Among these questions are the following:

1. Does the material focus on student inquiry and engage students in the process of science?
2. Does the material provide opportunities for students to gather and defend their own evidence and express their results in a variety of ways?
3. Does the material include a balance of student-directed and teacher-facilitated activities as well as discussions?
4. Does the material incorporate effective strategies for the teacher and/or students to use in assessing student learning?
5. Does the teacher's guide suggest opportunities for integrating science with other areas of the curriculum?
6. Do students have opportunities to work collaboratively and alone?

Teachers need to help deaf students think of ideas for experiments that will lead to the students' talking about, writing up, and internalizing all of these experiences into a greater understanding and appreciation of science. The overriding principle of teaching science is for the teacher to engage deaf students in their learning of science rather than to control their movement through passive science activities.

You too should become active in the process of learning new techniques to teach science. Throughout this chapter we have stressed the importance of emphasizing literacy skills in the learning of science. Engage the students in talking about science as a means of preparing them for reading and writing about it. Yore (2000) offers an interesting conundrum about this effort:

> The most difficult issue involved in explicit reading instruction and writing-to-learn activities in science is to convince teachers and professors who did not receive such instruction or experience that such activities are valuable (p. 119).

This assessment of the field's reluctance to incorporate literacy into teaching science may be correct and, if so, then it is a challenge that teachers of the deaf must face. Experimentation in the classroom and professional development are two ways of meeting this challenge.

As a teacher of deaf students, the more effort you put into teaching science, the better command of language your students will gain. Meet with other teachers and researchers (see, for example, the box titled, "Ten Important Emphases in Teaching Science to Deaf Students") in the area of science to discuss effective teaching strategies, attend conferences, read up on science related topics, and use the Internet to explore science-related ideas and to establish contact with other teachers interested in teaching science.

A Sampling from the Internet

We have talked about the value of the Internet as a tool for teaching and as a resource for both teachers and students. In this section we provide an example of what the Internet has to offer with a description of AESOP, which is a Web site (http://www.rit.edu/~ aesop-www/index.html) developed by Dr. Harry Lang, a deaf researcher and educator at the **National Technical Institute for the Deaf (NTID).** Lang codirected a National Science

Ten Important Emphases in Teaching Science to Deaf Students

Dr. Harry G. Lang is a professor and researcher at the National Technical Institute for the Deaf in Rochester, New York. He has conducted extensive research in the area of how deaf children learn science and how their teachers teach it. We asked him what he thought teachers should know when teaching science to deaf children. His thoughts were as follows:

Educational research and teacher preparation activities over the past thirty years indicate that the following are ten important considerations science instructors should keep in mind when teaching and developing curricula:

1. *Cognitive engagement.* Hands-on activities are very important, but more important are minds-on activities. That is, while manipulating materials and learning content, the students should be answering questions, formulating hypotheses, and developing other science process skills. Incorporate a variety of activities that will strengthen both short-term (working) memory and long-term memory, which are essential for effective reading.

2. *Critical thinking.* Ask students questions constantly and encourage them to make decisions based on their thinking about each question. Whether it is planning for an experiment or reflecting on a recent science class to identify the most important things learned, these decisions should be both frequent and varied in nature.

3. *Literacy.* Science literacy and English literacy should be developed together by incorporating informal writing-to-learn strategies on a regular basis and frequent reading activities that include course texts and related outside readings (magazines, newspapers, etc.).

4. *Content knowledge.* Research with both hearing and deaf students has shown that knowledge of content by teachers is perceived as the most important characteristic of an effective teacher. Science teachers who do not have a strong background in science or science education should seek out professional development activities (courses, workshops, networking with other professionals, etc.) to develop the appropriate knowledge and skills. The Internet (World Wide Web) is rich with resources for preparing for classes, and many available books and other materials offer excellent strategies for using inexpensive materials to teach science content and processes. National standards for science teachers are available, which serve as excellent guides for developing appropriate emphases in teaching and curriculum development.

5. *Self-esteem.* Help the students learn that many deaf men and women in history have made significant contributions and found fulfilling careers in the fields of science, engineering, mathematics, medicine, and invention. Increase student motivation in science by providing readings, inviting role model deaf scientists, and other activities that will inform and inspire.

6. *High expectations.* Biographical research has shown that one of the primary barriers to the success of scientists with disabilities is the attitude held by gatekeepers, including teachers, parents, counselors, and others. Establish high expectations for your deaf students. It will make a difference. The literature includes hundreds of stories of very successful deaf persons whose parents and teachers questioned their abilities in science or mathematics.

7. *Variety of experiences.* Avoid constant lecturing and provide a variety of activities (experimental, cooperative, experiential, relating science to their everyday lives, field trips, etc.). The more deaf students experience and the broader vocabulary they develop, the better readers they will be.

8. *Communication with students.* Learning as a process of dialogue may be enhanced by establishing rapport with the students and knowing how best to communicate with them. This also means identifying, as a starting point, the students' conceptions and misconceptions about science content. Once the dialogue rapport is there, the construction of meaning in science will improve.

9. *Use of technology.* Technology can bring access to science (content of films through captioning; distance learning through the Internet, etc.). It can be a learning tool (science journals through e-mail or word processing; personal captioning of a videotaped science experiment, etc.). And, importantly, the use of technology will prepare deaf students to be knowledgeable of the many complex roles technology plays in our world. But as with any instructional strategy in general, the use of technology should be based on evaluation of its benefits to learning.

10. *Action research.* Research, in its most general sense, is planned, systematic inquiry. Action research can take the form of a science teacher attempting new strategies and informally evaluating their effectiveness and following up with modifications in the process of seeking the most effective ways to educate particular students or groups. Teaching a course in such a way is much like a scientific method, whereby the teacher seeks to identify which variables (strategies, materials) have the most positive effect on student learning.

Foundation three-year grant titled "Access to English and Science Outreach Project" (**AESOP**). Its primary goals were to:

- Develop and deliver a coherent set of instructional strategies that may be used to teach the content and language of science to deaf students.
- Increase deaf students' access to information about the accomplishments of deaf women and men in scientific professions.
- Create a national network of science teachers of deaf students.

AESOP brings together research on the teaching of science to deaf students, extensive science-related references, strategies for teaching science, particularly in the area of hands-on activities with key emphasis given to the teaching of English in science, examples of actual lesson plans designed for deaf students, and notes about deaf people in science. The Web site developed during this project has been expanded on a continual basis and highlights some of the most critical variables in helping deaf students learn science.

For example, a teacher studying the central nervous system might wish to use a lesson titled "Pathway of a Nerve Impulse" (contributed by Chuck Bell, Vancouver, British Columbia), which is available in its entirety. AESOP also links you to a Web site designed by students at the Model Secondary School for the Deaf that provides a listing of deaf people in various areas of science along with a brief entry of their accomplishments.

Among the many listed are Anders Gustaf Ekeberg, a chemist who discovered the element tantalum, and Thomas Meehan, who is known as the Father of American Horticulture. The variety of selections that AESOP offers makes it a model for the design of other Web sites related to the teaching of a subject to deaf students.

Evaluation

In addition to science tests we would like to see teachers pursue **portfolio assessment** (also referred to as performance-based assessment) as part of their overall evaluation process. (See Chapter 9 for further discussion about testing.) A portfolio can be defined as "a container of evidence of a person's skills" (Hamm & Adams, 1991, p. 18). Many textbooks view portfolios as being student generated whereby students select the work that they feel best highlights their learning—in much the same way that an artist selects his or her best drawings and paintings for a portfolio. In science, a student's work can include written reports based on experiments, field trips, and observations; fictional stories related to a science theme; pictures of experiments conducted and models made; collections of science artifacts and student-made objects; and many more things that demonstrate a certain aspect of their understanding of a concept.

Newer science textbooks and programs are espousing the importance of portfolio assessment and their teacher guides will contain suggestions about what might be placed in a student portfolio. For example, the Teacher's Planning Guide found in the Macmillan/McGraw-Hill 4th Grade Science kit (1995 edition) included the following suggestions for a unit on plants:

- Draw and label the parts of a flower.
- Prepare a demonstration using visual aids about symbiotic relationships.
- Dry and press a flower and then glue it to construction paper.
- Research and prepare an illustrated booklet about plants that were domesticated by Native Americans.
- Write a paragraph on how to prevent soil erosion
- Prepare and record or videotape an oral report about the different jobs done by botanists.
- Write a story about what it would be like to live in Biosphere 2.

These activities illustrate both the specificity and the generality of the activities that can be included in a portfolio, all of which can be applied to the teaching of deaf students. The research aspect of some of these activities can help lead students through a wide choice of resources as they search for information that highlights the learning aspect of this type of portfolio assessment. Encyclopedias, library books, science magazines, science laboratories, and the Internet can all come into play. Take a research project on the Biosphere 2 as an example. Although many people have heard about this project, how many people can actually describe key aspects of it? Located thirty miles north of Tucson, Arizona, the Biosphere 2 is an enclosed research facility for studying how changes in the environment impact on seven different types of ecosystems. A rainforest, a 900,000 gallon ocean, and a desert are three of the wilderness ecosystems, and a human habitat is also a part of the research. Students can explore these ecosystems by taking a video tour on the Biosphere 2's Web site.

Creating a science portfolio will give deaf students the opportunity to invest in their education, because it encourages students to make decisions about what to collect and how to shape an image of themselves with this collection. Furthermore, it gives deaf students the opportunity to measure their understanding in nontraditional manners such as through the delivery of a presentation (signed and/or spoken) that is first captured on videotape or digital video and transferred to a CD.

In addition to students' deciding what should be placed in their portfolio, we suggest that teachers also select activities that can best tease out the knowledge and skills that deaf students have acquired in science. This can be accomplished if the teacher also creates a separate but parallel portfolio for each deaf student. Both types of portfolio assessment can be used for tracking a deaf student's academic progress and development of language skills, which is critical to ensuring that annual IEP goals are meaningful and are based on a comprehensive picture of a student's performance in school and not simply a test score or a page number in a textbook.

Portfolios, therefore, not only measure a student's past performances but also indicate the direction that future instructions might take. To this end, teachers should consider including the following indicators of student progress:

1. *Vocabulary chart*. Words and signs that have been taught directly to the student during a unit should be recorded for future reinforcement. As with any children, we do not anticipate that all deaf children will memorize all of the new words and signs they come across. This is, in fact, the reason we advocate a vocabulary chart, because it should help teachers make steady progress in a student's vocabulary growth as well as give the student a sense of where others have encountered certain vocabulary words. An example of a vocabulary chart is shown in Figure 2.2.

Obviously, if a student is not in a signing environment, the middle column in the chart would be deleted. For teachers who sign, the use of signing and the selection of appropriate signs is a constant challenge for many teachers. By containing information about the key words that were signed, a future teacher may use this information to help the student recall the meaning of a word or to create instructions to refresh students' understanding of the words based on their recall of the sign.

A vocabulary chart provides a form of accountability to teachers who can check to see how thoroughly they have covered a particular word and the number of activities in which this word was reinforced. Each teacher is also exposing elements of his or her teaching to a student's future teachers. If this chart appears to be a lot of work, it isn't. Most classes of deaf students only have four to seven students. If vocabulary expansion is one goal in the education of deaf students, then keeping track of vocabulary growth is an essential task for teachers.

2. *Writing samples*. Each portfolio should contain a collection of writing samples that highlight exemplary work by the student as well as illustrate the progress that a student has made over the unit and over the school year. The written work should be both unedited

Vocabulary Chart   Date:_____

Unit: How Plants Grow

Key words taught	Signed (S)/fingerspelled (fs)	Instructional activity/ reinforcement
shade	S, fs	taught, notes, report writing
photosynthesis	fs (abbreviated)	taught, notes, illustration
nursery	fs	notes, letter writing, field trip
evaporation	S	experiment, report writing
carbon dioxide	CO_2	taught, notes, chart, illustration
nutrient	fs + S (FOOD)	taught, experiment, report writing, student presentation

FIGURE 2.2   An example of a vocabulary chart relating to a unit on how plants grow.

prose as well as teacher-assisted edited work. The work should span a range of writing associated with science from observation notes, report writing, and experiment documentation to creative writing using a list of key vocabulary words. Writing taken from a science unit can help with language arts instruction. In thematic teaching, some of the vocabulary and language related to science could be covered in a language arts class. However, regardless of the subject matter in which science-related language and vocabulary is taught, assessment of this knowledge should still appear in the science portfolio.

3. *Concept maps.* **Concept maps** come in many forms, but basically they are a series of interlinked words that students use to "to convey to teachers the way(s) that they have constructed knowledge of a particular concept or idea" (Barba, 1995, p. 139). In other words, a concept map helps a teacher understand how a student is thinking about something. Perhaps more important, a concept map provides students with a strategy for exploring the relationship between concepts and facts about these concepts. Students typically use words or phrases and not sentences to key in on a concept or something about this concept. Concept maps or the strategy of mapping is based on schema theory.

A concept map works well with deaf students for a number of reasons, including the fact that it does the following:

- Overrides the concern for using sentences to structure thoughts.
- Is a simple method for helping students to organize their thoughts.
- Forces students to put their thoughts on paper.
- Helps students see relationships and patterns.
- Can be used to help recall information.
- Can be done as an individual or a group activity.
- Can be used to introduce new vocabulary.
- Provides a basis for writing a scientific report or a story about a concept (e.g., a report about "linking people through communication").
- Provides teachers with an insight to the way a student is thinking about something.

Thus, whether used in a cooperative learning setting or as an individual activity, mapping is an effective teaching strategy for helping students understand an array of scientific ideas, both simple and complex. Figure 2.3 shows a fourth-grade student's concept map of how plants grow, what types of plants are eaten, and the various names associated with plants.

Some students might lack the necessary words to build a concept map that adequately captures their thinking. You can listen to a student expressing ideas prior to or while creating a concept map. You can then suggest words to the student that match his or her thinking, but be careful not to give words simply for the sake of mapping—the words given must be based on what the student has said. You may wish to make a list of these new words and use them in a language arts exercise to reinforce a student's understanding of them.

If your students know how to sign, then their knowledge of sign language could be adapted to the development of a concept map. However, even deaf students who are fluent in ASL lack knowledge of the necessary English words to express themselves in print or speech. A teacher can adapt the student's knowledge of ASL to aid in the development of a concept map. For example, a student could explain in signs their understanding of a con-

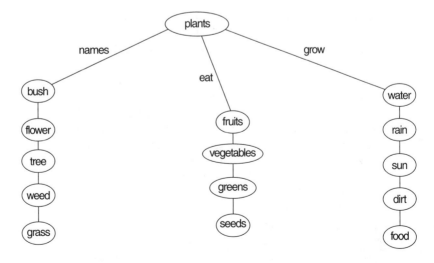

FIGURE 2.3 An illustration of a concept map of how plants grow created by a fourth-grade student.

cept. As the student explains, you build a concept map on the blackboard or overhead. When the student has finished explaining about a concept, you would then review the words and/or phrases shown on the map, pointing out that they represent the same idea that was expressed in signs. This is a good way to help students see the relationship between English and sign language.

4. *Presentations.* Presentations force students to organize their thoughts in a manner that is understandable to others. Videotape students' verbal presentations, signed and/or spoken and show them how to translate or transcribe this presentation into a written one. Include both the videotaped and written presentations in the student's portfolio as well posters and slide shows using software available on personal computers.

Because of the anxiety associated with presentations, some teachers may feel that this is an unfair manner for evaluating a student. Again, do not use a student's perceived inability to do something as an excuse for not doing that thing. There are many skills involved in making a good presentation, and they include the ability to organize thoughts in a logical sequence, to express these thoughts in language that is comprehensible to other people, to select words (and signs) that capture the meaning of what a person is trying to say, to be able to repair a line of thought when necessary, and to be able to evaluate the effectiveness of one's presentation. Teach deaf students the art of making presentations verbally and in writing. Use their presentations not only as a partial means of testing their knowledge of science but also of their command of language.

You should also consider allowing students to make a group presentation that can include all aspects of the experiment, from the planning stage through the experiment and to the presentation itself. This type of activity requires careful planning and assignment of responsibilities to ensure that one student does not do most of the work. Catching this presentation on videotape would make an excellent addition to a student's portfolio.

5. *Journal writing or student logbooks.* Get your students to write. It could be something as simple as a logbook in which whole sentences are not necessary. Or it could be a journal entry by which students describe activities they performed and reflect upon what they have learned. Barba (1995) stated that journal writing is a process of writing about learning, which encourages students to "(1) assess their prior knowledge, (2) think about the process of schooling, (3) formally state what they have learned in the classroom, and (4) integrate language arts and science skills in the classroom" (pp. 141–142). This activity could even be done after the class has shared their reflections about a science experiment because it encourages students to share and gain ideas from each other and also allows them further opportunities to engage in science talk.

Students who are not inclined toward writing are to be encouraged to engage in this activity. (See Chapter 4 for a discussion of journal writing.) With such students, teachers should emphasize the following:

- The purpose of the writing activity is to have them place their thoughts about science on paper.
- Their writing is not being graded for grammar and vocabulary.

- The teacher will help provide words and structure sentences when requested.
- The journal or logbook is especially for the student; something that the student can read to recall information.

At all times, the teacher needs to take care that the student views the writing activity as part of being a scientist and not as a chore.

Conclusion

So how should you teach science to deaf students? Teaching science is about giving deaf students the tools needed to explore and understand scientific phenomenon. In our teaching, we aim to help deaf students appreciate science for what it is and the impact that it has on their lives. We outlined instructional strategies in this chapter that require a dedicated teacher who is prepared to meet the challenge of teaching science. Without this internal motivation, teachers may be tempted to teach solely from a textbook.

Although there are many different approaches to how science can be taught, we have proposed that teachers can help deaf students by emphasizing hands-on learning and by creating opportunities for visual learning, such as having the students design concept maps. It is also important for teachers to be cognizant of the experiential deficit that deaf students might have when exposed to new concepts. In some instances, providing background information or experiences may be as important as the science lesson itself. At the same time, science must not simply be all hands-on. Deaf students need to become accustomed to the language of science and gain expertise in using this language to help them acquire new science-related knowledge. Thus, writing and talking about science are two important teaching strategies.

Finally, it is important for teachers to expose deaf students to role models, both deaf and hearing. We want deaf students to be interested in learning about science and role models can be used as a source of motivation. When deaf people are used as role models, opportunities may arise that help deaf students reflect upon their own deafness and how this affects their interests and desire to learn.

KEY WORDS AND CONCEPTS

AESOP: An acronym for Access to English and Science Outreach Project, which is a Web site designed to provide information about teaching the content and language of science to deaf students. The Web site is maintained by researchers at the National Technical Institute for the Deaf.

authentic learning experiences: Learning about things from life. Taking advantage of these opportunities yields authentic learning experiences.

concept maps: An illustration of connected words (and/or phrases) that shows the relationships of these words to a particular concept. A concept map shows teachers the way students are thinking about a concept. It is also called a conceptual map and the use of such maps as a teaching strategy is often referred to as *mapping*.

content standard: Items listed in a curriculum that describe what it is that students are supposed to learn in a particular subject.

curricular goal: A goal that breaks down the content standards into units that can be taught. Where a content standard might talk about students being able to describe the life cycle of a plant or animal, a curricular goal addresses whether the life cycle of a animal or a plant is going to taught. In addition, the curricular goal may even be about a specific aspect of the life cycle, such as the growth of a seed to a mature plant.

hands-on activities: Active participation in activities that will help deaf students grasp the meaning of a concept. Therefore, science teaching that is activity-oriented as opposed to textbook-oriented can be an effective means because this type of activity ties in well with deaf students' needs for visual learning experiences.

instructional objectives: Typically created by the teacher, objectives that are often stated in terms of outcomes: what it is that the teacher wants a student to be able to do after a lesson.

National Technical Institute for the Deaf (NTID): Situated on campus of the Rochester Institute of Technology, in Rochester, New York. It has about 1,200 deaf students pursuing postsecondary education at the associate and bachelor's degree levels.

portfolio assessment: Also referred to as performance-based assessment, an alternative to testing that relies on demonstrations of a student's knowledge and skills. A portfolio is often described as being something that the student generates. The key element is that whatever is included in the portfolio demonstrates in some way a student's understanding of a concept. Examples of what can be included in a portfolio are written or videotaped reports, science-related stories, pictures of experiments conducted and models made, and collections of science artifacts and student-made objects.

reading center: An area of a classroom that has been set aside for the sole purpose of reading. The design of a reading center will vary but some of the items that they might include are a selection of books related to the topics under discussion in the classroom, a range of reading levels, a computer with access to the Internet, posters, and other reading materials.

unit plan: A series of lessons that revolve around a common theme. One advantage of incorporating unit plans when teaching a subject is that they are conducive to a more comprehensive exploration of concepts, and they make it more convenient to incorporate critical teaching techniques such as engaging students in science talk, planning authentic learning experiences, and creating a reading center.

visual learning: Used in reference to the fact that deaf people rely on their sight to gain information and learn about things. The lack of access to complete auditory information makes the use of visual learning techniques critical in the education of deaf students.

QUESTIONS

1. Why should learning language be an expected outcome of learning science?

2. Other than being scientists, what did Thomas Edison, Robert Weitbrecht, and Charles Bonnet have in common? What inventions or contributions to science did each one make?

3. What elements of teaching science make it a suitable subject to teach deaf students?

4. What did the TIMSS researchers find out about the science curriculum in the United States that may be problematic for deaf students?

5. What did the National Science Education Standards say that students must do in order to acquire scientific knowledge?

6. What is the relationship between deaf students' exposure to authentic everyday experiences and their learning science?

7. Why is talking important for deaf students learning science?

8. What are the seven elements associated with developing a unit plan? Describe each of them.

9. Outline three strategies for introducing new vocabulary words in a science lesson.

10. Describe a reading center that you might create for a middle school classroom studying environmental science.

11. What are four ways in which a science teacher can use the Web site AESOP in planning unit plans or lessons for deaf students?

12. Provide a definition of portfolio assessment, then describe the benefits of using this type of assessment with deaf students in science.

13. What are the key elements of a vocabulary chart?

14. Define a concept map and give six reasons why mapping is a beneficial technique to use with deaf students.

15. Why is journal writing a good technique to use in a science class?

ACTIVITIES

1. Compile a list of five role models for a unit plan on the rainforest, biochemistry, weather, or some other field of science suitable to a grade level that interests you. These role models do not have to famous or well-known people. They can be someone local. If you are having difficulty coming up with role models, how might you use the Internet to help you?

2. Select a science-related theme for teaching to a specific grade level. Use a science curriculum for this grade level, and derive a series of complementary content standards and curricular goals. For each curricular goal, create at least two instructional objectives.

3. Select a topic that might be taught to students in one of the upper elementary grade levels. Draft a list of vocabulary that might be included in the instructional unit related to teaching this topic.

CHAPTER

3 Teaching Social Studies

CHAPTER OUTCOMES

After reading this chapter, you should be able to:

1. Use the basic principles of teaching social studies to guide the development of both individual social studies lessons and social studies units.
2. Integrate the teaching of a social studies topic or theme into other subject matter.
3. Design lessons that are educationally relevant in that they require higher level thinking. In addition, these lessons will provide deaf students with access to culturally relevant information.
4. Apply principles of cooperative learning into the design of a lesson plan.
5. Demonstrate that your instructional planning meets the challenges that deaf students face when studying social studies by
   (a) exposing them to the culture associated with many communities including the Deaf community; and
   (b) helping them access the language and resources associated with a social studies topic.
6. Incorporate portfolio or performance-based assessment throughout all social studies activities.
7. Infuse a study of deaf people into the social studies curriculum.
8. Discuss the role of the itinerant and resource room teachers who are teaching or helping deaf students learn social studies.

A lasting impression of the benefits of learning social studies was made on one of the authors when he was in the ninth grade. At this time, he was an avid reader who absorbed anything in print at all times of the day. But history was seldom a preferred choice of literature. It took a student teacher who was teaching social studies in a middle school to pique his interest in the connection between print and history. Here's the story:

> I was a teenager watching Neil Armstrong taking his first step on the moon. Sitting beside me was a 29-year-old university student named George who was preparing to become a high

school social studies teacher. George loved learning and talking about people and their ways of living. He had traveled around Europe, the Middle East, and Northern Africa, and his conversations were laced with tidbits about history and culture. While Neil was making his famous speech, I stated the obvious: "There's something for the history books. Don't you think that you will get to the moon one day?" With a gleam of mischief in his eyes, he responded: "How do you know that Armstrong is on the moon? Maybe the whole thing was filmed earlier in a Hollywood studio." An outlandish statement? Perhaps, but it made me pause for thought. How much of history is fact? How do we know that what is in print is in fact an imprint of something that had happened? I began to take a greater interest in reading books about history and comparing the information they contained with my understanding of the time period. In doing so, I became better versed in my understanding of human nature and the forces that shaped the culture of each society.

What's special about this experience? The student teacher was the biggest influence in this author's decision to become a teacher. George had a knack for asking thought-provoking questions. Following Armstrong's historic announcement, the two of them engaged in discussion about what is taught in social studies and how it is taught. The author in this study had always relied on reading to get him through school because his deafness precluded any attempt to participate in classroom discussions (this being a time before interpreters were available). Yet, he always wondered what it would have been like to listen to others speak about a subject and for him to speak his thoughts to his classmates. George helped him realize that learning social studies required much more than book knowledge. Just as social studies is the study of people and their interactions with one another and the environment, so too should social studies involve students interacting with one another.

Why We Teach Social Studies

There are a paltry number of journal articles about teaching social studies to deaf students. Textbooks and literature that discuss how we teach subject matter to deaf students are mostly devoted to the language arts. To our knowledge, there has never been a specific federal grant competition for research in the area of teaching social studies to deaf students. Perhaps most telling is the fact that the literature is essentially devoid of reports of deaf students' achievement in social studies. Social studies is part of the education of deaf children but more as a visitor than an integral part of their learning.

Yet social studies has the potential to be the most treasured of all the core subjects taught in schools. It is the only subject that encompasses elements of language, science, and mathematics, in addition to the social behaviors of people. It also touches upon health, music, and the arts. The many faces of social studies should be used as a guide for teaching it. Let's take a walk through the years of the Renaissance and see how all subject matter can be intricately woven into a single social studies unit.

There are many topics available for a social studies subunit on the Renaissance. There was the Hundred Years War (1337–1453) between the French and English monarchies. There is the inspiring story of Joan of Arc, the daughter of peasants, who was burned at the stake in 1431. She is credited with having saved France from certain defeat at the hands of the English. There were numerous explorations during the Renaissance that can be studied, such as Christopher Columbus's landing in the Americas and Sir Francis Drake's circumnavigation of the world.

No matter which topic you select, there is something to be said. In the area of social studies we learn that the Black Death made its way into European society in the fourteenth century. This single event speaks of the social consequences stemming from the death of many leaders, laborers, and peasants; of science because of the transmission of the bubonic disease by fleas and mites that were transported by rats from the Middle East to Europe and from one city to the next; of health for the unhygienic conditions of the people, homes, and cities that ensured that transmission would take place quickly and effectively; and of mathematics for the decimation of the population. For example, the Black Death killed a third of Europe's estimated 4.2 million people. Many towns lost more than 50 percent of their population. What would today's population in Europe be if the Black Death had never occurred? The hygienic concern is a potent reminder to students in a health class of the consequences of not being clean (see the box on "Making Scents of History").

Social studies is also a great subject for further development of a deaf child's literacy skills. The Renaissance ushered in many great writers whose writings are still subjected to the scrutiny of high school English students. William Shakespeare is perhaps the most famous and prolific of these writers. Chaucer on the other hand was one of the first Renaissance writers, and his *Canterbury Tales* (1385–1400) are still enjoyed by people of all ages. And how can you not talk about nursery rhymes? (See the box titled "What Was Mother Goose Thinking?")

There is also a Renaissance link to Deaf studies. This is a more difficult area to explore but one event that comes to mind is the documented teaching of deaf children. This came at a time when deaf children (and most other children) were not taught and therefore did not learn to read and write. Nor did they aspire to accomplish their own livelihood.

Making Scents of History

Teaching the facts of history is not enough. Good teaching helps students acquire a feel for the era and the people that they are studying. To say that most people were not clean (by our standards) during the Renaissance years means very little to high school students. Most of them have already developed a picture of life during those times from TV, videos, and the movies, and Hollywood doesn't make its money portraying reality. Therefore, teachers must search for stories or information that can enlighten students as to the lives of the people they are studying. Take the unhygienic conditions. What does this mean to a 15-year-old? Wearing the same socks for a week? Forgetting to wash your hands for a day? Drinking milk directly from the container then putting it back in the refrigerator? Try this. Having a bath just once a year in the month of May. Always getting married in June because the bride and groom have been without a bath for just one month and the smell of unclean bodies is beginning to be noticeable. In addition, flowers have blossomed in June and are carried close to the bride and groom, thereby masking some of the smell. This was the way some people lived during the Middle Ages. Few students will forget this story soon, and it can serve as a mnemonic device for reminding students about the conditions that led to the spread of the Black Death.

What Was Mother Goose Thinking?

Nursery rhymes or Mother Goose rhymes are a part of every child's early linguistic experiences. But how often are deaf children exposed to them? Some of their teachers (and parents) might be reluctant to read nursery rhymes because of the importance of rhyming in the verses. But there are many good reasons for reading them. One obvious reason is that they are everywhere in a young child's experience—they can be found in books, magazines, movies, television, at the dinner table, at bedtime, in the car, and other places as well. A second and not so obvious reason is that the origin of some of them goes back to a time when oral history and not print was used to pass stories and information down through the ages. No exact dates for many of the rhymes are available because they were used long before someone penned them in a book. But dates can be estimated. Try this activity. Have older deaf students collect different variations of a nursery rhyme and analyze them. For example, "Ring Around the Rosies" was created during the time of the Black Death. The line "We all fall down" is a reference to the fact that near the end of their lives, some of the people afflicted with the bubonic disease would run around and then drop dead. And the line before it, "Hatcha, hatcha"? This is a reference to coughing up blood. Or is it? Some children learn the line "Ashes, ashes, all fall down." Present students with both examples for analysis. "Baa, Baa Black Sheep" is another rhyme describing the plague. What do you think "The little boy who lives in the lane" is referring to?

They were viewed as being incapable of rational thought, and in many societies they could not inherit because they were thought to have no language. Then a monk, Pablo Bonet Ponce de Leon, came along. He sought to change how deaf people were viewed when he was challenged with the task of teaching two deaf brothers to read and write, a requirement in some places for those who wished to inherit their parent's estate. He wrote down his teaching methods in 1545. Furthermore, the fingerspelling he used is almost identical to the manual alphabet now used in American Sign Language.

This brief walk through the Renaissance illustrates how even a cursory investigation in social studies requires some understanding of most other subject matters. Unquestionably, social studies is a good platform for showcasing the application of skills learned in reading and writing, science, and mathematics. For this reason, it is prudent for teachers, and especially for those who espouse thematic teaching, to revolve their teaching around a social studies–related theme.

Social Studies and the Deaf Student

First of all, there is no consensus about what social studies is and why we teach it. Ross (1997) noted that some scholars believe that its purpose is **citizenship education**, which is "the preparation of young people so that they possess the knowledge, skills, and values necessary for active participation in society" (p. 6). This is a hard position to argue against because we want to teach deaf students about values, social behaviors, social issues, and how their individual behavior contributes to the growth of a society. We want students to gain a picture of their role in society and how this role came to be. We want them to be able to read the newspaper, interact with friends, and watch television knowing what's right and what's wrong.

Others argue that the purpose of social studies is to emphasize **cultural transmission**, especially with respect to the dominant society (Stanley & Nelson, 1994). This too is a valid position that values "stability and common standards of thought and behavior" (Ross, 1997, p. 7). However, more and more schools are emphasizing the need to teach students to be analytical in their thinking and to "question and critique standard views accepted by the dominant society" (Ross, 1997, p. 7). Within this framework, or perhaps as an adjunct to the critical analysis of cultures, comes the call for schools to take a multicultural approach, teaching students to respect differences in people (Banks, 1997; Delpit, 1995). This is an approach that has been translated in our field to include a study of deaf people and their ways of living. Whatever its role, scholars do agree that social studies must have an important part in the education of all children (Ross, 1997).

Teaching social studies to deaf students is buttressed with the need to teach them how their place in society has been influenced by factors such as societal forces, federal laws, and educational practices—factors that are unlikely to be described through the regular social studies curriculum. Most of these factors came into being since the 1960s. The beginning of these influences was marked by a growing awareness in professions and in society that people with disabilities were people first who should enjoy the same rights to education, employment, and accessibility that people without disabilities have—a set of rights that some ethnic minority groups such as African Americans have long fought for. From this awareness came a recognition that people with disabilities have their own characteristics and set of social behaviors that make them unique. This meant recognition of the culture of Deaf people and concomitant appreciation of the value and desirability of the **Deaf community**. One result of this recognition was the growing practice in the literature to refer to those deaf people who used ASL and were affiliated to some extent with the Deaf community with the term "Deaf." Today, this is now standard practice.

By the late 1970s many Deaf people all over the United States and Canada embraced this new sense of self with a growing degree of pride in being Deaf and in all that is associated with the Deaf community. They no longer viewed communication in a hearing and speaking society as their problem but rather as a situation that could be accommodated through the use of interpreters (Stewart, Schein, & Cartwright, 1998) and through technology. They gained access to a wider range of effective communication and with that access to better employment opportunities. They fought for the right for deaf people to represent the interest of their own population in a manner similar to the action of African Americans, Native Americans, Hispanics, Asians or Pacific Islanders, and other ethnic groups. This fight is exemplified by the **Deaf President Now** movement at **Gallaudet University** where deaf students successfully argued for the ouster of a nondeaf president in favor of a Deaf one, Dr. I. King Jordan (see Christiansen & Barnartt, 1995).

All of these events were preceded by linguistic research by William Stokoe that described American Sign Language as a language (Stokoe, 1960). This was a change from previous thinking that referred to the signing behavior of deaf people as being "broken English" or quite simply "Deaf signs." The realization that the Deaf community was anchored with its own language led to an upsurge in pride within the Deaf community, a linguistic empowerment in society as well as an enhancement of the stature of Deaf people in public activities, a redefining of how deaf children should be educated, and a slew of employment opportunities in the field of sign language teaching.

These events frame a unique social studies curriculum for deaf students. In their bid to learn more about society, deaf students can be helped by a thorough examination of their own being. These possibilities are numerous and range from a study of **Deaf culture** to a critical review of medical advances—for example, cochlear implants that strive to eliminate deafness or at least make deaf people more comfortable in their interactions with the hearing and speaking elements of society. We see the incorporation of a study of deaf people into social studies as a movement toward a more meaningful curriculum for deaf students. This modification of how we teach social studies should allow schools to better apply the concept of citizenship education and cultural transmission to deaf students.

In sum, there is much that deaf students need to learn about the world they live in. Deaf students have experiences in life that are not always comparable to others who are not deaf. Social studies can be used to help deaf students use these experiences to gain a better understanding of the similarities and differences between deaf and hearing people. This greater awareness can be used to enhance the overall well-being of deaf students. This is the job of a social studies teacher. This is not a call for the removal of the regular social studies curriculum from the education of deaf students. It is a call for a greater infusion of content that is relevant to deaf students into the curriculum in order to provide them with a template upon which an understanding of other groups of people and social forces in society can be built.

Methods for Teaching Social Studies

Self-expression is a key principle in the design of social studies instruction. Research shows that learning is best when students are actively engaged in the process (Perkins, 1992; Schmidt et al., 1999). Memorizing and repeating information in social studies is simply not enough. Students must be taught how to analyze the information they are receiving. This analysis is facilitated through discussions that hinge on ideas, for example, about why events occur and their effects on people's lives including the lives of the students. Thus, it is inadequate for students to know that the Civil War took place during the years 1861–1865. They have to learn to ask why the Civil War took place, how the war might have been averted, what were the long-term consequences of the war were, and what events in today's society are a reflection of the causes fought for during the war. This is the function of self-expression in learning social studies.

Similarly, knowing that the Deaf President Now (DPN) revolution in 1988 resulted in the appointment of a Deaf president at Gallaudet University is merely introducing information that tells us little about how well a student might understand the significance of the revolution. Understanding DPN requires that students examine the elements of the revolution as a concept and not data. This examination can be spurred by discussions about how the civil rights movements of African Americans in the 1960s impacted on the outcome of the DPN. Students can explore how the study of ASL prepared Americans to empathize with the student's demands. They can debate how the appointment of a Deaf president might have changed society perspectives about people with disabilities in general. This type of exploration gives greater relevance to the DPN events and forces students to engage in deeper levels of thinking.

You might be wondering how DPN can be taught when, unlike the Civil War, it is nowhere to be found in the curriculum. This is not unusual because, traditionally, minority students have been underserved by the social studies curriculum (Ladson-Billings, 1997). As important as DPN might be for the Deaf community, it is nevertheless a concept framed within the context of deaf people interacting with hearing people, which is a foreign concept for general education students.

Even if DPN did find its way into the curriculum, the way in which it would likely be taught is a cause for concern. **Conventional social studies** consists of a number of events and topics that are discussed in terms of dates, locations, and names of people or things. Such teaching breeds sterile learning that can only be demonstrated through regurgitation of information. Erickson (1998) offers an alternative in **problem-solving context** for "actively engaging students in the thoughtful application of knowledge" (p. 7). Perkins (1992) illustrates this concept as follows:

> Some students read about nutrition, water as a standard of density, solar-powered airplanes, and other matters in the usual textbookish way, with the intent to remember. Other students read the same items of information in the context of thinking about the challenges of a journey through a South American jungle. For instance, the students read about the density of water in the context of how much water the travelers would have to carry. (p. 22)

Some research has shown that students who learn using a problem-solving context are better able to transfer this knowledge to other tasks than students who learn in a conventional manner (Perkins, 1992).

Like the previous chapter on teaching science, engaging deaf students in the learning process is the goal. Teaching social studies using a concept-based curriculum, as opposed to a curriculum that is centered around the teaching of topics and events, achieves that goal (Erickson, 1998; Perkins, 1992, Schmidt et al., 1999). The conventional way of teaching social studies makes it difficult for deaf children to achieve. But teachers can make a difference, as we will address later in this chapter. We are now going to examine additional challenges for deaf students learning social studies and provide strategies for responding to these challenges.

Four Great Challenges for Teaching Social Studies to Deaf Students

The previous chapter described four challenges science teachers face when teaching deaf students are deaf students' lack of (1) authentic experiences that will help them relate to material taught in classes; (2) vocabulary that will give them greater access to writings and dialogue about science; (3) opportunities to talk about topics they are learning; and (4) knowledge of or exposure to deaf role models in the field of science. These considerations carry similar weight in the area of social studies. There are additional challenges that the social studies teacher faces when teaching deaf children. Four of the major ones are discussed below.

1. *Schools must address the different communities that deaf students have access to by providing culturally relevant instruction.* Content is not a problem in social studies. There are numerous topics that can be taught. Making them interesting is something that good teachers do. But an interesting topic does not mean that the topic will be meaningful to the students. For a topic to be meaningful, it must satisfy a number of conditions including "the classroom context" and the "physical and psychological characteristics of the students" (Shulman, 1987, p. 6). One obvious example of this is using classroom material that is relevant to the culture of the students.

The term **culturally relevant** has been used "to describe the kind of teaching that is designed not merely to fit the school culture to the student's culture, but also to use student culture as a basis for helping students understand themselves and others, structure social interactions, and conceptualize knowledge" (Ladson-Billings, 1997, p. 123–124). Not making topics culturally relevant to students has been seen as the reason why many ethnic students do not achieve as well as white students (Banks, 1997; Grossman, 1995). Volumes of literature on multicultural education have been built on this premise (see Miller-Lachmann, 1995, for an annotated bibliography about the education of ethnic groups in the United States), and while there does not appear to be a consensus on what works best, it is generally agreed that a "teacher who is sensitive and knowledgeable, regardless of his or her ethnic or racial group, can teach any subject effectively" (Banks, 1997, 532).

Likewise, there is a growing belief that deaf children will benefit if Deaf culture is incorporated into the curriculum (Erting, 1994; Lane, Hoffmeister, & Bahan, 1996; Mahshie, 1995; Moores, 1996), the primary reason being that the world of deaf children is a visual one, and for many of them their linguistic attachment to this world is through sign language. Therefore, these proponents argue, educators must take advantage of the visual nature of signing and of ASL in particular. Along with the learning of ASL, it is argued that deaf children's self-esteem will be enhanced if they come to learn about Deaf people's ways of living, their use of language, their organizations, and their celebrations—in short, if they learn about Deaf culture.

Culturally relevant instruction for deaf students is not an assertion that all deaf children are destined to be active members of the Deaf community, nonetheless, being deaf entails some amount of shared experience. The experiences of deaf people are varied, and the fact that some deaf children will communicate primarily with hearing people while others interact mostly with those who use sign language are just two aspects of these experiences.

The pivotal issue in the inclusion of information about deafness is the fact that just as all deaf children will have to associate to some degree with those in a hearing and speaking world, it is also true that using ASL and socializing within the Deaf community will always be an option for them. Therefore, it is important to teach things about the Deaf community, which can be done by discussing the reasons for its existence, the history of a local Deaf club, and the functions of some of its national organizations such as the U.S.A. Deaf Sports Federation and the National Association of the Deaf as well as some of the statewide and local organizations. In addition, deaf children need to be aware of organizations that cater to the needs of different groups of people who have a hearing loss, such as the Association of Late-Deafened Adults (ALDA) and Self Help for the Hard of Hearing (SHHH).

All of this can be taught as part of the social studies curriculum by incorporating information about how deaf people live and the workings of their social institutions. In this way, learning about deafness would be an integrated part of all deaf children's education and not an option offered by a few school programs.

It is the job of the school to help students get ready to become contributing members of their community, and when more than one community is an option, as is the case for all deaf children, then schools must address this in their teaching. Schools for deaf children and self-contained classrooms are likely to have teachers who have the requisite knowledge and pedagogical grounding to integrate information about deaf people into the social studies and other subject matter curricula. General education classroom teachers may not be similarly prepared, but teacher consultants or resource room teachers who are certified as teachers of the deaf can assist them.

2. *Teachers must rethink conventional methods for teaching social studies to deaf students.* The American curriculum is different from the curricula of many other countries, including those countries who achieve higher academically (Schmidt et al., 1999). The American curriculum emphasizes brief encounters with many different topics at each grade level. The unintended result of the curriculum is for students to learn a little bit about a lot of things and nothing in-depth about anything.

Teachers who are required to teach many topics and none of them in depth may seek ways to complement their teaching and assigning reading activities is one of them. To succeed under the American social studies curriculum, a deaf child has to be a good reader and especially so in the matter of social studies. Most deaf children are not good readers (Paul, 1998), and certainly by the time they are in middle school their lack of proficiency in reading is significantly hampering their ability to use textbooks in their efforts to learn material assigned in classes.

The disparity between reading levels of deaf students and the reading needs for subject matter learning has long been recognized by the field but solutions to bridging the gap are few (Moores, 1996). One of them is for teachers to write or rewrite materials to match the reading levels of their students. This method is manageable at the lower elementary levels but at the upper elementary, middle school, and secondary levels the value of this strategy is overwhelmed by the large amount of reading required by the various subject matters, and the changes in tone, structure, and intent that result from rewriting.

Another strategy is for teachers to only teach key concepts using textbooks as a reference rather than as a critical part of the learning process. Resource room teachers are able to do this because they are expected to provide supplementary support for deaf students, and assistance with reading is one type of support. This strategy may also be suitable for those teachers in self-contained classrooms and schools for the deaf because of their small class sizes and the fact that they generally have more control over the content they teach than do general education teachers. As long as teachers have the time necessary for preparing lessons, the idea of focusing on key concepts is feasible.

3. *Teachers should make social studies a cooperative learning affair.* A major reason why we teach speech to deaf children is that "They live in a hearing world and they have to learn to get along with hearing people." Similarly, a common reason for teaching signs to deaf children has the refrain, "When they grow up they will end up in the Deaf community where they will socialize with other deaf people who sign." But, being able to communicate is only one part of the larger picture of being able to get along with people.

Getting along means having a shared sense of values, respecting differences in other people, learning to come to mutual agreement on action that needs to occur, contributing your share of the work, assuming responsibility for your action, and more. These are things that social studies teachers will teach as part of the goal of citizenship education.

Thus, activities are needed to provide deaf students with experiences in how to get along with other people, and social studies teachers can do this by incorporating cooperative learning into their class activities. **Cooperative learning** is a teaching strategy that is possible in self-contained classrooms, resource rooms, schools for deaf children, and general education classrooms. It is a strategy that "enables students to experience firsthand many of the benefits of cooperation and of particular cooperative behaviors and abilities" that will allow them to "realize how their own academic and social growth is enhanced by working cooperatively with peers in structured academic tasks" (Stahl, 1994b, p. 3). The emphasis on social and academic growth is especially important for deaf students because it provides a much-needed alternative to traditional teaching methods that have not had much success in raising their achievement levels. Furthermore, it tackles the concern that deaf students tend to lack the social maturity of their hearing peers (Moores, 1996). Teachers can use cooperative learning activities to expose deaf students to models for learning successfully and behaving appropriately.

As for the evidence in support of cooperative learning, a review of the literature by Stahl (1994b) noted that students who have experienced cooperative learning over prolonged periods of time tend to:

- Achieve higher scores on academic tests, especially those aligned with targeted outcomes objectives.
- Have higher proficiency in critical reasoning abilities and strategies.
- Have higher levels of intrinsic motivation to learn.
- Be less disruptive as individuals and as group members.
- Engage in more and higher quality on-task, academic, and group interaction behaviors.
- Actually work cooperatively in small-group settings toward attaining a common goal.
- Possess many of the positive attitudes necessary for working effectively with others.
- Have more positive attitudes toward teachers, principals, and other school personnel.
- Be more willing to share and interact positively within group settings.
- Form greater numbers of friendships based on human qualities.
- Have more positive relations with individuals of different ethnic or racial groups.

- Voluntarily increase their personal contact with other students in a variety of contexts.
- Be more willing to state and discuss their own ideas in public.
- Have more positive self-concepts and self-esteem.
- Have greater feelings of psychological acceptance of themselves as persons.
- Have greater interest in and willingness to engage in academic study. (p. 9)

In many respects this foregoing list reads like a wishlist for teachers of deaf students. There have long been calls, for example, for these teachers to enhance deaf students' low self-concept and self-esteem (Meadow-Orlans, 1987; Stinson, 1994), to improve their critical thinking skills (Marschark, 1997), to increase their interactions with hearing peers (Kluwin & Stinson, 1993), to help them become sensitive to their own community as well as others (Christensen & Delgado, 1993), to help them overcome their low levels of achievement (Moores, 1996; Paul, 1998; Schildroth & Karchmer, 1986), and more. Cooperative learning strategies can help these teachers meet these calls.

The success of communities, societies, and all other types of groups is based on people cooperating with one another. Social studies provides an ideal platform for acquiring the knowledge and skills necessary to being a cooperative citizen. Teachers of deaf students must think beyond the challenges posed by communication concerns and delve into what it is that they can do to help deaf children shape desirable social behaviors.

4. *Incorporate performance-based assessment throughout all social studies activities.* If social studies teaches students about the world they live in and how their behavior affects such a world, then assessment needs to be versed in real-time, authentic activities. This means focusing on the quality of the information that a student knows rather than the quantity. Knowing the names of the capitals of all fifty states is a fine piece of knowledge but in a conversation that's all it is: a piece of data. Knowing the government, people, culture, and geography of several of the capitals is more than a piece of knowledge: It is information that can carry a conversation. In social studies, we want to know how well our deaf students can talk about the world they live in, and to do this, it helps to conduct **performance-based assessments** (also referred to as portfolio assessments and further described in Chapter 2).

The challenge for teachers is to give their deaf students opportunities to demonstrate their understanding of social studies concepts, opportunities that move from requiring students to read for the purpose of memorizing facts relating, for example, to the main agriculture products of each Southeastern state, to searching for information for a display case explaining how changes in climate affects the growth of crops in the state of Florida and the price that consumers have to pay when an untimely frost strikes.

This type of assessment gives deaf students more control over their learning. It allows them to use different modes of communication (print, graphics, signs, and speech) and, for some, language of communication (English and ASL) to express their understanding. It facilitates the infusion of language arts into the activities leading to the final assessment product. Finally, it can be used as a vehicle for helping students learn about themselves and other deaf people.

Helping Deaf Students Learn Social Studies

Learning social studies is a cooperative affair. Students helping students with guidance from their teacher is an enriched approach to learning about how communities and societies work. In this section, we review the applications of different types of cooperative activities with deaf students.

A. A Basic Setup Plan for Stimulating Cooperative Learning

Cooperative learning activities should be ongoing and run through the entire school year so that students get used to working with others and that they learn how to work interdependently in an effective manner. For this to happen, it helps to establish a routine and a set of expectations for the groups. An example of doing this is shown below. In the example, the teacher is always cognizant of the importance of modeling and monitoring communication behavior for their deaf students.

There are five basic steps to effective cooperative learning, and there are certain skills that are particularly relevant to participation in such groups. Johnson and Johnson (1994) have identified some of these skills as follows:

- Individual accountability: The performance of a student is assessed and this information is shared with the entire group as well as with the individual student. This strategy allows for the group to provide assistance to those students who need the support. It also ensures that students do not simply tag along while contributing minimal effort to a group project.
- Positive interdependence: This is the acknowledgment that each member of the group contributes to the group's success. It is the basis for people working together for a common goal.
- Face-to-face promotive interaction: This skill builds on the notion of positive interdependence. In face-to-face promotive interaction, students actively assist, encourage, support, and praise their fellow group members.
- Social skills: To act responsibly in a group, students must have adequate interpersonal and small-group skills. These skills must be taught, and they incorporate notions about trust building, decision making, communication, and conflict management.
- Group processing: Essentially, this skill refers to the group monitoring its own progress and relationships.

Other skills that are of particular importance with deaf students include the importance of accessing the communication of the group and preparing students for the language requirements of the cooperative activities. These latter skills are a major focus in the following description of the five basic steps to effective cooperative learning.

1. *Grouping*: **Grouping** for success is a critical factor associated with successful teaching (Kluwin, Moores, & Gaustad, 1992). In self-contained classes, including classes in schools for the deaf, the small size of the class might mean that the entire class forms just a single cooperative learning group. An example of such a situation is described later in this chapter where two team teachers instituted a cooperative learning strategy in a class of nine students. This class, however, could easily have been divided into two or three groups, with students regularly rotating from one group to another to allow generalization of the social skills that are developed from group activities. When such a division is made, the teacher needs to ensure that the students in the resulting group are compatible with each other from the perspective of the academic task at hand and the social skill requirement necessary for the group. In time, teachers develop a sense for how to group students in order to optimize the learning experience for the students.

In a general education class, a single deaf student will participate in a group with several hearing students. Although the dynamics of this situation are different from those in which only deaf students are interacting, grouping is still very much a key factor. Obviously, it would be beneficial if the deaf student was matched with students with whom he or she could communicate directly in whatever modality and language. Lacking this choice, a teacher might initially group a deaf student with those students who are sensitive to the communication needs of the deaf student and will help the deaf student be an active participant in all activities. In other words the teacher is grouping for success—a strategy that should be employed with all students, deaf or hearing, at the beginning of the year. As students gain familiarity with the routine of cooperative learning activities, they should be more receptive to being a part of a new group.

When an interpreter is involved, both the deaf and the hearing members of the group should discuss how this person is going to facilitate the communication of the group. The placement of the interpreter relative to the others in the group is one consideration and another one is the set of rules or strategies for talking to the group, talking to the teacher or others outside of the group, making presentations, and so forth. Also important is making it clear to the group the role of the interpreter. Although it is true that most interpreters simply interpret, it is also true that the presence of an interpreter alters the dynamics of the group (Stewart et al., 1998). Factors such as an interpreter's signing and speaking skills, ability to hear, demeanor, appearance, familiarity with the students, and knowledge of the subject being studied may contribute to how effectively the deaf student will interact in the group. Thus, knowing about the interpreter is an important part in the grouping decision of the teacher.

2. *Introductory activity*: Most group activities are preceded with a lecture or a description of what the students are about to do or both. This is where the teacher provides background information and prepares the students for what they are going to do in their group. To help deaf students at this stage, visual information should be provided that will guide them through the group tasks that lie ahead. This can be done by charting out a **cooperative learning schema** that outlines all of the fundamental activities that students are being asked to do. This helps the student know what is expected of the group and of him or her. This knowledge gives the student a sense of security when interacting in the group because it reduces the anxiety associated with not knowing what the group is doing.

The box titled "Sample Activity Chart" shows an example of a chart based on a **cooperative learning schema** (see Stahl, 1994a, for a comprehensive discussion of cooperative learning and Johnson & Johnson, 1994, for further explanation of cooperative learning schema) that describes the expectations for an activity about "The effect of British settlers in Australia," which meets one of the curricular goals for studying different people and cultures in the seventh grade. This activity could be conducted over five class periods or more depending upon the depth a teacher wishes the students to explore.

Although a deaf student might have an interpreter, the **visual information** that a chart provides (e.g., presented in print for those who can read fluently and in drawings and print for those who cannot, such as first- and second-grade students) acts as a security blanket when communication is about to become more intense and likely more chaotic once the activity begins. Note that a teacher can use the ten bonus points (shown in the Sample Activity Chart) for behavior as a means of tracking each student's meeting of targeted social behavior goals. Listening to others, acknowledging the ideas of others, and attempting to express oneself clearly are examples of possible social behavior for tracking.

Sample Activity Chart

Cooperative learning can be a confusing activity for deaf students even when all of the students in the group are deaf. The following is an example of an activity chart that is useful for helping guide deaf students through a cooperative learning activity. The chart puts deaf students in the position of knowing what to do and when to do it, thus reducing the dependency on others for assistance.

a. Grouping
   1. You will be placed in a group of three students.

b. Research activity: Your group will...
   1. Describe the type of people Great Britain sent to Australia.
   2. Explain why these people were sent to Australia.
   3. Describe the cultural characteristics of today's Australians.
   4. Plan how to present this information to the other groups in the class.
   5. Make sure each member of the group knows about this information.

c. Enrichment activity
   1. Guess (hypothesize) what type of signing Deaf people in Australia use today.
   2. Plan how you can research your hypothesis.
   3. Do the research.
   4. Follow the instructions in b.4 and b.5.

d. What did you learn?
   1. Make a presentation to the class.
   2. Listen to other presentations.
   3. Write down the best ideas that you hear from other people and add to your list.
   4. Group writes a one-page report about "The effect of British settlers in Australia" and gives it to the teacher.

e. Applying what you have learned
   1. Explore the following question: "What would people in Australia be like today if the early settlers had come from Africa rather than Great Britain?"
   2. Group plans how they will answer this question.
   3. Group conducts the activity.
   4. Group writes a one-page response to this question and gives it to the teacher.

f. Bibliography
   1. Use at least three to five different types of media to obtain information. Examples of media types are newspaper, magazines, encyclopedia, books, videos, and the Internet.
   2. Keep a complete record of each type of media used.

g. Assessment
   1. You will collate the material that your group made, then write a one-page summary of what you have learned. You can include information from the presentations of the other groups. (Note: Alternatively, you may want to offer students an opportunity to do an oral or signed presentation). The product of this performance-based assessment is worth one hundred points.
   2. You will receive ten bonus points if all members of your group scored ninety or above.
   3. You will receive ten more bonus points if you acted properly during the activity.

3. *Student preparations.* Have the students talk to other members of their group to ensure that they all understand what the teacher had explained during the introductory session. This includes going over the chart and making clarifications or asking the teacher for assistance in understanding what is expected of them. Students should be taught how to ask questions of each other that demand more than a simple "Yes, I understand" acknowledgment. They should aim for questions like "How might the paper and presentation be alike in part d of the Sample Activity Chart?" or "What are the countries that make up Great Britain?" This activity fosters positive interdependence and is designed to make everyone an active communicator.

4. *Conduct the activities.* Each group should have a copy of the activity chart, and one can be prominently displayed on an overhead. Activities should be conducted within a time frame that will allow all groups to complete their tasks. It is during this time that the students can earn ten bonus points for meeting certain targeted social behaviors, and therefore the teacher needs to be prepared to look for these behaviors. Some deaf students might feel uncomfortable about speaking in front of their group, or they might not have the language skills necessary to allow them to express their ideas effectively to their groups. These students should be identified early in the school year so that their teacher will be prepared to assist them and intervene if they are continually being ignored or finding it difficult to participate (e.g., some people are just shy). A most important concern is that all students are actively participating with no single student dominating the group's effort.

5. *Language arts component.* As mentioned earlier, one of the challenges in teaching social studies to deaf students is to rethink the conventional method of teaching it. One alternative is to teach more about fewer topics than less about more topics. Although some teachers might feel overwhelmed by the curriculum demands for facts (see box titled "But I Gotta Teach All of These Facts!"), the point remains that by teaching more about fewer topics it becomes easier to integrate learning across subject matter. Take the following question found in part e:

> "What would people in Australia be like today if the early settlers had come from Africa rather than Great Britain?"

In a language arts class the teacher might want to prepare students for this task by giving them opportunities to write about hypothetical ideas such as:

> "How does a group of people decide which language it will use?" or

> "People in different parts of Africa speak different languages. Imagine that people from different parts of Africa settled in Australia. Describe how you think they decided to communicate with each other."

In effect, this type of language arts activity is providing students with a model for how they might approach the question posed in part e. It also leads to a product that might be included in a student's portfolio.

In the area of reading, a teacher might have the students look up information about Australia in books, magazines, an encyclopedia, or on the Internet. This activity could be used, for example, to help learn several language arts curricular goals for the middle school grades including the following:

- The learner will be able to identify appropriate sources of information.
- The learner will be able to determine the best sources for finding specific information.
- The learner will be able to identify the type of information found in an almanac.
- The learner will be able to compare and analyze data displayed in a table.

All of these goals are conventionally taught using topics that are unrelated to anything that the student might already be learning about in school. It is more effective if teachers use the curriculum to establish a link between subject matter.

The five basic steps to cooperative learning with deaf students just described provide only one example of the cooperative learning strategies that teachers can use. The steps associated with grouping, the introductory activity, and the language arts components are especially critical when deaf students are a part of the cooperative learning group. Teachers aim to make it more comfortable for a deaf student to interact with others by attending to basic concerns relating to communication, language, and expectations.

B. Field Trips

Unit plans allow teachers to schedule **authentic field trips** that help deaf students give substance to what they see and read about in the classroom. For as long as we have been in the field we have heard many deaf children say that they do not get out of the house much when

But I Gotta Teach All of These Facts!

A carefully planned thematic unit can cover large amounts of "facts." Let's suppose that you are feeling the pressure of having to teach everything from the Civil War until the Depression of the 1930s. You might tackle this challenge by creating a thematic unit titled, "Becoming America: One Citizen at a Time." You then design cooperative learning activities centered around four Americans:

1. White farmer on the frontier
2. African American sharecropper in Alabama
3. Italian immigrant in New York City
4. Urban poor

Some of the activities that the students can engage in are the following:

- Create a family history for each of the listed Americans.
- Create a time line of events that impacted the lives of these Americans.
- Design charts that contain facts that were pertinent to the era associated with each of these Americans.
- Do displays and collages of images for each of the Americans.
- Write letters for each of them depicting a day in their life or their immediate concerns in the face of hardships.

they are at home. A part of this is a result of ineffective communication between the family and the deaf children. Another part of it is that too many parents are opting for television, video games, and computer games over museums, walks, and libraries. As a result, deaf children are not given many opportunities to expand their world knowledge.

It might be said that parents must become more accountable for their child's learning experiences. This is true, but schools must also acknowledge that parents of deaf children might not be offering many experiences that will help their children in school. To counter this deficit in real-world experiences, schools should design programs that will help deaf children see and interact with more of the world outside of the classroom. Although not all schools have the resources to take many field trips, teachers of deaf students should make the effort to take field trips when the experience will assist deaf students in their learning of class materials. The small sizes of classes in schools for deaf children and self-contained classes certainly give them traveling advantages over general education classes. With parental involvement, the use of volunteers, pooling of resources between classes, and a resourceful teacher, field trips can become a more important factor in planning social studies for deaf students.

Teachers should also explore the IEP process as a means for gaining support for field trips. There are many justifications for field trips, including the fact that they will help students gain critical experiences to expand their social behavior skills, language and communication skills, and world knowledge. Each of these can be stipulated as an IEP goal. One teacher moved from a single field trip one year to a weekly field trip the next year through her wise use of the IEP process. She noted that her students' vocabulary levels were too low to allow them access to many parts of the curriculum. She also noted that past school practices had not succeeded in significantly improving this access. She came to the IEP prepared to argue that to learn social studies the students require hands-on experience to understand such concepts as the dependency of a community on industry, the value of different types of transportation to the community, and the contributions of social agencies to the welfare of the community. These were translated to IEP goals and the Intermediate School District Special Education office picked up the tab for those trips that required extra funds.

C. An Integrated Social Studies Theme-Based Unit Plan

What would we get if we joined the basic plan for cooperative learning, as described in part A, and field trips? This was done by Stewart and Hollifield (1988) with a class of nine boys aged 13 to 16 years, all of whom used signs as their major means of communicating. They created a unit plan that had a common theme across their social studies and language arts classes. Their school year was divided into four units of five to eight weeks' duration. Figure 3.1 shows the social studies and language arts components of one of the units.

Class activities for each week were devoted to meeting specific curricular goals and to preparing the students for the field trip. For Week 1 in Figure 3.1, two of the language arts goals were as follows:

1. Students will practice using the newspaper as a source of reference.
2. Students will learn the format of a newspaper article and the function of the headline, lead paragraph, accompanying photograph, and photograph caption. (Stewart & Hollifield, 1988, p. 17)

For the same week, two of the social studies goals were the following:

1. Students will learn to identify the five types of Pacific Coast salmon.
2. Students will discuss the different ways the salmon influences the lives of coastal people. (Stewart & Hollifield, 1988, p. 17)

The two teachers also developed two goals for the field trip taken during the first week that involved students gaining an appreciation for recreational fishing and appropriately interacting with nonschool people during the field trip. At the end of the unit plan, the students had an all-day Open House and made presentations to other classes in the school.

The unit plan and field trips were cooperative learning affairs. Students conducted work by themselves and in groups. The same type of work was required throughout the year

Social Studies Lecture/Discussion Topic	Language Arts Reading Assignment	Field Trip
Week 1: Pacific Coast salmon	"Most Salmon This Fall" (newspaper article)	Angling fishing trip
Week 2: Life cycle of the salmon	"Life Cycle of the Salmon" (encyclopedia article)	Visit to a salmon hatchery
Week 3: How fish swim	"The Boy in the River" (Aesop's fable)	Visit to an aquarium
Week 4: Migration behavior of the salmon	"Why the Salmon Came to the Squamish Waters" (Indian myth)	Visit to salmon spawning grounds
Week 5: The salmon industry	"Danger in Our Rivers" (newspaper article)	Visit to a canning factory
Week 6: The impact fish and humans have on each other's lives	"Red and Green" (poem)	Shopping trip and salmon lunch (cooked and eaten at school)
Week 7: The role of fish in Indian folklore	"How to Smoke Salmon" (story about Indian customs)	Visit to the Museum of Anthropology
Week 8: Methods of fishing	"Skana the Killer Whale" (Indian myth)	Commercial fishing boat trip
Week 9: Open House		

Source: Stewart, D. A., & Hollifield, A. (1988). A model for team teaching: Using American Sign Language and English. *Perspectives for Teachers of the Hearing Impaired, 6*, 15–18. Reprinted with permission.

FIGURE 3.1   Outline of a nine-week unit on the salmon.

so that students developed a sense for routine. Thus, on field trips the following duties were assigned: "photographer, reporter, interviewer, map reader, brochure collector, artist, and letter writer" (Stewart & Hollifield, 1988, p. 17). The photographer was responsible for captioning the pictures, which, along with the results of the reporter's story and the interviewer's report, fitted nicely into the portfolio assessment that was used to grade student performance. Students rotated through all of these activities. In the classroom, the social studies component had activities that complete a language arts component. Students were required to take notes during the lecture, complete question-and-answer assignments, and complete written examinations. The emphasis in social studies was always on content knowledge. In the language arts activities the teacher keyed in on grammatical features and tested for vocabulary, reading comprehension, grammar, and the ability to follow instructions.

Now, let's look at the integrative aspect of the unit plan. In the chart below, there is a listing of some of the actual social and academic goals identified by Stewart and Hollifield (1988) that is arranged by subject matter, along with some other possible goals that we have identified.

Social Studies
1. Social goals
   - Social interactions with classmates during cooperative learning activities
   - Social interactions with classmates during field trips
   - Social interactions with other people during field trips
   - Using an interpreter during the interactions with hearing people during the field trips
2. Academic goals
   - Importance of an industry (fishing and canning industries)
   - Interdependence of the salmon and the Indian community
   - Interdependence of the salmon industry and workers in society
   - Exploration of different cultures (Coastal Indians) including their customs
   - Historical relevance of the salmon (e.g., visiting the museum)
   - Geographical relevance of the salmon (e.g., mapping out migration routes)
   - Signing in a clear manner so that the interpreter can correctly and smoothly interpret what is being said

Science
1. Social goals
   - Acquiring a sense of social responsibility (e.g., exploring the life cycle of the salmon)
   - Debating the social consciousness of citizens toward natural resources based on an understanding of the interdependency of humans and natural resources
2. Academic goals
   - Studying the life cycle of the salmon
   - Investigating the motion of a fish when swimming
   - Exploring the migration behavior of salmon

Language Arts
1. Social goals
   - Working cooperatively for reporting and interviewing tasks before, during, and after field trips
   - Making a presentation that is understandable to younger deaf students at the end of the unit plan that includes answering questions
2. Academic goals
   - Studying the poetry of Coastal Indians
   - Using an encyclopedia as a reference material for looking up information
   - Reading newspapers for the purpose of gathering information
   - Writing reports, captions for photographs, tests, and other materials
   - Listing the new signed and spoken vocabulary related to each of the weekly topics studied

Mathematics
1. Social goal
   - Understanding the financial impact that the fishing industry has on a community of people with the ultimate aim of developing greater sensitivity to the preservation of natural resources
2. Academic goals
   - Calculating the economic value of the salmon industry
   - Calculating the time it takes a salmon to swim each mile during its migration
   - Calculating the cost of feeding the class before and after going on a shopping trip then comparing it with the actual cost

Undoubtedly, there are more social and academic goals that can be added to this list. But the key point is that field trips can be used to help deaf students *access* the curriculum and to show how a common theme can be woven through different subject matters. Notice how information relating to signing is infused into the unit plan itself rather than taught out of context.

Infusing a Study of Deaf People into the Social Studies Curriculum

In Chapter 5, three different models for teaching about deaf people in schools are presented. Infusing information throughout the kindergarten to grade twelve social studies curriculum is one option for teaching about deaf people. This information could be presented in a manner that allows it to be studied in conjunction with other similar topics. For example, people who serve the needs of deaf and hard of hearing people such as teachers, rehabilitation counselors, and interpreters could be taught as part of a study of community workers that includes nurses, doctors, police officers, and meter readers.

The emphasis on infusion is to foster the impression that deaf people are normal and experience life much the same way that their hearing peers do. Focusing on infusion is an idea endorsed by many proponents of multicultural education. It used to be that teachers would spend a week studying about the accomplishments of famous African Americans and reading literature written by African American authors. Posters of African Americans would be displayed in the school hallways and perhaps someone wearing African theme clothing would visit the school. Today, more and more educators view such practices as being an inadequate, piecemeal approach to helping all children appreciate the significance of this large American community (Banks, 1997; Grossman, 1995). Although it might be easier to teach about a specific culture intensively for a short period of time, a long-term infused teaching method is more likely to garner the understanding and empathy that we want children to acquire about themselves and other groups of people. Thus, there is need to infuse information about deaf people throughout the curriculum.

Table 3.1 displays an example of the kinds of infusion that can take place at the elementary through secondary school years.

TABLE 3.1   An Example of Infusing Concepts Related to Deaf Studies Throughout the Social Studies Curriculum

School Level	Key Concepts to Be Infused
Lower Elementary	1. Introduce people who serve the needs of deaf and hard of hearing people: teachers of deaf and hard of hearing children, ASL instructors, interpreters, audiologists, hearing aid dealers, rehabilitation counselors, etc. 2. Describe the work of these people. 3. Introduce some basic technologies that are used to help deaf and hard of hearing people access communication and sounds (e.g., TTYs, alerting devices).
Upper Elementary	1. Introduce different groups of people with disabilities (e.g., blind and visually impaired, deafblind, wheelchair users, etc.). 2. Describe the services that these people receive from their communities. 3. Make comparisons with the services that deaf people receive. 4. Explore the various technologies that help deaf and hard of hearing people communicate and access services (e.g., e-mail, Web sites for government agencies).
Middle School	1. Introduce consumer organizations for deaf and hard of hearing people (e.g., National Association of the Deaf). Describe how these organizations serve a community. 2. Introduce service organizations for deaf and hard of hearing people (e.g., Michigan Division on Deafness). Describe how these organizations serve the needs of a group of people. 3. Discuss the historical development of these organizations. 4. Make selected comparisons with organizations serving the needs of people with other disabilities. 5. Discuss value orientations that are specific to deaf and hard of hearing people.
Secondary School	1. Examine laws that have impacted the lives of deaf and hard of hearing people (e.g., Americans with Disabilities Act, Vocational Rehabilitation Act of 1973). 2. Examine the concept of "access" as it applies to deaf and hard of hearing people as well as to people with other disabilities. 3. Debate society's obligation to ensure that all citizens have access to basic services and information. 4. Compare the principles associated with access to those associated with the civil rights movements of African Americans. 5. Discuss the dynamics of social change as it pertains to deaf and hard of hearing people and the responsibilities that students have to ensure progress in improving the lives of deaf and hard of hearing people.

Information about most of the topics listed in this chart can be found in books, magazines (e.g., *Deaf Life*, *Odyssey*), and the Internet, although the volume of such material is small relative to the size of this community. When possible, deaf or hard of hearing people should be brought to the class to serve as role models as well as to provide information that cannot be found in the literature. State agencies such as the Division on Deafness are excellent sources of information about state and national laws affecting deaf and hard of hearing people, employment practices, and other matters pertaining to the lives of deaf and hard of hearing people. Directors of these divisions regularly give lectures to police officers, hospital staffs, and employers to teach them about deaf and hard of hearing people, including suggestions as to how to communicate with them. If you look hard enough, you will find the resources you need to teach about this community of people.

Connecting with Deaf Students from Other Places

No matter what philosophical approach you take to social studies your students should connect with deaf students from other schools in the state or country and even in the world. The cyberworld of e-mail and online dialogue technology can make this happen in a manner that is convenient and timely. Letters sent through the mail are a slower process but nevertheless a valuable means for establishing a connection between deaf students. Even faxed letters can be used to make connections. In fact, the means for connecting is not as important as the actual link between students.

Teachers should help deaf students communicate with other deaf students on a social studies–related theme for many reasons including the following:

- To motivate students to learn more about a particular topic. The more knowledge a student has about a topic the more confident that student will feel communicating about it. Knowing that one is communicating with a fellow deaf student in a distant land could be powerful source of motivation.
- Communicating in an appropriate manner with peers contributes to citizenship education. Communication is not a free-for-all affair. Students need to be coached in the art of speaking to others in different modalities (e.g., signs, speech, or print)
- Differences and similarities between cultures can be explored to supplement in-class instructions. More so, contact between students from different cultures might reveal cultural characteristics that are not easily understood from in-class instructions. This would be true for those deaf students who might give an account of their place in society that is far removed from textbook accounts of their culture.
- Information gleaned from such communication can be enlightening. Most deaf students in America fare far better than their deaf counterparts in other countries. They have access to many support services in school and in their community that are not available elsewhere. While interpreters and message relay services are taken for granted in many parts of the United States and Canada, they are nonexistent in many other countries. American students have available to them many assistive listening devices, and most of them have access to a computer in their home and/or their schools. This is not true for deaf students in Poland, Zimbabwe, Thailand, and many other countries.

- There is much disparity in the rights of deaf people from one country to another and in their access to visual communication and support services. Again, American deaf students have a strong advantage because of laws such as the Americans with Disabilities Act of 1990, which gave deaf people the right to full access to communication in schools, the workplace, and in most places where services are provided. Deaf students face far fewer barriers to a quality education and gainful employment in the United States. They might, however, take the notion of access and equal rights for granted. By communicating with students from less advantaged countries, American deaf students may acquire a better appreciation for what they have, which may lead them to contemplate actions that may help their less fortunate peers in other countries—an excellent example of how social studies can benefit the overall humanistic character of a student.
- Students will gain many hours of practice in the area of reading and writing.
- Students who sign will gain many opportunities to improve their ability to convey and receive messages in the sign modality because videophones and online videocameras are already a reality, waiting for marketing conditions to make them affordable.

This list is not exhaustive, but it does show the variety of benefits that can stem from linking deaf students from different regions or countries.

So how do you go about linking students from different regions and nations? You can start simply by contacting another school program for deaf students in your state or elsewhere. The *American Annals of the Deaf* contains an up-to-date directory of school programs serving the needs of deaf students throughout the United States and Canada. It also contains the same information for over 600 mainstream programs. This listing includes names of a contact person, phone and fax numbers, addresses, and for many people, e-mail addresses. You can also try searching the web. There is actually a Web site for pen pals—try a search for pen pals and deaf pen pals and see what you find.

You might even create a home page for your classroom, which is becoming a relatively simple thing to do. Include information about your students and their school program. Invite visitors to your Web site to contact you for information about becoming a pen pal with one of your students. It would be helpful to ensure that prospective pen pals are in fact students with sincere interests in corresponding with your students. Check with your school Internet policy for information about how to guard against contact with unwelcome people in cyberspace.

You can contact the Laurent Clerc National Deaf Education Center for help in reaching students. Located on campus at Gallaudet University, the Clerc Center, as it is popularly known, is charged with developing and testing innovative and exemplary courses of study for deaf and hard of hearing students from preschool through twelfth grade. It puts out a publication for deaf teachers called *Odyssey* (previously called *Perspectives in Education and Deafness*), which can be used to gather ideas or to tell others about your goal for making contact with deaf students.

Encourage your students to write to people from other nations. Most libraries will have a reference book that lists the names and addresses of embassies in the United States. Where no embassy for a nation exists in this country you might be able to contact that country's tourist office. Most embassies can be found in Washington, DC, while tourist offices are usually found in New York City. For example, the Embassy of Portugal is at 2125 Kalorama Road, NW, Washington, DC 20036, and the Egyptian Tourist Authority is at 630 Fifth Avenue, New York, NY 10111.

Resource Room and Itinerant Teachers

Much of what has been described in this chapter focuses on teachers of the deaf teaching in a separate classroom either in a public school (i.e., self-contained classroom) or in a school for the deaf. Obviously, general education teachers who have one or more deaf students in their classroom can also use the principles described in the chapter. This is especially true with respect to the application of principles associated with cooperative learning.

For the resource room and itinerant teachers, social studies raises other concerns. The planning and teaching of complete social studies units is often not an option. There are, however, several strategies that these teachers can use for helping their deaf students access the social studies curriculum. This section overviews these strategies using real examples from a teacher of the deaf who has worked as both a resource room teacher and as an itinerant teacher.

Diane Little has been a teacher of the deaf for over twenty years. During this time she first worked in a high school as a resource room teacher with up to nineteen deaf students in her room at a time. Later, she became an itinerant teacher (teacher consultant) for deaf students in a large city school district. All of her students were mainstreamed in general education classes. Although she was able to provide assistance with all subject matter, she often focused on a single subject. Her rationale was that the knowledge and skills that the students received in this one subject area would translate to better overall performance in other subject matter. She used the subject to improve her student's study skills, reading and writing skills, ability to use multiple resources to do research, and more.

The subject she often selected as her focal point was social studies. One reason for this selection is that she felt her deaf students feared facing new knowledge. Social studies is loaded with new information for students, and she strove to help her students overcome this fear so that they would have a better opportunity of handling the social studies curriculum (which included related subject matter such as history, geography, and civics) and consequently other subject matter as well.

As a resource room teacher or as an itinerant teacher, she was not able to teach the entire social studies curriculum but she was able to pull out students for assistance. Her first step in teaching social studies obviously began with a meeting with the general education teacher to determine if extra support was needed in this subject matter and, if so, then a discussion of possible reasons why support was needed followed. These reasons may be related to vocabulary enhancement, understanding of particular concepts, assistance with study skills, or some other learning needs.

However, when the extra support required was quite general, Diane was able to design activities that aimed to help students do better overall in their regular social studies class. This approach differs from the approach of those resource room and itinerant teachers who viewed their role as helping students just do the work that they were assigned in their general education classes or to help the students without pulling them out of their general education classroom—for example, monitoring the students progress and providing support only as needed to the general education teacher. Diane took a global approach that aimed to spur student's interest, to show them how to research a topic, and to relate social studies information to their own lives. Following are three ideas that she felt helped her be effective in this endeavor.

A. *Tie in social studies themes across all subject matter.* Social studies is not to be taught as an isolated subject. Social studies not only touches upon many other subject areas but also that it is related to many aspects of a student's life. **Thematic teaching** is one way of teaching across subject matter. But resource room or itinerant teachers are limited in the time that they can spend on a certain social studies theme. Diane overcame this limitation by taking a multisubject approach to the way that she assisted students with social studies. For example, she once had a deaf student in an elementary school who was studying about pioneers in the West. She saw this student three days a week for one class period (about forty minutes). Following is a list of what she studied with her student, much of which was in addition to what the general education teacher was doing:

1. Clothing: What type of clothes did the pioneers wear? Do we wear any of these clothes today?
2. Food: Where did the pioneers cook their food? How did they cook it? Were their cooking utensils the same as we use today?
3. Housing: They designed a home using hay and rocks. They discussed what homes are built of today and if it was possible for the pioneers to build a similar home where they were living.
4. Music: They made a musical instrument using gourds and pebbles (i.e., a shaker).
5. Games: They talked about games that the children probably played back then using cowpies, clay, wood, and other materials that were available.
6. Writing: She helped the students write a journal of a 9-year-old deaf girl living in the country far from other people during the early years of pioneering. Each journal entry had to contain at least three to five target vocabulary words.
7. Geography: The student plotted a map showing how a pioneer family got from their house to a river.
8. Mathematics: The student made a list of things that needed to be counted when living in the country (e.g., days, animals, and food for the winter).

Diane supplemented the above activities with low-vocabulary, high-interest books about pioneering. She said that although she was not able to do so herself, the general education teacher had taken the class, including the deaf student, to a fort that was built over 150 years ago.

B. *Spend time exploring current events.* Although many teachers spend some of their class time doing **current events**, it is doubtful that many deaf students in a general education class are actively participating in this activity. Factors working against their participation include the large number of students in general education classes, the lack of direct communication, the incidental use of vocabulary words that the deaf student might not understand, and the logistics of participating in a lively discussion that is largely speech driven. Yet, current events help stimulate students interest in learning, and current events make relevant much of what is studied in school.

Therefore, Diane regularly shared newspaper or newsmagazine articles with her students. She would briefly explain the story to the students, have them read the story, circle words and sentences that they did not understand, review reading strategies such as identifying key words and concepts, asking oneself questions, and re-reading, and discuss the story along with anything else that might arise from this discussion. This entire activity took no more than ten to fifteen minutes of class time for most stories. If a story was long, then she would have the students read it at home and be prepared to discuss it the next time she met with them. Over time, Diane felt that the current events activity that she did helped her students become more inquisitive about what was happening in the world around them.

C. *Develop projects to initiate creativity and imagination and to develop experiential background for later learning.* No one ever said that a resource room teacher or an itinerant teacher has to do just what the general education teachers are doing. Nor do they have to spend all of their time on activities directly related to improving deaf students' language skills. With a little bit of creativity these teachers can embark on their own projects. We asked Diane to give us some ideas of what she might do if she was seeing a couple of deaf students three times a week who were studying about the Renaissance. Diane responded with the following suggestions:

1. Design a coat of arms using the students' surnames. On the coats of arms they could make references to their favorite colors, interesting facts about themselves, things they love to do, and best friends. Pose the question to the students that if their family and relatives are mainly deaf and use signs to communicate, what would their coats of arms look like? Alternatively, they could actually research their family surnames and relate them to their present lifestyles.

2. Design a tapestry for a surname using a variety of materials such as news magazine, colored paper, and fabrics. The information contained in the tapestry can be similar to the coat of arms, or it could be thematic, relating to an aspect of life. Again, this might be a good area to tie in deafness and communication. If some students do not want to make an point about deafness, perhaps feeling that to do so will only heighten the difference between them and others, then this feeling must be respected.

3. Design a book cover with a Renaissance-related theme on it. Have the students compose simple poems relating to this time period to be written on the cover. If possible, use Carolingian manuscript or a calligraphy style script for all lettering.

4. Compose a short play to show an aspect of a peasant's lifestyle or that of a landowner. A peasant's life was a harsh one and in sharp contrast to those who lorded over the peasants. Explore themes within this framework of lifestyles looking, for example, at marriages, eating habits, and shelter. Look also at how a deaf child's life might differ depending upon the social status of his or her family.

D. *Write biographies of famous deaf people.* There is much value to doing biographies of famous deaf people. This activity fulfills curricular objectives for social studies and the language arts, gives students opportunities to practice reading and writing, exposes students to different resources that can be used to locate information on people that might not be easily available in print, and shows how deaf people have overcome barriers to succeed in life. Diane does not wholly emphasize the deafness aspect of the person. She has her students show that deaf people are people first who have goals in life just like everyone else. This activity should be followed up with a biography of a deaf person who is still living. Find out where this person was born, what schools he or she attended, what type of communication was used at home and at school, what social sphere he or she grew up in and what present social group he or she is now in, what postsecondary educational and vocational training was received, what jobs were held, and what their family was like, and so forth. Then compare the two biographies.

Notice how each of the above activities combine elements related to literacy with social studies. In several of these activities, art has a prominent role. All of these activities serve to make the temporary placement of the deaf student out of the general education classroom a pleasant and productive one.

Conclusion

Some people might argue that social studies might be too daunting of a subject for deaf students because of the exposure to many new things, such as new words, new names, new dates, and new countries. And each of these new things are found with each new topic taught. Still, this is not a novel approach. Hearing students, too, are exposed to many new things in their encounters with social studies.

The key to teaching social studies is to make it relevant and exciting. Teachers must consistently reinforce social studies concepts with examples from everyday life in today's society. Providing experiential background knowledge is essential to give deaf students a better chance at succeeding in social studies.

In this chapter, we showed that for deaf students to succeed in social studies, they must have knowledge and skills related to language arts, science, and mathematics. Likewise, to successfully teach social studies teachers must use other subject matter to help teach various concepts or to help students access knowledge relating to these concepts. This cross-curriculum connection is also necessary for helping to show students that the conceptualizations that they gain from their work in social studies can be applied to things that are happening in their lives everyday.

Finally, it seems reasonable to say that the better reader a deaf student is the greater access to social studies resources that student will have. Although this might be true, there are other ways to help deaf students access these resources. One way in particular is the use of cooperative learning strategies, examples of which were provided in this chapter. Whatever strategies one uses, it bears recalling that social studies is an all-encompassing subject that touches upon all aspects of our lives—past, present, and future. Use this knowledge to make social studies relevant and exciting for deaf students.

KEY WORDS AND CONCEPTS

authentic field trips: Based on the notion that educational field trips should be designed to provide students with meaningful learning experiences. Students are prepared before going on such trips. When they are on a field trip, activities are planned beforehand so that students are engaged in authentic learning experiences such as recording observations, interviewing people, making measurements, gathering data, analyzing a series of events, and so forth.

citizenship education: The belief by some scholars that citizenship education is one of the reasons why we teach social studies. It means to instill knowledge, skills, and values in children and youth so that they are prepared for participation in society.

conventional social studies: Until recently, the teaching of social studies as a subject that consisted of a number of events and topics that are discussed in terms of dates, locations, and names of people or things. This method of teaching social studies is thought to be especially challenging to deaf students because neither the topics nor the events are covered in-depth, and little time is involved in their study. This makes it hard for some deaf students to absorb the new terminology and language associated with the topics and events.

cooperative learning: A teaching strategy that groups students together to work on various class assignments.

cooperative learning schema: A list of expectations associated with the activities that students in a group are conducting. Such a scheme presents students with a clear picture of the sequence of activities that they are going to do and the outcomes of each activity. When presented in the form of a chart, a cooperative learning schema provides visual information for deaf students that reduces the amount of uncertainty that he or she might have when interacting with other students, and especially when interacting with hearing students.

cultural transmission: A rationale for a social studies curriculum that aims to pass on to children and youth the culture of society and, in particular, of the dominant society.

culturally relevant: In the context of planning a social studies lesson or unit, the incorporation of information and concepts derived from the student's culture. The incorporation of information relating to the passing of the Americans with Disabilities Act is an example using culturally relevant information in a lesson for deaf students because of the impact that this act has on the lives, education, and employability of deaf people.

current events: A popular instructional strategy that typically selects an event from the newspaper or a newsmagazine that has just occurred or is presently occurring in the real world.

Deaf community: In one sense, a group of people who have some degree of hearing loss and identify with other Deaf people who use sign language as a means of communication. Typically, Deaf people participate to some degree or extent in the activities and events of the Deaf community. These activities might include sports, social interactions, religious affiliations, and so forth. Events include local ones sponsored by Deaf clubs and associations as well as national ones such as those sponsored by the National Association of the Deaf and the USA Deaf Sports Federation. In a broader sense, the Deaf community includes hearing people who have either an intimate connection with Deaf people (e.g., hearing children of deaf parents) or a professional connection with them (e.g., teachers of the deaf, interpreters).

Deaf culture: Refers to the language and activities of a group of people who have some degree of hearing loss and use sign language as their primary means of communication when interacting with one another.

Deaf President Now: A famous revolution that illustrated the solidarity of Deaf people in their fight to place Deaf people in position of authority in educational institutions and elsewhere. In 1988, Gallaudet University appointed as its president a hearing woman who had no experience in the education of deaf people or more generally, experience working with deaf people in any professional area. She was selected over two other applicants, both of whom were

Deaf and at that time presently employed as administrators at the university. The students at Gallaudet shut down the university in protest and in the process gained national recognition through numerous television, newspaper, and newsmagazine reports. Their slogan was "Deaf President Now" or DPN as it is commonly referred to in the Deaf community. The students were successful in their protest, and I. King Jordan became the first Deaf person to be appointed president of the university.

Gallaudet University: The only liberal arts university for the deaf in the world. Situated in Washington D.C., it has approximately 2,000 students in its graduate and undergraduate programs.

grouping: In cooperative learning strategies, refers to the placement of a small number of students together for the purpose of pursuing a learning experience.

performance-based assessment: An assessment requiring students to demonstrate their knowledge and understanding of a concept. Some of the ways in which this can be done include projects such as creating a video or compiling information and objects for a display case, preparing information and materials for a presentation, and creating a portfolio a particular topic. One of the advantages to this type of assessment is that it provides a fairer opportunity for those students whose language and communication skills might penalize them in a closed-end test or an essay format test. Often used interchangeably with the term portfolio assessment.

problem-solving context: A method of teaching that uses meaningful contexts for framing questions relating to the concepts and knowledge that students are actively analyzing. Applying this technique in social studies is thought to be one way of making the curriculum meaningful to students.

thematic teaching: The selection of a common theme that cuts across more than one subject matter. A school that endorses thematic teaching might have all of its same grade students learning about a common theme such as "Exploring the West" that is touched upon in all subject matter.

visual information: The range of ways in which information can be presented in a visual form that is accessible to deaf students. Visual information can be presented through signing, print, illustrations, demonstrations, and other means.

QUESTIONS

1. Suppose you are an itinerant teacher who had a upcoming meeting with a general education social studies teacher to discuss the performance of a deaf student in the class. What would you tell this teacher about the importance of teaching social studies to deaf students?

2. What might you tell general education social studies teachers about incorporating into the curriculum information about societal forces and federal laws that have affected the lives of deaf people?

3. What useful purposes for deaf students would a study of the Deaf President Now revolution in 1988 serve?

4. What is meant by the phrase "Schools must address the different communities that deaf students have access to by providing culturally relevant instructions"?

5. Identify at least eight possible beneficial outcomes for students who experience cooperative learning over prolonged periods of time.

6. Describe why performance-based assessment is useful for evaluating deaf students' understanding of social studies concepts.

7. Describe the similarities and differences for setting up a cooperative learning activity in a separate class for deaf students and in a general education class where there is only one deaf student present.

8. What considerations are there for the use of an interpreter in a cooperative learning situation?

9. Why should teachers plan field trips that present authentic learning opportunities for deaf students? If you were planning a field trip to the state legislature building, describe two activities that you might do there that will make the trip especially relevant for a deaf middle school student.

10. Describe the process by which Stewart and Hollifield (1988) integrated a social studies unit across two subject matters and the role of field trips in this process.

11. Describe four activities that a resource room or an itinerant teacher might do to assist a seventh-grade deaf student learning about the agricultural industry in the south in the middle of the nineteenth century.

12. Select two deaf people from the twentieth century about whom you would like ninth-grade deaf students to write a biography. How would you explain to the deaf students the importance of doing these biographies?

13. What are the advantages of infusing a study of deaf people into the regular social studies curriculum? Compare this method with that of teaching about deaf people in a separate curriculum (i.e., Deaf Studies curriculum).

14. Describe the process that you would use to link your deaf students with a group of deaf students in Poland to study one of the following topics:

   ■ a comparison of educational practices with deaf students in the United States and Poland
   ■ the prevalence of TTYs among deaf people and the effects of its use in both countries
   ■ special laws that effect the employability of deaf workers

A C T I V I T I E S

1. Select two of the following social studies topics, and describe how you could use other subject matter—language arts (i.e., reading and writing; English grammar), science, and mathematics—to teach or supplement the teaching of items and issues related to these topics:

   a. environmental responsibility
   b. acceptance of other people's culture and ideas
   c. ancient Egypt (i.e., during the times of pharaohs and the building of the pyramids)
   d. any other topic that you might wish to use

2. Reread the chart outlining a unit plan put together by Stewart and Hollifield (1988). For each of the social and academic goals listed by subject matter in this chart provide an example of a performance-based assessment.

3. Design a cooperative learning activity for a class studying a deaf person who has contributed to improving the lives and hence the community of deaf people. This deaf person should be someone with whom the students can contact in person or via an alternative means such as the Internet. Include in your design each of the following activities:

   a. identification of the aspect(s) of the community that this person is helping
   b. a research activity requiring the students to look up information
   c. a written report
   d. a presentation to the class based on the report plus anything else that the students might wish to include
   e. any other activities

4. Look up information explaining the basic tenets of the Americans with Disabilities Act (ADA) and describe five ways in which ADA has made it easier for deaf people to obtain employment. Use real examples of work situations in your description.

CHAPTER

4　Teaching Literacy

CHAPTER OUTCOMES

After reading this chapter, you should be able to:

1. Describe text-based, subject-based, and interactive models of language processing.
2. Plan a lesson that incorporates strategies for enhancing the literacy skills of deaf students.
3. Use a multitude of teaching strategies to encourage literacy at different stages of the development of a deaf child's reading and writing skills.
4. Organize a meaningful dialogue journal project.
5. Use a six-step approach to help students use I-Search as a means to improving their research and writing skills.

At the dawn of the twenty-first century, the hottest word in deaf education is *literacy*. High hopes are riding on a reading and writing platform that is being embraced by educators from all corners of the field. We, too, feel that literacy instruction is a crucial part of a deaf child's education. But let's pause for a moment and put the task at hand in perspective.

Literacy is about words. Reading them and writing them. There are 10,000 words or so that circulate in our everyday speech. And the average adult can recognize between 70,000 and 120,000 words. If you are ever stuck for a word, then the *Oxford English Dictionary* has thousands of them standing by. In fact, it has over 450,000 entries in a set of volumes that is about three feet wide standing side by side. A new edition is in the works, when many more entries will be added. With steady injections of ingenuity and a few decades of leisure time, you can use affixes and other linguistic tools to expand this number to over 2,000,000 words. In sheer volume, no other language in the world comes anywhere close to having a vocabulary half the size of English.

Learning words is just a part of the task that deaf children face. Words are strung together to form meaningful sentences, and to do this our deaf child needs a command of a syntax. And wouldn't you know it, English syntax is complex, too.

So what do these numbers tell us about teaching literacy to deaf children? They make it very clear that the practice of introducing ten vocabulary words on Monday, writing their definitions out on Tuesday, writing sentences about them on Wednesday, and reviewing them on Thursday for a spelling test on Friday is a woefully inefficient means for teaching deaf children about words. So too, is the practice of trying to learn English by only using the Fitzgerald Key. Or by just translating from American Sign Language (ASL) to English and visa versa. Ditto for creating signs for English morphemes and for spending hours reading to a child.

How about that all-time staple of the elementary classroom, the **basal readers**? Then there's the basal reader's best friend, phonetics, which is currently being pushed as a must for hearing children. Should these also play a prominent role in the education of deaf children? And how about whole language? Now that it has taken a beating in the research literature after nearly two decades of experimentation in public schools, should teachers of the deaf still hang on to this philosophy as a way of bypassing the emphasis on phonetics?

The answer is that *no single approach* to the instruction of reading and writing will be adequate. Indeed, the complexity of English is such that no one method of instruction will be efficient enough to allow a deaf child to gain control of this language. With what we know today about how deaf children learn to read and write, the best approach to the development of literacy skills in deaf children may well be an interactive one—an approach that chooses from a wide array of literacy teaching strategies including those mentioned above.

Teachers should use many instructional methods in an interactive approach to give deaf children a set of linguistic tools that will help them steadily increase their command of English. Language instruction is the most prolific topic in the literature on the education of deaf children, and no chapter can do justice to covering all that teachers of the deaf need to know. For that matter, it is doubtful if a single book is sufficient. Thus, we urge our readers to explore language instruction through further readings of other textbooks on this topic. Peter Paul's *Literacy and Deafness*, Barbara Luetke-Stahlman's *Language Across the Curriculum*, and Barbara Schirmer's *Language and Literacy Development in Children Who Are Deaf* will give you a good start.

In this chapter, we focus on (1) providing a general overview for teaching literacy by describing the basic principles of text-based (bottom-up) and subject-based (top-down) approaches to language development and (2) a description of instructional techniques that can be applied to an eclectic-interactive approach to language processing that emphasizes the engagement of the deaf student in the reading and writing process.

What Is Literacy?

There are different definitions of literacy that range from a focus on the processes of reading and writing to one that looks at how print is used in various aspects of our lives. Carol Padden and Claire Ramsey stressed the need to distinguish reading and writing using a global perspective of literacy that encompasses the practical uses of writing within a social and personal milieu:

> Literacy focuses on practices outside the individual, whereas reading and writing focus on processes occurring inside the individual. Literacy moves away from the idea that knowledge of basic skills resides in individuals' heads and towards groups of people who interact using print, who accomplish career, social and personal ends with print, and who hold sets

of values and attitudes about print. Literacy also shifts our view away from the classrooms and methods to a range of communication activities human beings engage in over their life spans. (Padden & Ramsey, 1993, p. 96)

In this chapter, we focus on the reading and writing aspects associated with being a literate person. We provide teachers with practical suggestions and examples to help them engage deaf students in activities designed to develop their overall literacy skills. Moreover, throughout this section of the book we stress the importance of engaging students in meaningful discourse, exposing them to authentic experiences, and helping them access the language associated with various subject matter learning; all of which are practices that contribute to a deaf student's overall development of literacy skills.

Models of the Process of Reading and Writing

The process of reading and writing divides into three approaches: bottom-up, top-down, and interactive. LaSasso and Metzger (1998) used a roughly parallel system when they characterized models of the fluent reading process as text-based, subject-based, or interactive. Figure 4.1 illustrates the relationship of each of these approaches to language processing.

What Is a Text-Based (Bottom-Up) System?

Text-based or **bottom-up** theories of language processing start with the minimally but not necessarily the smallest distinguishable units of language, such as morphemes, in speech or letters in print. Text-based theorists argue that words are assembled into sentences and sen-

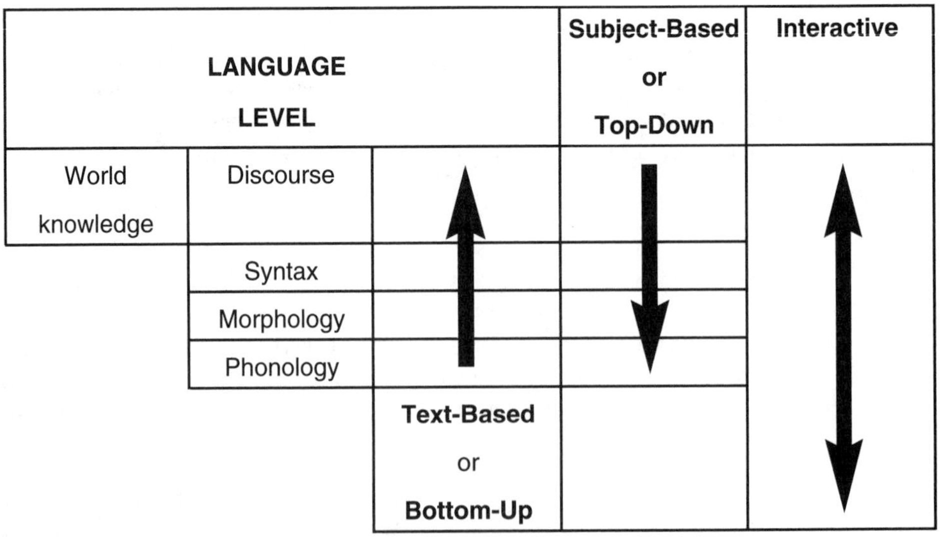

FIGURE 4.1 Approaches to language processing.

tences into discourse. Failure to process the lowest levels results in higher order misunderstandings. For example, such a theorist would argue that deaf children cannot read well because the printed word is a code for the spoken word. Since the deaf child has problems decoding speech, this carries over to problems in reading. Intuitively, this argument appears reasonable because of the generally low reading levels of deaf adults and because the usual progression for most hearing children is to move from decoding letters to words to sentences (Calfee & Pointkowski, 1981).

Text-based or bottom-up approaches seem to have a logic that matches how the typical reader learns to read. However, about 10 percent of normal hearing children do not use a bottom-up approach in learning to read (Calfee & Pointkowski, 1981). In addition, some skilled readers apply a top-down approach to reading to such a degree that they can be distracted by material that deviates slightly from their expectations.

What Is a Subject-Based (Top-Down) System?

Subject-based or **top-down** theorists note that you need context in order to interpret even simple sounds (Anderson & Pearson, 1984). For example, sound spectrographs are able to recognize variation in the same individual's production of single phonemes. How then can people compile discrete units into larger wholes if they do not already have some sense of what the intent of the utterance is?

A simple demonstration of this is to ask several people to finish the following sentence:

I just finished reading Ham____.

Most people will supply "let" to complete the name "Hamlet." A very few would supply "Hamilton's Federalist Papers." Subject-based theorists argue that prediction is an essential trait of language processing, thus context and prior knowledge are key parts of language processing. Using a top-down approach, the challenge that deaf children face when reading would appear to be a lack of context and prior knowledge imposed by the communication limitations of being deaf in a hearing society.

What Is an Interactive System?

Both text-based and subject-based theorists vary in their acknowledgment of the degree of permeability between layers of language processing (i.e., phonology, morphology, syntax, and discourse). In other words, will a person use one level in order to interpret or process a unit from another level? This leads to another approach to language processing, the **interactive approach to language development** (Just & Carpenter, 1987; Rumelhart, 1977; Stanovich, 1980). This approach is also referred to as the compensatory-interactive model. In this model, the direction in which processing tends to occur is irrelevant because the layers are permeable and one layer can compensate for another's lack. For example, a deaf child will use context clues to interpret words he or she does not know in a sentence. Studies of deaf readers have shown both the use of text-based and subject-based strategies (Kelly, 1995; LaSasso & Metzger, 1998), thus making an argument for an interactive system as a model for deaf students' reading process.

What is particularly interesting about the interactive model and actual teaching practice is that teachers will use basal readers within a text-based or language experience approach or use language experience methods along with a basal reading series (LaSasso & Mobley, 1998). This approach is often referred to as "eclectic" or selecting what seems to work best. In practice many teachers of the deaf appear to teach based on an interactive model because they are not particularly wedded to a text-based or a subject-based approach. Instead, they select teaching strategies that they feel will be successful with their students.

Text-Based Approaches to Literacy Development

The fundamental hurdle in a text-based approach to the teaching of reading to deaf children is a child's lack of knowledge of the English phonological system; hence, the propensity of some teachers of the deaf to place a great deal of emphasis on speech training as a means of enhancing a deaf child's reading and writing skills.

Teaching deaf children to read and write in English is not that great a problem theoretically. However, the consensus in the field is that the child has to have a first language (L1) before literacy skills can be adequately developed.

For oral students, speech and hearing are used to develop English as the first language. For students who sign there are a number of alternatives. In total communication programs (i.e., those program that stress the use of signs, speech, and hearing) English is usually the designated L1. However, there are some total communication programs that espouse the use of ASL as the L1, and a form of English signing is used to create a basis for English as the L2 (Stewart, 1995). Luetke-Stahlman (1999b) and many others have proposed that learning a manually coded English system such as Signing Exact English gives deaf children direct access to English, which becomes their L1. In some bilingual education programs, ASL is accepted as the first language, and reading and writing provides the only access to L2, English. LaSasso and Metzger (1998), on the other hand, argued that phonological information is critical to understanding differences in a language. Their suggestion is to use Cued Speech as the basis for teaching phonological information essential to learning to read and write while using ASL as the primary means of communication in the classroom. Once the child has mastered Cued Speech, the child would be able to map the L2 (English) structure against the L1 (ASL) structure and could then be ready to learn to read. Reading instruction would then proceed in the same fashion as it does for hearing children. Obviously, there is a diversity of approaches to communication and first language issues in our field, and no single approach is successfully meeting the language needs of all deaf students.

Among the variety of communication methods used, there are many teachers of the deaf who rely on a text-based approach to reading instruction, which traditionally has meant that they use a basal reading series. Basal readers are a series of books and related materials built on several premises of which the first and most obvious is that reading is a bottom-up process. Supporting materials can include workbooks for the children, word charts, or tests. Each series will vary on the degree of emphasis placed on the initial learning of phonics. Phonics is always taught at the start but the amount of phonics instruction and the length of time devoted in later levels of the series to the teaching of phonics will vary.

Lessons in basal readers tend to be highly structured around a story and reflect a general plan that includes the following elements:

- Preparation for reading the story
- Presentation of new vocabulary and practice with the new vocabulary
- Guided reading and interpretation of the story
- Follow-up activities

The structure of the process reflects the general bottom-up approach in that words rather than stories or ideas come first. The stories tend to be the focus of the activities with little connection to reading or experiences outside the classroom.

In the teaching of a lesson, there is a heavy emphasis on teacher control and on understanding the story, that is, on comprehension skills. Generally, the teacher presents the materials, directs the reading, and monitors comprehension. Students are not expected to independently engage the material. Follow-up activities continue the bottom-up approach in that the reader is encouraged to move from the decoding of specific elements toward a general comprehension of the overall text.

Basal reading systems are sequential in that as a child progresses through the series the vocabulary becomes more sophisticated and the sentence structures become more complex.

If composition is taught within the context of a basal reading system, it is generally taught after the fact—that is, a child is taught to write a less complex structure than the child is assumed to be able to read, and writing is used as the servant of reading. In other words, children write the answers to questions or they write descriptions of events similar to what they are reading. Writing is not used to support an interest in reading. For example, children generally do not write to each other as members of an audience.

Currently, larger public school programs for the deaf and schools for the deaf primarily use basal reading series over other methods (LaSasso & Mobley, 1998). At the moment the most popular series used to teach deaf students is *Reading Milestones* that, along with two Scott Foresman series, account for about two-thirds of the programs that LaSasso and Mobley (1998) surveyed. Programs used basal readers because it was felt basal readers provided the best organizational framework for reading instruction; basal readers were required by the state or school district; or basal readers were selected for program specific reasons.

One of the often unspoken reasons for using basal readers in early reading instruction is that they are both highly structured and come with a quantity of supporting materials. Teachers who are not specifically trained to teach reading or who feel their skills lie in other areas prefer the security of the highly structured and material-rich series. Teachers in the early grades tend to see the attempt at meeting the interest level of the children, the supplementary materials, and the flexibility of use with deaf children as advantages to using basal readers (LaSasso & Mobley, 1998). However, teachers of the deaf find the inappropriateness of the vocabulary, insufficient repetition of the vocabulary, complexity of the syntax, and the amount of idiomatic or figurative expressions to be a problem (LaSasso & Mobley, 1998).

We did not include in this section an explanation of the underlying principles of phonetic approaches to teaching reading because phonetics is a complex issue in the teaching of speech, an area that does not fit into the purpose of this book. However, the teaching of speech can be beneficial to some deaf children if it is approached from the perspective of learning to read. These children will benefit from undergoing speech training so that they develop a form of "inner speech" that can help them decode written words. Thus, for some deaf children, the teaching of speech is not necessarily aimed at producing intelligible speech. Rather, the goal is to give these children another tool for tackling the task of reading.

Subject-Based Approaches to Literacy Development

We are not including a separate section on subject-based approaches in literacy development. Instead, in our following discussion we have focused largely on an overview of teaching literacy to deaf children that essentially covers subject-based or interactive techniques.

Principles of an Interactive Approach to Literacy Development

This section explains the underlying philosophy of an interactive approach to literacy development (see Figure 4.2).

All Forms of Language Are Related

Reading, writing, speaking, and listening are variations on the form in which a language is expressed and received. They have formed the basis for most of the English language cur-

Principles	Some Practices
All forms of language are related.	Using writing to teach reading.
Meaning is drawn from authentic context.	Reading trade books to pique interest.
Classrooms are communities of learners.	Writing dialogue journals to encourage expression of thought.
Literacy is acquired through use.	Guiding students through the process of writing.
Children should own their language.	Publishing student's writing as a mean or motivating them to write.
Emphasis is on process not product.	Teaching through thematic units.
Literacy development and content should be integrated.	

FIGURE 4.2   Principles and practices of an interactive approach to literacy development.

ricula in the United States for almost all of the twentieth century in general education. In the education of deaf children, two other forms for conveying English are fingerspelling and various types of English-based signing.

Meaning in Authentic Context

There is a general psychological principle that you cannot learn what you do not already know. In other words, to learn something new you have to have a structure on which to hang the new information. Depending on the psychological theory, the terms *schema* or *scaffolding* are sometimes used to describe this phenomenon. The basic principles of a schema were described in Chapters 1 and 3. When a teacher engages in **scaffolding**, she or he is providing deaf students with whatever assistance they need to do the task at hand. Assistance is broadly defined as a range of instructional support that includes initial explanations, the provision of relevant experiences, key vocabulary, and examples of what a product should look like.

In practice, reading instruction in **authentic context** means that children are taught using real pieces of language: books, magazines, advertisements, and so forth. The 500-word composition is replaced with writing recipes or job descriptions because these exist in the real world and are connected to the experience of the students. In the context of authenticity, the two tests for including an item in the curriculum are whether it has relevance for the child's learning needs and if it has a real-world significance.

Classrooms Are Communities of Learners

Language is a tool of the individual, and it is also a social device. It is in the community that language is learned. Thus, the classroom needs to be a community in which language is exchanged in meaningful ways about meaningful topics. As we will show later, the use of dialogue journals is one way of exchanging language in meaningful ways.

Literacy Is Acquired Through Use

Driving a car is a complex physical and intellectual exercise, but it is probably simpler to learn than it is to learn to walk or to speak or to write continuous discourse. While many people probably first learned to drive in a classroom, ultimately they learned to drive on a road while going someplace. Similarly, hearing children acquire language for the most part without much direct instruction during the process of interacting with other human beings. Literacy development with deaf children should parallel these situations and involve a high degree of purposeful reading and writing.

Emphasize Process Not Product

Studies of both first and second language learning show patterns of evolving language structures as well as the interference of old rules with the new ones. In other words, for most individuals language learning is not a smooth curve but a jumbled path toward a general standard. Further, language use is dynamic. It consists of components such as vocabulary, syntax, discourse rules, and schema. These components interact with each other, which sometimes allows one component to compensate for deficiencies in another. Consequently, children should not be expected to produce perfect examples of language. "Correctness," while important for precision and efficiency is *not a trait of developing language*; it is a trait of develop*ed* language. Children who are becoming literate should focus on working and experimenting with language rather than on being proficient in all of its forms.

Literacy Development and Content Should Be Integrated

Try to write twenty-five words on a topic you know nothing about. Try to stay interested in an event such as a rugby game or an opera of which you might have no understanding. You will find that these are difficult tasks to do. The same principle applies to language development. Language develops when an individual is interested in an area of knowledge and desires the linguistic proficiency to talk about it. This interest and desire should be carried throughout the entire curriculum.

To give a real-world example, if you want to elect a political candidate, you will likely engage in a variety of activities like writing letters, making phone calls, putting up posters, and making coffee at rallies. Important things in our lives are complex and contain many forms of expression. Artists don't just simply paint or sculpt; they look at, talk about, and often write about art. Language in all its forms is part of a complete literate person. This is the basis for thematic teaching. If the material to be learned is important, then students should read and write about it as well as communicate the information to each other in other forms as well. This is the same point we made in Chapters 2 and 3 in our discussions about teaching science and social studies.

Some Practices of an Interactive Approach to Literacy Development

We have headed this section "some practices" because we do not insist that every practice be used nor do we assume we have described every possible alternative. Teachers of the deaf face unique situations even to the point of having classes in which no two children have identical literacy needs. You will need to pick and choose among text-based and subject-based techniques to support your students in their attempt to become literate. This will also help your students respond to the demands of a curriculum and the instructions of other teachers.

Using Writing to Teach Reading

Isn't that backwards? Not really, because children who are just about ready to read will start to make scribbles on a piece of paper and declare that they have written something very important. In the mind of the preliterate child, both reading and writing are wondrous and only vaguely understood. Reading is probably taught first because it is easier to talk about writing if the person can read. For example, a teacher might say the following:

You wrote r-e-e-d, but it should be r-e-a-d.

Furthermore, if writing correct English is the goal from the beginning, then it is necessary to have a vocabulary in order to talk about mistakes; hence, the early emphasis on teaching reading first. But when fluency is the goal, then producing something on paper is an important goal and even a misspelled word is better than not writing anything at all.

Process Writing. It has been over twenty-five years since Janet Emig (1971) did the first study of the writing process of adolescents. However, the basic outline of the process of composing remains the same. Overall, writing as a process is not a linear sequence of steps but a recursive process with identifiable subprocesses such as planning, translating, reviewing, and revising.

Kluwin and Kelly (1991) have modified the process slightly for deaf students and field tested the method. The basic components of the process are shown in Figure 4.3.

Planning is a thinking process during which the writer begins to form an internal representation of the finished product. Planning also involves the expansion or reduction of the content and the setting of goals. It is the quality of the goal setting that is one of the initial differences between more able and less able writers. Better writers create a complex network of goals and subgoals that in turn not only control but also generate content. This stage may include some rehearsal for actual writing such as taking notes, forming outlines, or physically acting out a sequence of events. For an example of the planning process see the box titled "An Exercise in Planning to Write."

Translating covers several related activities such as actually writing or drafting the composition. It is the transformation of meaning from thought to print. It is also a major block in the minds of many writers who become reluctant to put words on paper. As explained later in this chapter, there are many techniques for helping writers. The practice of prewriting is one such technique.

Reviewing is the process of going back over what has been written to determine if the previously established goals have been met. Reviewing may be an ongoing process occurring during the drafting of the composition, or it may take place at the end. Individual differences are apparent during this part of the process and can influence the overall quality of the production.

The biggest difference between more able and less able writers at this stage is not the pacing of the review but the subject of the review. More able writers temporarily ignore

Generic Categories for Designing a Process Approach to Writing	Modified Categories for Deaf Students
Planning	Prewriting
	Organizing
Translating	Writing
Reviewing	Feedback
Revising	Revising

FIGURE 4.3   Steps in a process approach to writing modified for deaf students.

errors and rethink the structure of the composition. Less able writers do not focus on structure, purpose, or audience but instead tend to merely monitor for errors. This reviewing can be ineffective because the less able writer appears to read what he or she intended to write and not what actually appears on the page.

Revising occurs continually throughout the writing process and not merely at the end. Revising involves changing one's mind as well as changing the text. Revising includes editing as well as major reorganization of the composition.

The difference between the more able and the less able writer during this subprocess is that the able writer views revising as a process of structuring and shaping the content to

An Exercise in Planning to Write

Molley Sheridan of Sam Houston High School developed a lesson that illustrates the planning process in a lesson designed for deaf students. The lesson is titled "Deaf Abby Revisited" and is based on the popular advice column found in newspapers across the country. The activity is intended for ninth- through eleventh-grade deaf students who have fifth- through sixth-grade reading levels. The purpose of the activity is for students to use writing to request advice from an organization.

Initially, the teacher provides the students with samples of advice columns, which are read and discussed. Students are then required to collect samples of advice columns on their own, which are then added to the previous collection of samples. All of these samples are posted on a bulletin board for the duration of the project. Repeating expressions and vocabulary should be highlighted.

The next step is for the students to brainstorm their own imaginary problems and then to list creative responses to these problems. For example, a girl might want to get rid of a boy's unwanted attention. All responses as to how to do this problem are accepted.

The students select one of the problems and go through the list of possible solutions using a Problem Solution Form like the one below:

PROBLEM: Pam likes Shirley's boyfriend

Solution	Steps To Be Taken	Limitations of Solution
1. Pam tells Shirley.	Get Shirley in a good mood.	Shirley might get mad.
	Pam explains her feelings.	
2. Pam steals boy from	Dress nice.	Boy may misunderstand.
Shirley.	Do what the boy likes to do.	Shirley might get mad.
3. Find another boy.	Go to dances.	Nice boys don't grow on trees.
	Go to the mall with a group of friends.	

Finally, the students order the solutions from best to worst based on the outcomes of each option.

be appropriate for a particular type of audience (e.g., classmates, the manager of a store, newspaper editor). The less able writer merely changes individual words or fixes grammatical errors when revising.

For deaf writers, the following modifications of the foregoing approach can prove to be a helpful teaching technique:

1. *Prewriting.* The practice of prewriting involves much discussion (i.e., creating opportunities for self-expressions). The purpose of the discussion is to clarify or stimulate ideas, to motivate a person to write, and to establish and enhance the community of writers and readers that the classroom should be.

To do this, the teacher presents the students with a stimulus for writing. The writing stimulus usually consists of a topic, an audience, and a form. A part of the prewriting stage is to define the limits and possibilities of the topic, to teach or clarify the particular form the writing is to have, and to define the audience for the writing and the type or style of writing that is appropriate to that audience.

Students often fail to write because they have no clear idea of the purpose of the assignment. One part of prewriting is to define the topic and thus motivate students to write. The other part is to directly motivate the students by piquing their interest in the assignment. For example, you can prompt students by taking them through steps that will help them decide upon a topic, the audience to whom they are writing, and the form of the writing. The benefit of this type of prompting is that students get an opportunity to express their thoughts and obtain feedback prior to the actual writing. Prompting also allows the teacher to introduce vocabulary that students can later use in their writing.

Clarification and motivation go hand in hand during the prewriting stage. Free association, recall of anecdotes, reference to vicarious or real experiences, and teachers asking questions to create verbal models of complex sequences are essential parts of the prewriting activity. The point of the prewriting activity is to expand the volume of ideas about the topic, that is, to create an excess of information. This is done primarily through extensive teacher and student communication.

A concrete example of a good prewriting activity is for the teacher to take a topic and to ask the students to free associate about the topic. All student ideas are accepted and are not criticized by the teacher. The only intrusion the teacher makes is if the student presents an idea that the teacher sees can be divided further into more information.

Throughout the entire process the teacher might be writing down each idea on small pieces of paper or creating a list on the board. At the end of this activity, there is a large quantity of unorganized information. It is this information that will be used in later stages of the writing process. This stage is important as a group activity for deaf students because collectively these children may have extensive stores of information. When prewriting is done as a group activity, any "holes" in the experience of individuals may be compensated for.

2. *Organizing.* Organizing is the next step in the writing process, and two types of activities occur at this juncture: conceptual and rhetorical organizing. *Conceptual organizing* involves recreating the logical, chronological, or natural structure of a concept or an event. Devices for organizing include written lists, semantic or concept mapping, priorities, and mechanical or physical aids for organizing. It also helps to create an overall organizational chart.

As a first approximation of an organizational structure, simple lists can be developed on the basis of criteria that are obvious to the deaf students. For example, during the prewriting stage words can be written on small pieces of paper. Different lists of these words can be structured. If the topic is the preparation of a food item, lists could be organized on the basis of ingredients, qualities of the finished product, and so on. A more elaborate variation on this idea is semantic mapping or a similar procedure in which spatial diagramming is used instead of the formal outlines familiar to all of us.

An important activity at this stage is for the teacher to provide students with criteria for the creation of lists and to carry out the logical conclusion of the application of the criteria. The role of the teacher at this point is to assist the student in thinking about alternatives.

One elementary form of organization for writing a description of an object is the physical representation of the object. In the case of a process, the temporal sequence can be reproduced spatially. If you have asked the students to describe the best pizza they have ever had, they can generate a list of ingredients and then structure this list by identifying which ingredients they would bite into first. If the teacher stays with the familiar and the concrete at the beginning, students will be able to transfer known information to a new procedure. An example of how to create a list from brainstorming ideas and then organize these ideas into a structure is shown in the box titled "From Brainstorming to Structure."

From Brainstorming to Structure

Following is an example of an original list of brainstormed ideas related to writing about "The Best Pizza Ever." In the first column, the items listed are simply anything that comes to mind related to what the students like about a pizza. In the second column, the basic parts of a pizza are listed under the heading "Pizza Structure." The students should suggest names for the structure with prompting from the teacher. In the final column, the ideas from the original brainstormed list are organized according to the parts listed in the Pizza Structure column.

Original Brainstormed List		Pizza Structure	Materials and Qualities	
cheese	tomato	toppings	ham	onions
ham	pineapple		pineapple	sausage
sausage	feta cheese		mushroom	
cheddar cheese			olives	
golden	warm	cheese	cheddar	mozzarella
olives	onions		feta cheese	
pepperoni	deep pan	sauce	tomato	
buttered		crust	buttered	warm
mozzarella			deep pan	garlic
			golden	

Rhetorical organizing involves making decisions about the general form of the composition. For example, will this be a five-paragraph essay and what information will be highlighted in each paragraph?

3. *Writing*. Being able to write one form does not guarantee success in writing a different form. There are clear hierarchies of assignments based on the cognitive demands of the writing assignment, and failure to provide students with clear initial directions for writing lowers the quality of the final product.

Topic complexity depends on the person's knowledge and intellectual abilities and the concreteness of the topic. First-person writing such as diaries and personal narratives are generally easier than third-person topics like essays. Concrete topics that the writer is familiar with will be easier than abstract topics.

Writing is the physical act of putting words down on paper. There are two types of barriers to writing: physical and psychological. Physical blocking means that the student has not assembled the needed materials for writing, which include not only paper and pencil or a word processor, but the notes and plans that have been made prior to writing.

Psychological blocks are motivational blocks and can come from opposite sources. One source is a complete lack of interest in the topic; the other is an excessive concern with correctness of grammar that can destroy the will to write. Both types of psychological blocking can be eliminated or at least alleviated by adequate prewriting activities, particularly lots of discussion during prewriting. For deaf students the lack of practice in writing and the lack of confidence in their English skills may serve as a formidable psychological block. Creating a structure for writing and engaging the students in extensive prewriting activities are ways to overcome this block.

During writing all writers will stop. One of the toughest decisions in writing is deciding when one has written enough. Good prewriting planning reduces some of the uncertainty of this decision, but stopping or stalling is a natural part of the process.

4. *Feedback*. In process approaches to the teaching of writing, feedback can be either a self-directed or a group activity. It will require a varying degree of teacher involvement depending on the writing ability of the deaf student. At all times, feedback must be a positive and constructive step like the other steps in the process approach to writing.

Less able writers already know that they make many errors in their writing, so the teacher does not have to point this out to them in detail. The teacher should correct only one or two errors in the composition, such as tense agreement, that the teacher wishes the student to work on.

The errors most destructive to the overall meaning of a composition are conceptual or rhetorical errors. That is, some essential piece of content is missing, or it has been presented in an inappropriate structure. The communication fails because the writing did not convey the intended meaning.

The next level of errors are the structural errors that are a function of the form of the communication. For example, a business letter has five essential parts: inside address, heading, salutation, body, and closing. Failure to include one of these components means the communication fails in the sense that a needed piece is not there.

Grammatical and mechanical errors are the types most familiar to teachers of deaf students, but are generally the least essential to the success of the communication. These types of errors may reduce the impact of a communication, but they do not necessarily destroy the essential content of the communication. Overcorrection of grammatical errors by a teacher can destroy a child's willingness to compose.

During feedback the teacher stays within one level and addresses those particular problems. Many teachers have reported that by working at the highest level of errors (i.e., conceptual and rhetorical errors), simple grammatical errors by deaf students disappeared (Kluwin & Kelly, 1991, 1992).

Trade Books

The process of becoming a good writer includes garnering an interest in reading. Readers are inspired to write well because of books and other literature that they have read. In an interactive approach to literacy, reading goes hand-in-hand with writing. Therefore, exposing deaf students to literature is a goal for all teachers. Trade books are one way of doing this.

Go into a drug store and walk down the racks of magazines or stand in front of a sidewalk magazine seller and look at the range of material available in print. Every conceivable topic has its own publication that people will spend money on. There is also an entire industry devoted to writing and publishing books for children. The appeal of these publications is evident from the financial success of writers such as Dr. Seuss, Judy Blume, and R.L Stine. Adults love magazines pitched to their interests, and children love books about themselves and their lives.

The world of a child contains velveteen rabbits and bears made from corduroy and fanciful monsters and worries about moving to a new house or the death of a grandparent. These books are good to use with deaf children because they have meaningful contexts for the children and they are intrinsically interesting, thus encouraging engagement in the process of becoming literate. Examples of some popular trade books used for teaching deaf students are *Curious George*, *Blueberries for Sal*, *The Little Engine That Could*, *Madeline*, *Where the Wild Things Are*, and *Runaway Bunny*.

Deaf Role Models in Literature

The ultimate reading goal for deaf students is that they attain a level at which they are comfortable reading their school textbooks, magazines, newspapers, Web site information, letters from their parents, the how-to-assemble instructions on a kit, and much more. The point is not how much they end up reading but rather that they have the ability to do so.

When deaf students are in the process of learning to read, it is important that they be encouraged to read on a regular basis and be allowed to choose from a wide selection of reading materials. To this end, every classroom should have a reading center that contains a selection of reading materials covering a wide range of reading levels. Included in this selection should be books written by deaf authors. Just as it is important for deaf children and youngsters to meet and interact with deaf role models it is also important that they be exposed to the products that deaf people have created. A book is one such product.

For teachers who have a long-term commitment to developing a well-stocked reading center, it is highly advisable that they search catalogs and Web sites of publishing companies who actively seek to publish the works of deaf people. Gallaudet University Press and DawnSignPress are two such companies. See the box titled "Deaf Authors and the Reading Center" for a listing of possible book selections by deaf authors.

Deaf Authors and the Reading Center

Ivey Wallace is a former teacher of the deaf who now works as the managing editor of Gallaudet University Press. She has had much contact with deaf authors and has compiled a list of books written by them. This list is not comprehensive but does represent a good proportion of those books available that are suitable readings for students at different school levels. Note that some books were authored by more than one person, one of whom is hearing (Jerome Schein).

Author(s)	Title
High School Level	
Emmanuelle Laborit	*The Cry of the Gull*
Albert Ballin	*The Deaf Mute Howls*
(Edited Book)	*No Walls of Stone: An Anthology of Literature by Deaf and Hard of Hearing Writers*
Leo Jacobs	*A Deaf Adult Speaks Out*
Mary Wright	*Sounds Like Home: Growing Up Black and Deaf in the South*
Bernard Bragg	*Lessons in Laughter: The Autobiography of a Deaf Actor*
Philip Zazove	*When the Phone Rings, My Bed Shakes*
Steven Schrader	*Silent Alarm: On the Edge with a Deaf EMT*
Cheryl Heppner	*Seeds of Disquiet: One Deaf Woman's Experience*
Raija Nieminen	*Voyage to the Island*
Hannah Merker	*Listening*
Jack Gannon	*The Week the World Heard Gallaudet*
Jack Gannon	*Deaf Heritage*
Stephen Baldwin	*Pictures in the Air: The Story of the National Theatre of the Deaf*
Jerome Schein and David Stewart	*Language in Motion: Exploring the Nature of Signs*
Carol Padden and Tom Humphries	*Deaf in America: Voices from a Culture*
Bonnie Poitras Tucker	*The Feel of Silence*

Continued

Deaf Authors and the Reading Center   Continued

Author(s)	Title
Middle School Level	
Virginia Scott	*Belonging*
Virginia Scott	*Balancing Act*
Lois Hodge	*A Season of Change*
For All Grades	
Christy MacKinnon	*Silent Observer*

Dialogue Journals

A dialogue journal is a physical device to permit the student to record thoughts on a topic and to let the teacher or another student respond to those thoughts. As the name suggests, there is a dialogue between two people about topics of mutual interest. Because the practice developed in the late 1960s, the physical form of the communication was the paper journal or notebook. The idea began as a variation on the traditional diaries kept by many professional writers or journalists. However, with today's access to e-mail, the journal process can be simplified and made even more effective because the burden of trading journals back and forth can be eliminated and responses can be more rapid. The use of dialogue journals has grown popular in the field of deaf education over the past two decades (Kluwin, 1996).

The goal of dialogue journal writing is to encourage writing by creating a realistic writing situation between the writer and audience (Kluwin, 1996). It involves personal and reflective writing that includes narration, explanation, and description. It is always written at the language and interest levels of the deaf students involved in the process. It can encourage extensive writing while reducing social isolation if the participants become involved with each other as individuals.

An important aspect of dialogue journal writing is that each journal develops its own life (Bailes, Searles, Slobodzian & Staton, 1986), which can serve as encouragement for deaf students to write. By its very nature, dialogue journal writing is a free-form writing exercise intended to stimulate interest in writing as an activity by emphasizing:

1. Student-selected topics
2. A focus on meaning over form (e.g., grammatical correctness)
3. Writing to a specific audience in a nonevaluative, private, or nonthreatening climate

Dialogue journal writing is self-generated, interactive, and conversational (Staton, 1984). It encourages an interest in writing by creating something that approaches a "real" writing situation—in that there is a real audience that dictates the form and content of the communication (Applebee, 1984).

Student-Teacher Dialogue Journals. The student journal should be a personal statement. At the same time, it has to be manageable logistically for the teacher. The usual compromise is for the teacher to require or provide a standard notebook. Decoration or personalization of the notebook is at the latitude of the teacher, however, banning of any personal expressions on the covers runs contrary to the idea of the dialogue journal. Nonetheless, racist, sexist, pornographic, or other offensive material defines the limits of what cannot be on the covers. The age of the children will also control the content of the journal cover. Younger children usually opt for stickers while high school students often draw rather elaborately on their journal covers.

To start students writing, teachers initially will have to assign topics. Simple, personal, interesting, and nonthreatening topics are good starters. Numerous topics are available, and simple ones such as the student's favorite kind of food and why, favorite place for a holiday, or the most interesting thing that can be seen out the window can be used to get deaf students started with the writing. However, these simple topics can also lead to simple sentences that just answer the question the teacher poses. When necessary, teachers must be prepared to help students elaborate their writings by talking to them about the topics—a strategy that is especially critical to deaf students because of shortcomings in their experiential backgrounds.

Also, letting students comment on topics in the newspaper or things they have seen on TV or in the movies are other ways to get started. Obviously, topics have to be tailored to the background and interest of the students. Teachers' knowledge of the students goes a long way toward helping students maintain an interest in writing.

Dialogue journals are intended to be read and commented upon, therefore the more the teacher responds to the student, the more frequently the student will participate. The pedagogical and linguistic goal of the dialogue journal is to encourage fluency because fluency contributes to the development of language skills. It's like dancing or rollerblading; the more a student practices the better he or she will get.

The content of the response for the teacher is important in encouraging students to write. Questions, praise, and involvement are the hallmarks of good teacher responses. When in doubt, a word of praise, and an indication of interest on the teacher's part followed by a question will keep things rolling. For example, "I enjoyed your description of Mama Mia's Primo Pizza. I've tried it myself. Where do you think you can get the best cheeseburger in town?" or "Your description of how you feel when watching a movie that you can't hear was very good. What would you like to see happen in movie theaters that will make going to a movie a more enjoyable experience?"

Unpleasant topics will occasionally appear. Stories of drug use, child or sexual abuse, marital discord, suicidal thoughts, death threats, and Satanism can appear in the dialogue journal. You will need to know your district guidelines on how to handle topics like suicide, drug abuse, or sexual misconduct. When you encounter this kind of situation, it is necessary to redirect the student to a different topic and to report the information to the proper authorities in a discreet way.

Peer Dialogue Journals. One of the authors had over 500 pairs of deaf and hearing students exchanging dialogue journals in ten cities around the country for two years (Kluwin, 1996). He used the following structure:

1. A general education teacher was paired with a teacher of a self-contained classroom.
2. Journals were distributed to the deaf students at the start of a Monday class.
3. Students were allowed about fifteen minutes to make their entries.
4. Teachers assisted and encouraged students to write.
5. Teachers monitored what was written to prevent misuse of the system.
6. Journals were then exchanged with the general education class.

The peer dialogue journal worked much the same way as the teacher-student journal. Initially, teachers provided topics to get things rolling, but after that the students were sufficiently interested in each other to keep the discussion going. In the process of doing the project the following general guidelines were developed:

1. Encourage students to take a conversational approach to resolving misunderstandings that arise from different language skills.
2. Do not tell hearing students that deaf students have language problems.
3. Suggest topics only in the beginning.
4. Don't be surprised by what students write, but don't let any pairs get out of hand.
5. Try to find compatible partners at the start by using age and gender matching.

Electronic Journals. Using e-mail, it is now possible to have dialogues without having to physically pass the journals back and forth. This can occur between students in the same school, district, state, or nation. It could even occur between students from different countries. Deaf students can be paired up with hearing students or with other deaf students. It would be an interesting classroom project to have students strike up an electronic journal with both a hearing student and a deaf student. Comparisons that could be made between the journals could lead to some interesting insight as to the language forms used (e.g., does the deaf student attend to greater grammatical correctness when corresponding to one person than to another?) and for what purposes the journals were used (e.g., do deaf students talk about things with their deaf partners that are different from what they talked about with their hearing partners?). Online discussions can also be interesting supplements to teaching.

Student Publications

One of the most enjoyable places in the Kendall Demonstration Elementary School, which is on the campus of Gallaudet University, is a section of the library where the books written by the children are kept. If there is a group of children in the library, inevitably there is at least one child reading through the books written by other children.

Most writing is done for some kind of publication. Since composition is a physically and intellectually demanding process, very rarely do individuals write books not to be published. Publication in some form is the logical end point of most composition. Obviously, the exception is the personal diary.

Think about the psychology of writing something for a teacher and then getting it back only to throw it away. Why commit to the process if it is only going to be thrown away? Yet children will spend endless hours in practice throwing free throws with a basketball. They see some logical end point to the effort; those that do not, won't practice. If we write, we write to see it in some form of print at some point in the future. We research because we want the information to be correct or we need an idea. We write to get a logical structure down or to find the right motivational device. We revise because we want to communicate our ideas to others clearly.

Children do not have to publish everything they write, but student publications—not just books, but newsletters, magazines, advertisements, plays, news reports—give students a sense of power over the printed word. In addition, generating student writing in this manner can be used for portfolio assessment. In fact, students should be encouraged to select material that they think should be entered into their portfolios.

Invented Spellings Accepted.   Let us make a simple historical point. Chaucer couldn't spell, and Shakespeare was not much better. Chaucer can be forgiven because he was a literary genius, and he was writing in order to standardize and legitimate his language, which was Middle English. Shakespeare was too busy writing for money in the early era of the printing press to worry about spelling. Caxton, who printed the first book in English, would be the first to standardize spelling. In order to achieve clarity and efficiency in print, publishers since Caxton have standardized English spellings.

What do the earliest and the best writers in English have to do with an approach to teaching literacy to deaf students? Spelling a written language follows a developmental process, but it is a process that follows rather than leads the need to communicate. No one says, "I will learn to spell *confabulation* because it is an important word." The writer starts with the need to express an idea. The idea requires a word. Eventually, the writer wishes to unambiguously communicate a certain idea, thus spelling becomes critical. As precision and clarity of communication become important to the young writer, spelling will improve.

Special Methods in Teaching Literacy

In Chapter 9, we talk about how computers can be used for instructional purposes. In this section, we focus briefly on using the computer to teach language skills.

Word Processor–Based Methods

In our chapter on integrating technology, we give an example of using templates to develop a classroom newsletter. Such a project is valuable for several reasons:

1. It informs parents, staff, or children of important information.
2. It uses an authentic piece of writing.
3. It teaches about how word processors work.

Other templates that are now a standard part of any word-processing package can be used to reinforce not only specific language skills but can make topics more interesting and engaging. For example, some of the templates available in some word processing programs are listed in Figure 4.4 with possible uses in the curriculum.

Template	Example	Skill or Use
Business letter	Request for a refund for a defective product.	Logical organization Business letter format Persuasive skills
Friendly letter	Describe an experience you recently had.	Tone Clarity Descriptive skills
Memo	Send a memo to the superintendent about a school problem.	Logical organization Memo format Appropriate tone
Resume	Applying for a job.	Chronological organization Personal direction
Greeting card	Birthday card to a literary character.	Personal response to literature Creativity
Sign	Advertise a school event.	Creativity Logical organization Planning

FIGURE 4.4   Examples of templates available on a word processor.

A template in a word-processing package should not be used frivolously or simply to keep students busy. Working with word processors in language arts gives the children opportunities to practice logical skills and creativity, operate in a real world language environment, and learn important lifelong skills. In the long run, it is a more effective use of the student's time than using a computer for drill and practice of subskills.

Document Sharing

Trent Batson (1993) developed a method of sharing documents on a computer network that would allow multiple contributions to the text. Named English Natural Form Instruction (ENFI), it was developed in the English department at Gallaudet University as an attempt to explore the potentials of computers as communication devices within the context of teaching language skills. Although it is no longer used at Gallaudet University, we are mentioning it because the principles for using ENFI are valid in today's technology-oriented classrooms.

ENFI involved students and teachers simultaneously in work on a shared document through a local area network in the classroom. The pedagogical issue is group work on a

Actions on the Document	Example	Alternative Example
Generate	Group writing of an essay.	One student's paper.
Display	Use an interactive web-based software.	Use a single computer with a projector.
Discuss	Brainstorm ideas.	Ask for revisions based on a specific goal.
Side issues	Discuss tone and word choice.	Correct grammar, spelling, or mechanics.
Revise	Students suggest changes.	Students suggest changes with prompting from teachers.
Publish or save	Print a copy of the paper for all participants.	Save for future revisions if topic will be ongoing.

FIGURE 4.5   General procedures involved in document sharing.

single document, which interestingly enough mimics a common form of work in business. The document is available to everyone in the class who can then make contributions to its "improvement." Students are exposed to language concepts, and grammar is addressed at the level of the student's immediate need. The exact procedures involved in document sharing will vary depending on the hardware and software available to you, but the general procedures are shown in Figure 4.5.

From the perspective of instructional goals, this approach is similar to the older techniques of making an overhead of the paper or passing out multiple copies. The benefit here is the opportunity for group participation and immediate change to the document, which is a critical skill because today much of business and governmental communication involves the handling and revision of documents. While individuals still do write reports, much work involves a group effort. Therefore, students learning in a group setting more than improve their individual writing skills; they learn communication and thinking skills that are valuable to the enhancement of their social skills.

Matching Methods with Teaching Situations

Teaching situations vary because both the classroom structure and the developmental level of the students can vary. Preliterate students are chronologically younger children who are ready to begin to read but who do not read as yet. The important goals are to foster an interest in books, to develop a sense of the structure of a story, to teach basic book handling, and to recognize symbols and print.

Becoming literate usually takes place in kindergarten through second grade among hearing children. At this stage the emphasis is most often on basic decoding skills and on being able to write single words and simple sentences. Narrative cohesion is stressed for the nonliterate story but is not necessarily required of written stories.

Becoming an independent reader occurs around third grade for hearing children. Children who fail to develop the skills to pick up a book and read it for themselves begin the slide towards school failure. Composition at this stage begins to emphasize the coherent narrative and other forms of writing such as the friendly letter.

The critical author stage can begin as early as seventh grade for hearing students and continues on through graduate school. By now the fundamental reading skills are established. Instead of simply reading to extract information, the student is challenged to compose independently and to examine what is in print.

Remedial or adult programs begin at any point at which a student fails to master age appropriate skills; however, remedial programs below the third grade are questionable because of the possibility of developmental variation among beginning readers and writers.

Matching Methods with Development

Figure 4.6 illustrates how the literacy level of a deaf child can be matched with the skills that are typically being developed at that level along with potential instructional strategies. This section highlights the key points of these matchups.

Preliterate Students

Children love to be read to, and they especially love predictable stories where they can see what is happening as it unfolds. In this section, we will focus on sharing books with children.

Literacy Level	Grade	Skill	Method
Preliterate	Pre–K	Print awareness Book handling	Shared reading Big books
Becoming literate	K–2	Decoding Sentence composition	Interactive language Predictable books
Independent reader	3–4	Read independently Coherent narratives	Process writing Word processor–based writing Metacognitive skills
Critical author	7–12	Read for information Critical evaluation	Dialogue journals I-Search reports Document sharing Study circles

FIGURE 4.6   **Approximate relationship between literacy level, reading skills, and reading instructions.**

Shared Reading. There are several benefits to reading with children including learning important concepts, providing a source of enjoyment, encouraging imagination and creativity, and learning how a book "works" both in the sense of how to physically handle a book but intellectually as in the structure of narratives (Ewoldt & Saulnier, 1995).

Many of the ideas related to **shared reading** were initially developed for parents. But the principles for doing the reading can be applied to the classroom as well. Some of these principles are the following:

1. A physical location should be selected in the house or classroom, where everyone can see the book.
2. Stories should be pretaught by connecting the ideas in the book to what students already know before beginning to read.
3. It may be necessary to engage in scaffolding or providing information about the parts of the story with which the students are not familiar.
4. Students need to be monitored for comprehension.
5. Reading the story more than once is critical to the acquisition of meaning, vocabulary, and syntax.

A Shared Reading Project was developed by teachers and researchers at the Clerc National Deaf Education Center at Gallaudet University. The basis of this project can be found in *Reading to Deaf Children: Learning from Deaf Adults* by David Schleper (1997). This project relies heavily upon the use of ASL and fluency in signing as well as a knack for reading in signs, which is one of its key components. The project is based on fifteen principles (see Chapter 14 for a full listing of these principles) that were gleaned from the literature and from observations of how deaf adults read to deaf children. These principles emphasize the importance of dramatization, connecting the English sentences with their ASL renderings, and engaging the students in the reading process.

Reading to a single deaf child is different from reading to a group of deaf children in that the child can have more control over the book and the pace of the story. But the message for both group and individual shared reading is that it has to be fun.

Guidelines for what books to use in shared reading situations are helpful, and one such guide is found in Figure 4.7. This guideline was assembled by Stewart, Bennett, and Bonkowski (1992), and it contains a "Signability Index" for children's books. It uses sentence length, quantity of text, word imagery, complexity and concreteness of passages, literary style, and plays on words in the story to categorize children's books as being good or poor candidates for shared reading. Teachers who read a lot to their students will benefit from creating their own list of books that they feel comfortable reading—in signs and/or speech.

Big Books. Big books are children's storybooks that are literally big. Big books can fold out to as large as a two-foot by three-foot size or even larger. They make it possible for groups of students to sit in a group near the teacher and share the text and pictures at the same time. With an easel and big clips, it is possible for the teacher to point and sign at the same time as he or she reads the story.

Big books are popular in many early literacy situations. In addition, they can be used with older children with vision or other forms of disabilities. Many of these books are nonfiction photo essays with text although most of the information is communicated through

Level 1 Criteria	Level 1 Books
a. No restrictions on reading rate; pace of reading does not affect student.	*Brown Bear, Brown Bear, What Do You See?* Bill Martin Jr.
b. Simple sentence constructions.	*Sitting in My Box*, Dee Lillegard
c. Complete thoughts expressed in short sentences.	*I Am Eyes—Ai Macho*, Leila Ward
d. Concrete, basic concepts (farm animals, things to play with).	*Little Gorilla*, Ruth Bornstein *Who Goes Out on Halloween?* Bank Street Reading Series
e. Repetition of key phrases.	*The Gum on the Drum*, School Zone Reading Series
f. Simple language, appropriate to beginning readers.	*A is for Angry*, Sandra Boynton
g. Only basic skills needed for translating text into ASL.	*Quick as a Cricket*, Audrey Wood *Just Like Jasper*, Nick Butterworth and Mick Inkpen
h. Easily articulated in sign.	
Level 2 Criteria	**Level 2 Books**
a. Flexible reading rate; slow pace may affect comprehension or interest.	*Snow*, Roy McKie and P.D. Eastman
b. Expanded simple sentence constructions.	*It's Not Easy Being a Bunny*, Marilyn Sadler
c. Complete thoughts expressed in short sentences.	*You and Me-Me*, Peter Curry *Indian Two Feet and His Horse*, Margaret Friskey
d. Concrete basic concepts.	*In Our House*, Anne Rockwell
e. Repetition of key phrases.	*Hello, Cat, You Need a Hat*, Rita Golden Gelman
f. Longer text than Level 1 books.	*Wait, Skates*, Rookie Reader Series
g. Basic to intermediate skills needed to translate text into ASL.	*Noisy Nora*, Rosemary Wells
h. Easily articulated in sign.	*The Very Busy Spider*, Eric Carle *My House*, Patricia F. Frakes

FIGURE 4.7   An example of a guide for ease of reading and signing books.

the photos. Other books are on topics such as science, technology, and multicultural issues, which makes them useful for language experience approaches as well as for integrated units of teaching.

Becoming Literate

Many of the principles of the interactive approach to literacy that were described earlier in this chapter can be applied to this level. In addition, the use of **predictable books** is a

Level 3 Criteria

a. Specific reading rate needed to maintain story cadence; slow reading may affect interest or comprehension.
b. Mix of simple and complex sentences; some fairly long.
c. Abstract as well as concrete ideas.
d. Repetition of some language patterns.
e. Longer text than Level 2 books.
f. Basic to intermediate skills needed to translate text into ASL.
g. Expanded sign vocabulary needed.
h. Sign practice may be needed before presentation.

Level 3 Books

Who Sank the Boat? Pamela Allen
Just Me, Marie Hall Ets
Green Eggs and Ham, Dr. Seuss
Madeline, Ludwig Behelmans
Where the Wild Things Are, Maurice Sendak
Is Your Mama a Llama? Deborah Kellogg
Lost, David McPhail
The Snowy Day, Ezra Jack Keats
When Sheep Cannot Sleep, Satashi Kitamura
Much Bigger than Martin, Steven Kellogg

Level 4 Criteria

a. Specific reading rate needed to maintain story cadence.
b. More complex sentences than in Level 3; many long sentences.
c. Abstract ideas common.
d. Story builds through complex plot, conversations.
e. Longer text than at Level 3; may require up to fifteen minutes of reading time.
f. Intermediate ASL skills needed to translate text into ASL.
g. Expanded sign vocabulary needed.
h. Sign practice may be needed before presentation.

Level 4 Books

Sadie and the Snowman, Allen Morgan
Love You Forever, Robert Munsch
Caps For Sale, Esphyr Slobodkina
The Runaway Bunny, Margaret Wise Brown
Five Minutes' Peace, Jill Murphy
The Little House, Virginia Lee Burton
The Snail's Spell, Joanne Ryder
Benjamin's Barn, Reeve Lindbergh
Frog and Toad Together, Arnold Lobel
Amos's Sweater, Janet Lunn

FIGURE 4.7　Continued

Level 5 Criteria	Level 5 Books
a. Specific reading rate needed to maintain cadence of the story.	*I Heard My Mother Call My Name*, Nancy Hundal
b. Many longer, complex sentences.	*Knots on a Counting Rope*, Bill Martin,
c. Abstract, often difficult concepts.	Jr. and John Archambault
d. Strong dependence on verbal imagery.	*The Mitten*, Jan Brett
	Owl Moon, Jane Yolen
e. Longer text than Level 4 books.	*Foo*, Richard Thompson
f. Intermediate to advanced skills needed to translate text into ASL.	*The True Story of the Three Little Pigs*, Jon Scieszka
g. Proficient signing skills needed to hold interest of deaf students.	*The Little Engine That Could,* Watty Piper
h. Sign practice needed for presentation.	*Blueberries for Sal*, Robert McCloskey
	The One in the Middle is the Green Kangaroo, Judy Blume
	The River Dream, Allen Say

Level 6 Criteria	Level 6 Books
a. Specific reading rate required to maintain story cadence.	*Wild Robin*, Susan Jeffers
b. Many long, complex sentences.	*A Day on the River*, Reinhard Michl
c. Abstract, often difficult concepts.	*The Velveteen Rabbit*, Margery Williams
d. Strong dependence on verbal imagery.	*Moses the Kitten*, James Herriot
	Thumbelina, Hans Christian Andersen
e. Longer text than Level 5; may require more than one reading session.	*The Tale of Jemima Puddle-Duck*, Beatrix Potter
f. Advanced skills needed to translate text into ASL.	*Mufaro's Beautiful Daughters*, John Steptoe
g. Proficient signing skills required.	*Puss in Boots*, Susan Saunders
	Lon Po Po, Ed Young
h. Signing practice required before presentation.	*Annie and the Old One*, Miska Miles

Taken with permission from D. Stewart, D. Bennett, & N. Bonkowski. (1992). Books to read, books to sign. *Perspectives in Education and Deafness, 10* (3), 4–7.

FIGURE 4.7   Continued

valuable component for students at this age (and younger too). Although routine may be boring in an adult's job, it is the essence of a good story. We understand and process language, either sentences or novels, because we have a template or a story grammar or schema already in our head that we are using to keep track of the information as it comes in. These patterns are learned, and until children learn them they are helped in processing longer pieces of text through readily recurring patterns.

Elements that contribute to a predictable book include rhyme, repeated phrases, repeated episode structures, and catch phrases that signal what is going to happen or that recall what already has happened. Children's books like *Madeline* with its twelve little girls in two straight lines are predictable books.

Predictable books are good as beginning books because they teach the structure of narratives, but they can also be good as first readers because of the reduced vocabulary size and repeated structures. The principle of the *Dick and Jane* basal readers was to use limited vocabularies and repeated structures. The difference with trade books that are "predictable" is that the stories they contain are more interesting to children, and the art work is usually better.

When selecting a predictable book, consider the obvious by selecting familiar sequences of events, ideas, and situations. If the book is not within the child's experience do not include it. Rereading books is a concept that is missed by teachers of the deaf who may become frustrated with reading for any number of reasons. Perhaps they get little positive feedback that their students are understanding the story. Or they might not feel comfortable signing stories because of their lack of fluency in signing or their limited sign vocabulary, aversion to fingerspelling, and other reasons. Nevertheless, whatever reading skills a teacher has, it is still better to have twenty books that you feel comfortable with to read over and over again than to have two hundred books that you read only once.

Becoming an Independent Reader

At this stage the deaf child has some understanding of decoding skills, and it becomes useful to stress larger or what are sometimes called "metacognitive" skills such as inferring, predicting, analyzing, attending, associating, synthesizing, and so on.

These skills extend beyond reading and writing into other common language situations, thus the teacher can use a variety of materials to help students develop these skills. For example, in the previous section we mentioned predictable books. The process of making predictions can be reinforced through activities such as drawing pictures, writing endings, or telling a similar story from home that show that the student understands the extension of the idea presented in the text to a time or place outside the text. Another early literacy material is to use wordless stories to practice making predictions. In addition, students can be asked to write dialogue for these stories, which calls for associating or synthesizing ideas.

Clearly, simple stories that appeal to the children can also be used to stimulate thinking about the larger structures and ideas behind the narratives. Writing letters to characters, book character parades, book character posters, writing alternative endings to stories, or even supplying a story without an ending all involve working with text at levels larger than the individual symbols.

Becoming a Critical Author

As the deaf student moves closer to becoming a critical author, **study circles** are a technique that can be used to stimulate thoughts about what to write. Study circles are an attempt to create a community of learners through meaningful interaction about books (Schleper, 1996). The procedure, like many other language experience approaches, stresses meaningful use of language, several modes of communication, and the use of materials that are self-motivating, such as selections of children's literature.

Some of the traits of study circles are as follows:

1. Students choose their own reading materials.
2. Students form small temporary groups based on book choice.
3. Each group reads a different book.
4. Regular meetings are held to discuss books.
5. Students generate written notes or drawings to guide reading and discussion.
6. Discussion topics come from students.
7. Group meetings are open, natural conversations about books.
8. Students take on diverse roles.
9. The teacher serves as facilitator.

When finished writing, students share their books with their classmates, and new groups are formed (Schleper, 1996).

This is not a simple method to use, and deaf students have to learn how to do it. Preparation for these groups can involve several months of modeling and practice before turning the groups loose on their own. This method is also an opportunity to teach group work skills and study skills in preparation to starting the book circles.

Another valuable instructional technique for assisting students in the writing process is the creation of **I-Search reports.** These reports are a variant on traditional term papers, but the difference is that a first-person approach is used (Reed, 1990). Instead of an impersonal task, the student's curiosity is stimulated by the personal nature of the topic.

One of the authors received a letter from an eighth grade student in Los Angeles who was conducting an I-Search report. She was using his book, *American Sign Language the Easy Way* (Stewart, 1998) to learn to sign and became curious about the author. We will call her Colleen, and taking up on her topic, we have designed an example of what an I-Search project might look like. We use a description of the six basic steps for creating an I-Search report in our illustration of this example:

1. *Clarifying the task.* The student selects a topic of interest and is told to become an expert on that topic. In addition, a model of an I-Search report is provided so that students have a sense of the final product, which will be a visual-verbal presentation. This could, for example, take the form of a poster, an explanation (or presentation), and a written report. Colleen's general topic of interest was:

Why do people write books about sign language?

2. *Choosing topics.* A funnel approach is used in prepping students for the topic. The first step is to frame the topic of interest with a researchable question. Colleen was learning how to sign, which influenced her decision to learn more about the author of the book

American Sign Language the Easy Way. Her central search questions aimed to find out more information about the author and why he wrote the book:

> Why did the author write this book?

Colleen then developed a list of questions that would help her answer this central question:

> When did the author learn to sign?
> How did the author learn to sign?
> Who influenced him the most when he was learning to sign?
> Has he taught ASL in classes?
> Why did he write this book about American Sign Language?

   3. *Exploring research possibilities*. Students are encouraged to research their own topics. However, the I-Search paper is also a good way to teach basic research skills, and guidance from the teacher can ensure that the activity does not become an exercise in frustration. In addition to the usual library sources, other forms of media and the Internet can become resources. Colleen approached this part of her I-Search by writing a letter to the author. She did not know how to contact him directly, so she sent her letter to the publisher, Barron's Educational Series, with instructions to forward the letter to the author.
   4. *Developing note taking, research, and organizational skills*. A challenge for deaf students when doing an I-Search paper is that they may rapidly gather more information than they can handle. A notebook is one solution but a workbook with examples of organizers is also an alternative. A very simple organizing table is shown in Figure 4.8.

Research Questions	Responses Found from the Research	Sources/References
1. When did the author learn to sign?		
2. How did the author learn to sign?		
3. Who influenced him the most when he was learning to sign?		
4. Has he taught ASL in classes?		
5. Why did he write this book about American Sign Language?		

FIGURE 4.8   An organizational chart for an I-Search report: Central question: Why did the author write this book?

Frequent meetings with the students to discuss progress are useful. A mechanical solution is to design a set of specific worksheets like the one above and have the students turn them in at specific points. This, however, takes the personal element out of the process. If possible, individual contact is preferable. Furthermore, personal contact will help the teacher monitor the gathering of data. Deaf students who are learning to read and write might overlook material that they did not fully understand or might not have the language skills to write down information in a manner that can be used later on. All students can benefit from frequent discussions about their research. Such discussions allow the teacher to model the language that the student might use to record information.

5. *Visual-verbal capsule presentations.* The visual-verbal presentation should be the most creative part of the project. This is the representation of the idea and as such it should also capture the mood of the project. Students should be encouraged to make a multimedia presentation and to use all of their communication skills. One simple option is to have the students make a poster and explain its significance. Outside speakers, pamphlets, videos, or other media can also be used if they encapsulate the idea of the project.

Colleen elected to make a poster with her questions and answers displayed. She surrounded her written part of the poster with enlarged copies of sign illustrations, examples of signed dialogues with their English glosses, and fascinating facts about ASL, all of which were taken directly from the book. Finally, she got the author to agree to be interviewed online, using the Internet to transmit a real-time video so that the students in her class see what ASL looks like.

6. *Writing the report.* The report includes a cover page, table of contents, body of the work, and a bibliography. It provides authentic opportunities for the students to engage in writing. However, since this report is written in the first person, students have greater latitude in their expression and can afford to be more creative in their discussion of the topic. The format gives the teacher the opportunity to make the distinction between first-person and third-person writing as well as concepts such as tone and voice in writing.

Conclusion

Regardless of the situation one is in, or the language processing model one prefers to use, teaching literacy to deaf students is a challenging task. In our discussions, we focused on the processes of reading and writing although literacy encompasses far more than just the act of creating and understanding print. Literacy includes, for example, a functional aspect related to how print is used to accomplish personal and social goals such as obtaining employment and planning for retirement. We did not provide a comprehensive overview of theoretical issues related to teaching literacy because that was outside the scope of this book. Instead, we described a number of strategies for teaching reading and writing, and we urge teachers to select those that fit the learning needs of their deaf students. In fact, teaching literacy is very much an eclectic affair, given what we know about how deaf children acquire and use language. Paul (1998) commented on the teaching of literacy in the following passage:

> As most teachers and practitioners know, it is counterproductive to espouse one literacy philosophy or perspective for *all* of these children and youth. Perhaps the focus should be not

on finding the best or most effective method for all children but on possible literacy techniques to use with each child in an interactive, custom-made manner. In light of the abundance of *either-or* paradigms that exist in literacy and deafness, I would hope that educators and other professionals see the need to create a deeper paradigm or a composite paradigm—one that focuses on the development of critical, logical, and reflective thinking, and this should be the ultimate educational goal for all students who are deaf. (p. 308)

The strategies that we described for teaching literacy are similar to those for teaching other subject matter to deaf students. Authentic activities must be incorporated into the learning experience, the students must be provided with opportunities to talk about what they are reading and writing, and modeling and guidance must be provided to help them overcome their lack of proficiency in the English language.

Most important is that the students come to appreciate the function of reading and writing and use literacy as a means of communicating with others and learning more about the world around them. Research has not identified a definitive method for teaching literacy that will help all deaf students but it has revealed that there are some instructional strategies that can succeed with some of them. We described some of these in this chapter but at the present time teaching literacy is every bit as much a learning experience as it is a teaching experience.

KEY WORDS AND CONCEPTS

authentic context: Instructional material that is of immediate relevance to a student.

basal readers: A series of books and related materials that are built on several premises, with the primary one being reading is a bottom-up process. Instructions in phonics at the beginning of a basal reading program is important to the success of the program.

interactive approach to language development: An approach where language processing is assisted by elements of both text-based and subject-based skills. In other words, good readers use text-based skills to overcome subject-based language-processing limits or vice versa.

I-Search reports: Reports where students select a topic to research, conduct the research, and write their reports in the first person.

predictable books: Typically picture books for young children that have a high degree of predictability built into their stories and/or sequences of pictures.

scaffolding: The practice of providing assistance to the students so that they can engage in a learning activity. The amount of assistance is reduced as the student becomes better able to work on a task independently.

shared reading: Typically, adults reading a book to a group of children in an interactive manner using such techniques as elaboration and dramatization to engage the student in the reading process.

subject-based or **top-down:** An approach to language processing that assumes that context and prior knowledge is the key to language processing. Deaf children's difficulty in reading, then, is attributable to their lack of context and prior knowledge.

text-based or bottom-up: An approach to language development that assumes that processing begins at the phonological and morphological levels and eventually moves to the processing of words in sentences and finally sentences in discourse. In this approach, deaf children's difficulty in decoding speech is translated to difficulty in reading.

QUESTIONS

1. What are the three models of language processing?

2. What are the educational implications of using a bottom-up approach to reading? What support service would be of help for a teacher who wishes to implement this type of approach in her classroom?

3. Describe at least three general principles of the interactive approach and give a concrete example of a practice for each of the three principles you select.

4. In process writing a lot of time and energy is devoted to generating ideas before you start to write. How could you help deaf students produce ideas, and how could you help them organize those ideas?

5. What is a possible administrative problem you could expect when implementing a dialogue or other form of journal writing? What is a personal or student problem that might come up from a journal writing project? How would you cope with each?

6. Student correction is a common form of teaching composition that involves having them read and comment on each other's writing. How would you manage such an approach in a self-contained class of deaf students?

7. What are the main purposes of shared reading between an adult and a deaf child? What are some of the obstacles to shared reading?

8. What are the benefits of reading predictable books?

9. Describe a strategy for establishing study circles in a typical self-contained class of deaf 13-year-olds.

10. What components of an I-search report can benefit a deaf student's overall literacy development and why?

ACTIVITIES

1. Select a picture book from Level 1 or 2 in Figure 4.7. After reading the book, make a list of what you think the challenges are for you to read the book to a group of deaf children. Practice reading the book to a group of adults (e.g., teachers of the deaf, preservice teachers, deaf adults, etc.) and have them provide you with feedback on various aspects of the reading. Depending upon the mode(s) of communication used (e.g., signs, speech, signs, and speech), you might receive feedback on the ease with which you can be lipread, the strategies you use to enhance comprehension of certain vocabulary words, clarity and appropriateness of signs and fingerspelling, pacing, and so forth.

2. In groups of two to four people, engage in a brainstorming session, then structure the ideas that are generated during this session. Relate your topic for brainstorming to teaching a sub-

ject matter to deaf students (e.g., science, social studies, and mathematics). See box titled "From Brainstorming to Structure" for a framework to organize the material generated from the brainstorming session.

3. Authentic language experiences are a critical aspect of language development. Plan a field trip experience that will be used to generate stories for a classroom-produced newsletter. Identify the stories that will be written, and describe how the students will be prepared for writing each story. Include in your planning a selection of writing strategies.

4. Add to the list of books shown in the box titled "Deaf Authors and the Reading Center."

5 Teaching Deaf Studies

CHAPTER OUTCOMES

After reading this chapter, you should be able to:

1. Distinguish between a traditional, global-interactive, and integrated approach to Deaf studies and to determine which approach would be most suitable for a particular classroom.
2. Use resources to help plan units and lessons that distinguish between the various groups of people who have a hearing loss.
3. Design a resource center for information relating to deaf people.
4. Structure Deaf studies units and lesson plans that provide the information and experiences necessary to help deaf students evolve generalizations about different ways of living as a deaf person.

The first **Deaf studies** program was established in the unwritten curriculum of residential schools for the deaf. These schools played an integral role in the local Deaf community. They produced Deaf leaders, brought together Deaf adults for social affairs and sport events, and served as a treasure trove of Deaf history with their collection of graduation photographs, trophies, yearbooks, annual reports, Deaf newspapers, newsletters from other schools for the deaf, furniture and artwork made by their students, and much more. Regardless of a school's communication policies, outside of the school building deaf children used American Sign Language (ASL) as their social lifeline. The legacy of ASL was that, in the dormitories and in conversations among the students and Deaf teachers, it gave students access to information about the community in which they lived.

More than that, ASL was the tool by which many deaf students were prepared for participation in the Deaf community when they became adults. Thus, going to a school for the deaf initiated students into a lifetime of learning about deaf people. Deaf studies was an experience and not a subject to be written about in IEPs.

Today, most deaf students attend public school programs. Deaf immersion is not an option for them at these schools. Schools must purposefully provide students with a study of the language, culture, and social affairs of Deaf people. Even at schools for the deaf, a growing body of knowledge about deaf people is making Deaf studies an indispensable part of their education program.

There are at least three reasons to justify the teaching of Deaf studies in the curriculums of educational programs both in the United States and Canada:

- Community building
- Self-image or self-awareness
- Diversity

There is a Deaf community, and any deaf child has a right to know its rich history. As a society, we are struggling with the issues of African American children being raised by white parents or how to explain to adopted Korean children their "other" heritage. In the same vein, deaf children have a right to know about how successful Deaf adults achieved success and in the process built a functioning community. In addition, there is both the need and the historical precedent for teaching children about the Deaf community so that they can develop a sense of themselves. The successful deaf adult is likely to function in both the Deaf and the Hearing world; therefore, deaf children need to be taught about the possibilities of both communities.

Finally, in not only the United States and Canada but throughout much of the world, the concept of the nation–state is being revised from one people/one language to societies that embrace more than one language and more than one ethnic or cultural group. Consequently, deafness as a cultural phenomenon needs to be taught to nondeaf children for the same reasons that we include African American authors in literature anthologies. In this chapter, we will cover all three reasons.

In response to these three motivations for teaching about deafness, we will present three approaches to presenting content about deafness.

- Traditional
- Global-interactive
- Integrated

What Is Deaf Studies?

There are various groups that comprise the deaf population. These groups are typically delineated on the basis of degree of hearing loss, onset of deafness, community affiliation, and preferred means of communication. There are Deaf people who use ASL and identify with the activities of the Deaf community. There are hard of hearing people who prefer to communicate using speech, are able to use their hearing to some degree, and function primarily in the general society. Similar to the hard of hearing is a group of people identified as being oral deaf—those who normally were either born deaf or became deaf early in their life. **Oral deaf** people favor speech communication but their degree of hearing loss is such that it is difficult for them to hear with or without a hearing aid, and therefore speechreading is important for communication. The **late-deafened** are a group of people who have lost their hearing as adults, and they tend to try to carry on with their lives as they always have with the support of assistive listening devices and perhaps some adjustments in the way they conduct their daily affairs. But all of these labels carry some degree of ambiguity and confusion as demonstrated, for example, in the fact that some late-deafened people call themselves hard of hearing.

One might be tempted to put all of these groups together because they share the characteristic of having some degree of hearing loss. In a way, we do that in this book with our use of the term deaf. But hearing loss by itself tells us little about a person. A late-deafened adult may have the same degree of hearing loss as an adult who was born deaf. The customary distinction between the groups is that each one of them can be identified with a particular way of living associated with certain linguistic and sociocultural implications. This distinction serves the purpose of facilitating discussions about these groups and allows for labels to be attached to them. It also underscores the tenuous lines of separation between the groups. Some people who can function adequately in the speech and hearing domain while wearing a hearing aid and speaking see themselves as being Deaf. These people come from a variety of backgrounds, but one in particular is someone who has Deaf parents and is sent to a school for the deaf.

We could go further and identify more subgroups of people for whom Deaf culture is a critical part of their lives. This can be done, for example, by looking closely at their shared experiences such as those who are products of public school programs, are college graduates (especially from the National Technical Institute for the Deaf or Gallaudet University), or are employed as professionals. In whichever way we divide and label groups we can rest assured that new groups and new labels or new characterizations of existing groups will appear in the future. At the time of this writing, we are witnessing the emergence of a new group of deaf adults with cochlear implants. Will this group begin to identify with one another or will they be satisfied with their affiliation with some existing group of deaf people?

This begs the question: Who are the "deaf" people referred to in "Deaf studies"? Deaf studies as a formal course of study is a recent occurrence in the field of education. Its appearance in schools followed closely the growth of awareness of the cultural and linguistic heritage of this community. No other group of people use ASL as their primary language for face-to-face communications. Schools for the deaf, Deaf clubs, organizations of Deaf people, Deaf churches, and Deaf sport are the pillars of the Deaf community, and they exist only because there are Deaf people. These entities and the people associated with them are examples of what comprises Deaf culture. Thus, by historical precedence the "deaf" people referred to in Deaf studies have been those "deaf" people who identify with the **Deaf community**. In fact, some authors use the capitalized word "Deaf" to refer to those people who are the focus of study in a Deaf studies course. To them, Deaf people have some degree of hearing loss, use ASL, and identify with the activities of the Deaf community.

A Deaf studies course that focuses mainly on Deaf people might appear to be too limited given the diversity of experiences and identity that people with a hearing loss have. This is readily evidenced in the brief description of various groups of people with a hearing loss that was provided at the beginning of this section. Moreover, public school programs do cater to a range of deaf students.

Thus, if Deaf studies is going to find a place in schools, then alternative approaches to teaching it are necessary. Each approach can have its own set of instructional goals and objectives that are meaningful to a particular group of students. We call the type of Deaf studies program alluded to above a **traditional approach to Deaf studies,** which primarily investigates Deaf people. We also propose a second approach to teaching Deaf studies that carries with it an eclectic flavor that allows teachers to select concepts about deaf people that closely approximate the backgrounds and interests of the students. We are calling this a **global-interactive approach to Deaf studies.** There is a third approach to studying about deaf people that looks beyond the lives of deaf people to include that of hearing people too. We are calling this the **integrated approach to Deaf studies.** This approach infuses information about deafness into the regular curriculum in public schools.

The content of the three approaches will overlap because there will be similarities between deaf people no matter what degree of hearing loss they have, what home environment they were raised in, or what language and communication system they prefer to use.

A Traditional Approach to Deaf Studies

One definition of Deaf studies states that it is "the study of language, education, history, arts, literature, sociology, and anthropology of deaf people" (Miller-Nomeland & Gillespie, 1993, p. 4). Invariably this approach has a strong focus on the lives of Deaf people. Teaching is marked by what's different about Deaf people when compared to the lives of hearing people in society. Schein (1989) commented on the lives of Deaf people in this way:

> Deaf people have demonstrated their talents for adaptation, for finding ways to work with and move around barriers. Their adaptations and accompanying folkways and values form Deaf culture. It reflects the differences from the majority culture that enable Deaf people to adjust to a world that frustrates them, not out of malevolence, but because the majority has naturally structured the environment for their convenience. (pp. 66–67)

This notion of adaptation is a succinct summary of the essence of what a *traditional approach to Deaf studies* attempts to teach.

Padden and Humphries (1988) related the differences between Deaf people and others to the notion of a "center" of the way Deaf people see themselves. In this perspective, Deaf people view their lives and their use of sign language as being the norm—that is, the center. This perspective contrasts with the longstanding practice, evidenced in the literature, of viewing the lives of people who are deaf, including their use of sign language, as a deviancy from the norm established by people who hear. Padden and Humphries observed that Deaf people, in trying to make sense of the world in which they live, "have created systems of meaning that explain how they understand their place in the world" (p. 121). This is an apt description of what a course on Deaf studies can be about. Thus, a Deaf studies course that focuses on people in the Deaf community is what we call the traditional approach.

The "Deaf Studies Curriculum Guide" developed at the Kendall Demonstration Elementary School (KDES) is an example of this traditional approach to Deaf studies, which will be discussed later in this chapter. This type of curriculum lends itself to being taught as a course. This is an option that is most likely available in schools for the deaf and self-contained classrooms where the teacher can devote a period of time during the day to teach it. Although most public school programs do not offer Deaf studies as a formal course, components of the Deaf Studies Curriculum Guide can be taught in a resource room, as part of an ASL course, and even by an itinerant teacher.

A Global-Interactive Approach to Deaf Studies

Most teachers of the deaf teach in public schools and the students they teach range from those who typically identify themselves as being hard of hearing to those who see themselves as being Deaf. Sign language is not a crucial language to all of these students, and many of these students do not participate in any Deaf community activities. For these students, the traditional approach to Deaf studies might not be meaningful enough to warrant its implementation—at least at this time in their lives. Yet, discussions about all types of deaf people, including the hard of hearing, and how they live should still be a part of their educational plan.

For these students, we recommend a *global-interactive approach to Deaf studies*. The approach is *global* in the sense that students study the different ways that people with all degrees of hearing loss live. In this approach, a comparative study of the role of speaking and signing, English and ASL, seeing and hearing, and the Deaf community and the community at large would be undertaken. No aspect associated with having a hearing loss is deemed unimportant.

The approach is *interactive* because the way in which Deaf studies is taught will reflect, in part, the characteristics and interests of the students. In other words, the background of each deaf or hard of hearing student in the classroom will influence the content of the Deaf studies instruction. Consider two classes of deaf students. One class has five 8-year-old deaf students, four of whom have cochlear implants. Another class has five 8-year-old deaf students, two of whom have Deaf parents and three others who have hearing parents who communicate comfortably in ASL. Both of these classes present a different challenge for a teacher teaching about deaf people.

Figure 5.1 illustrates the major components of the global-interactive and traditional approaches to teaching about deaf people.

An Integrated Approach to Deaf Studies

The *integrated approach to Deaf studies* differs from the other two approaches in that it is intended for use with both deaf and hearing students in public schools. It also does not consider Deaf studies to be a separate field of study. In the integrated approach, as with the global-interactive approach, information about deafness or deaf people is spread across the curriculum and inserted where it is appropriate. Therefore, the role of the teacher of the deaf in the integrated approach can be as a curriculum consultant or resource person or even a guest lecturer.

Martha Gonter Gaustad and her colleagues at Bowling Green State University (Gaustad, 1997, 1999) designed an infusion approach to including information about deafness in

	Traditional Approach	Global-Interactive Approach
Main focus	Deaf population; Deaf community	All groups of people with a significant degree of hearing loss (e.g., Deaf, hard of hearing, late-deafened)
Instructional module	Typically taught as a separate course but can be infused into the social studies and language arts curricula	Content infused in other subject matter classes (e.g., language arts, science, social studies)
Curriculum	Formal curriculum (e.g., KDES Deaf Studies Curriculum Guide)	Goals and objectives aligned with those of other subject matter
Content	ASL, American Deaf culture, history, communication, identity, social change (as stated in the KDES Deaf Studies Curriculum Guide)	Variable and can include topics relating to communication, technology, history, Deaf culture, development of self, social dynamics, community dynamics, multiculturalism (e.g., ethnic), education, language (e.g., ASL, English), sociolinguistics, audiology, medicine, and more
Key feature	Availability of curriculum and resources	Content can be influenced by the characteristics of the students

FIGURE 5.1   Features of the traditional and global-interactive approaches to teaching Deaf studies.

the regular K–6 curriculum. The purpose of their project was to lessen the impact of additional content on an already burdened curriculum while at the same time showing the relevance of the deafness-related information to the everyday life of hearing children.

The curriculum was built on four content areas: science, social studies, health, and language arts. Within each area, subtopics were defined—for example, the study of the senses within the science curriculum. From conferences with teachers, extended units of study were developed that included both the standard content and the expanded information related to deafness woven throughout the unit. From these units, a cumulative K–6 curriculum was developed (see Figure 5.2).

At each grade level, specific objectives were developed under the headings of Deaf Culture and Sign Language. These objectives covered knowledge of hearing, deafness, amplification, and so on. Age appropriateness and other curriculum concerns guided the selection of supporting materials. The goal of cumulative outcomes was maintained throughout the curriculum so that each year's content would build on what had been learned previously as well as provide an opportunity to review and reinforce earlier taught material.

When the material was actually taught, deafness specialists came into the classrooms to teach the material with a large degree of participation by Deaf adults from the community.

Grade Level	Content Area Topics	Deaf Culture Components
Kindergarten	Science/Social Studies: Sound awareness and Deaf awareness	Basics for interacting with Deaf people
First grade	Social Studies: Family life of the Deaf	Deafness and communication
Second grade	Social Studies: Deaf people in the community	Sensitivity activities ASL as a language
Third grade	Science: Sound, hearing measurement, and amplification	Deaf vs. hard of hearing Social interaction norms
Fourth grade	Reading: Biography and history of Deaf people	Deaf history Deaf identity Interview Deaf adult
Fifth grade	Health: Hearing and deafness	Deaf community Organizations and recreation
Sixth grade	Science: Communication and assistive devices for the Deaf	Deafness and literature Deaf values

FIGURE 5.2   **A curriculum overview of an integrated approach to Deaf studies.**

The Deaf adults served as guest speakers as well as technical experts. In addition, they gave students the opportunity to interact with an interpreter and to learn appropriate interactive behavior in that situation. Hearing students were encouraged to use their newly learned signs as well. Cross-grade events were scheduled as the culminating activity for each unit for each year.

Hearing students particularly enjoyed the opportunity to use their sign language skills and to have personal contact with Deaf adults. The general education teachers found the units informative, motivating, and necessary adjuncts to the instructional program. The frequent refrain throughout the evaluation of the project was the opportunity for human contact.

A less curriculum-driven version of this approach is practiced by the Mantua Elementary School in Fairfax, Virginia, and some other center-based public school programs for deaf students. This approach takes advantages of opportunities to create activities such as "Deaf Fair" or "Deaf Town." Again the idea builds on the standard K–6 curriculum with its emphasis on family and community awareness but showcases the Deaf community as exemplified both by the Deaf students in the school and by Deaf adults from the community who come in as resource support for the event.

The obvious advantage of the integrated or infused approach is that it is harder to drop it out of the schedule and requires only a single professional in a deafness-related field to bring it into a local school program. A major barrier to the approach, however, is convincing schools that such infusion of deafness-related material into the curriculum is worthwhile.

What Should Be Included in a Study of Deaf People?

There are many topics that can be touched upon in a study of deaf people, some of which have been listed in this section. The basic premises of such a study are as follows:

- Deaf people are individuals first.
- The thoughts of a deaf person are shaped by a unique set of experiences that occur inside and outside of the classroom.
- A variety of information about deaf people is available from a variety of resources.
- There are diverse perspectives about deaf people that are related to their use of communication, interactions with deaf and hearing people, cultural affiliation with different ethnic groups, social patterns, use of technology, educational experiences, participation in the workforce, and more.
- Studying about deaf people is an opportunity for gaining knowledge about and appreciation for these perspectives.
- Deaf studies is a means for helping deaf students discover their own identity.

The emphasis on teaching Deaf studies is to expose deaf students to a variety of information pertaining to people who are deaf. We, their teachers, should approach this task from the point of view of enlightening the students. Our job is not to indoctrinate by praising certain perspectives and disparaging others. Rather, we should ensure that deaf students are exposed to information that is presented fairly. Students should rely on their knowledge and experiences to then formulate their own thoughts about topics and issues relating to being deaf.

Teaching topics per se, however, should not be the goal of a Deaf studies program. For that matter, it should not be the goal of any core subject teaching. Instead, comprehension of concepts embedded in the teaching of these topics is a goal; derivation of principles and generalizations is another worthy goal (Erickson, 1998). Thus, what we teach in Deaf studies is ultimately going to contribute to helping deaf students learn about themselves. For example, on the one hand, we teach about the TTY so that deaf students understand both how to use it and the protocol for carrying on a TTY conversation. More importantly, the study of the TTY is an opportunity for a deaf student to learn about the effort to have TTYs accepted by society in general, the long struggle to enact legislation that protects TTY users and expands their access to all services provided by a telecommunications company, and the psychological benefits that stem from increased independence (i.e., not having to depend upon a hearing person to make a phone call). [*A Phone of Our Own* by Harry Lang (2000) is an excellent source of historical information relating to the development of the TTY.]

This is the basis for the eclectic nature of the global-interactive approach to Deaf studies. From the multitude of topics available to teach, the teacher should select a few of them each year with the purpose of challenging deaf students to a deeper understanding of who they are as deaf individuals and what it means to be deaf.

Furthermore, as teachers we must not presume the nature of the understanding that each deaf student will achieve. It is not our job to help students identify with a particular community. Our role is to provide the students with information and experiences from which the student will evolve generalizations about different ways of living as a deaf person. If a student eventually embraces the values of the Deaf community, then that is her or his choice. If a student comes to treasure the use of hearing aids and interacts mostly in a hearing environment, then that is another acceptable choice.

So what should we teach? Figure 5.3 shows a list of possible topics with a few statements of desired learning principles to encourage higher level thinking at the lower elementary school, upper elementary/middle school, and high school levels. The principles are based in part on Bloom's taxonomy of educational objectives, which is a systematic procedure for progressing through a series of six successive levels of thinking. The six levels can be described as follows (Evans & Brueckner, 1990):

i. *Knowledge*: Student recalls facts, information, or processes.
ii. *Comprehension*: Given the appropriate information a student is able to use materials or explain ideas.
iii. *Application.* Student applies abstract ideas or thoughts to a particular concrete situation.
iv. *Analysis.* Student identifies explicit relationships of individual parts, recognizes patterns, and explains the significance of those parts.
v. *Synthesis.* Student relies on creative processing to assemble parts into a whole.
vi. *Evaluation.* Student uses thinking skills of five previous levels to make quantitative and qualitative judgments.

The topics in Figure 5.3 are not listed in any order of importance because the age and grade of the student along with the subject matter curricula will have a strong influence on what is taught in your school.

KDES Deaf Studies Curriculum Guide

There might be times when a course on Deaf studies is the most effective way to teach to a group of deaf students. Schools for the deaf and separate classrooms in public schools offer programming that is amenable to the inclusion of a self-contained block of time for teaching about deaf people. Parts of the Kendall Demonstration Elementary School KDES Deaf Studies Curriculum guide[1] are described here as an example of a framework for a Deaf studies course. All quotes in this section are taken from the Guide (i.e., Miller-Nomeland & Gillespie, 1993).

The KDES Deaf Studies Curriculum explores six areas of interest and is designed for teaching deaf students in the elementary through middle school levels (1st–9th grade).[2] A

Topic	Early Elementary School and Learning Principles	Upper Elementary/Middle School and Learning Process	High School and Learning Principles
1. Dimensions of society	• There are different groups of people that share simularities and differences. • There are similarities and differences in the way people live in society.	• Cooperation between groups is important for a harmonious society. • Different groups of deaf people share similar attitudes toward living in society.	• A society's attitude toward a group of people is a collation of the thoughts of many people. • Societal attitudes are impacted by the economy, family values, the education system, and more.
2. Social dynamics	• Deaf and hearing people live in the same communities. • Getting along with people is important in social relationships.	• People tend to get along with others who share common characteristics with them. • The presence of deafness can influence a social relationship.	• The actions of a deaf or hard of hearing individual will influence how society views other deaf or hard of hearing people. • The actions of the Deaf community will influence how society views deaf people.
3. Communication	• All forms of communication serve useful purposes. Sign language, other forms of signing (e.g., contact signing, English sign systems), speech, and print are purposeful ways of communicating. • Literature is one means of communicating ideas.	• Deaf people (and all other people) should have equal access to information. • People have beliefs about why different types of communication are used. • There are some literature and Internet sources that are dedicated to the providing information relating specifically to the lives of deaf people.	• Understanding why people use different types of communication is one step toward nurturing respect toward differences in people. • Deaf people can be proactive in shaping their access to information. • Deaf people can use the literature and the Internet as a means of informing others about their beliefs activities, and organizations.

Continued

FIGURE 5.3 **Examples of instructional topics and accompanying learning principles in a Deaf studies program.**

Topic	Early Elementary School and Learning Principles	Upper Elementary/Middle School and Learning Process	High School and Learning Learning Principles
4. American Sign Language	• ASL is a particular way of communicating that is unique to the Deaf community. • Good signing skills will make it easier to socialize with others who sign.	• ASL defines a particular way of living. • ASL can use different linguistic devices to express a thought (e.g., number incorporation, facial expressions, nonmanual markers such as sticking out the tongue to show sloppiness or inattentiveness).	• ASL can evoke images that are unique to a visual language and not readily duplicated in a spoken language.
5. Deaf culture	• Groups of people do things together. • Activities deaf people do are a part of Deaf culture. • Specific activities are unique to Deaf culture. • Deaf culture has its own language, traditions, history, legends, humor, and values.	• Deaf culture is transmitted by deaf people in different ways (e.g., schools, storytelling, social events, sports, Deaf clubs). • Awareness of Deaf culture influences people's attitudes about deaf people.	• Deaf culture is affected by changes in society. • Demographics of the deaf population influence the cultural activities of the Deaf community.
6. Multiculturalism	• There are similarities and differences among groups of people in society. • We can learn about people by meeting them and reading about them.	• Different cultures make different contributions to society. • Ethnic deaf groups have made contributions to the Deaf community.	• The impact of ethnic deaf groups on a Deaf community is sometimes related to their location in the United States. • Each ethnic deaf group may face different barriers to accessibility (e.g., access to information, schools, and jobs).

FIGURE 5.3 Continued

7. Technology	• There are special devices for alerting deaf people to sounds. • Technology help deaf people watch TV and talk on the phone.	• Certain skills are required to use technology effectively. • Deaf people can use technology and computers to make changes in their lives.	• Deaf people can use technology to advocate for changes to laws that will benefit them. • Technology can be used for the transmission of culture.
8. History	• With no schooling deaf people could still communicate thousands of years ago. • There are famous deaf people.	• Deaf people have always had a role in the education of deaf children in the United States. • Changing attitudes toward deaf people have changed the opportunities for deaf people in society.	• Acceptance of ASL paralleled recognition of Deaf culture. • Deaf people's place in society has improved over time.
9. Education	• Deaf children can learn in different ways (e.g., signs, speech). • There are similarities (e.g., reading, science, and math) and differences (e.g., use of technology to assist in learning) in the things that deaf and hearing people usually learn in school.	• Deaf children need accommodations to learn in public schools. • Schools can socialize deaf children into the Deaf community.	• Schools can be microcosms of the relationship between deaf and hearing people in the working world. • A deaf person's selection of a career goal could depend on their opportunities to go to certain schools such as public colleges, Gallaudet University, and the National Technical Institute for the Deaf.

Continued

Topic	Early Elementary School and Learning Principles	Upper Elementary/Middle School and Learning Process	High School and Learning Principles
10. Audiology	• Deaf people have different degrees of hearing loss. • Different instruments can bring sound to the ear.	• A person's hearing loss will affect their communication skills. • Using a hearing aid has educational and social implications.	• The benefits of audiology services are related to the age of a person and his or her degree of hearing loss. • The identity of a person may affect his or her use of auditory listening devices such as hearing aids and cochlear implants.
11. Medical	• There are different reasons why a person is deaf. • Special doctors specialize in the care of ears.	• There is a medical viewpoint of deafness as a pathology and not a cultural minority. • A cochlear implant is a medical response to deafness.	• All people have a right to medical help with their hearing. • Changing technology and medical practices will influence how people view deafness in the future.
12. Development of self	• People belong to different groups. • Deaf children may belong to more than one group of people.	• How a person communicates influences how that person views himself or herself. • Language, schooling, friends, family, and other things contribute to a person's identity.	• Identity is shaped by how a person evaluates experiences. • How a deaf person views life as a deaf person influences his or her self-concept and self-esteem.

FIGURE 5.3 Continued

124

spiral curriculum format is used so that all areas or strands are repeatedly covered in each of the nine years of study. For each area and year of study, the Guide provides a list of sub-objectives such as the following two found in Year 5 of the History strand:

> Discuss the attitudes, beliefs, and laws that the Romans had about deaf people and their education. . . .
> Discuss probable modes of communication among deaf people during this time period. (p. 167)

A list of activities is then provided. The following two activities prescribed for Year 1 of the ASL strand give a sense of the strong role that Deaf culture has in this curriculum guide:

> Invite deaf adults to visit the class to share ASL stories, poetry, puns, jokes, etc. with the class. The stories and poems can be adapted from literature, from experience, or [be] original creative stories and poems. Videotape the visits to share with other classes and the school. . . .
> Teachers and students can plan an ASL and Deaf culture fair. Learning centers can be designed where students and teachers observe creative stories, poems, jokes, riddles, puns, etc. told by deaf adults in ASL. (p. 51)

The activities described in the Guide can be modified to meet a variety of educational goals. For example, a teacher who has adopted a global-interactive approach to teaching about deaf people might prefer to fit the activities to the type of students in the classroom. Although in the long run, it might make sense that all deaf students learn something about ASL, it is unlikely that elementary age oral deaf students would have the opportunity to acquire ASL. Therefore, these oral deaf students would lack the skills to fully appreciate an ASL storytelling experience. But an alternative activity that celebrates deaf people's use of English to express poems, stories, songs, jokes, and other ways of expression would be a valuable learning experience for these oral deaf children.

To gain a better sense of the Curriculum Guide a brief summary of each strand of study is now presented:

1. *Identity.* Students learn about who they are by examining their experiences growing up and comparing themselves with others. This is followed by experiences and discussions to help students develop a positive group identity. The notion of a positive group identity is accompanied with a strong recommendation that the "students have contact with the Deaf community" (Miller-Nomeland & Gillespie, 1993, p. 25).

2. *American Deaf culture.* Students acquire an appreciation for Deaf culture and the accomplishments of deaf people. The Guide encourages students to examine deaf people from various ethnic backgrounds such as Hispanic, African American, Asian American, and Native American. Deaf people's accomplishments in the arts, literature, and especially in their use of ASL along with the work of organizations of deaf people play a major role in the activities associated with this strand.

3. *American Sign Language.* ASL has a crucial role throughout the Guide but the purpose of this separate strand is to develop students' awareness of ASL as "the primary

language of deaf people" (p. 91). The assumption is made that culture and language are intricately related and the culture of any group of people cannot be studied without also studying the group's language. This strand does not directly teach ASL signing skills but may indirectly foster better skills through a study of various aspects of ASL grammar, such as how the production of some signs indicates pluralization and identification of the qualities associated with the distributional aspects of some ASL verbs. ASL signing skills are also promoted through the strand's heavy reliance on exposing deaf students to fluent adult ASL signers.

4. *Communication.* Deaf people have a right to access information and deaf students need to know their rights to such access. In this respect, visual communication is of paramount importance in deaf people's lives. This strand explores the various ways in which visual communication aids deaf people and includes a study of the role and use of interpreters, visual alerting devices such as flashing lights, and various means of communicating in stores, restaurants, and elsewhere when an interpreter is not available. There are also activities about how students can educate others about the importance of visual communication.

5. *History.* In studying the history of deaf people, the Guide offers two caveats. First, little is known about the history of deaf people in other parts of the world. Second, most of what we know about the early history of deaf people was written by hearing people and therefore has a hearing perspective embedded in it. What we do know mostly comes from the field of education and therefore this strand "deals primarily with the history of the education of deaf children in Europe and in America from the 1600s to the present" (p. 155).

6. *Social change.* Deaf students need to "look at the changing ways society views deaf people, and discover how these changes in attitude influence their daily lives through both legislation and the expectations of society as a whole" (p. 183). This strand wraps up the study of deaf people. The sense is that although much has changed to make society a better place for deaf people to live in, more changes are still needed. Thus, a critical message that deaf students learn in this strand is that they should be in touch and involved with the Deaf community to help make the changes.

The KDES Deaf Studies Curriculum Guide provides a sound structure to the study of deaf people who are intimately associated with the Deaf community and who use ASL as their primary means of communication. It might be best suited for use by those teachers who have students who already know ASL because many of its activities involve the use of ASL in some way, whether it be through discussions or through listening to deaf adults tell stories in ASL.

How to Facilitate a Study of Deaf People

Teachers may need support when it comes to teaching about deaf people. For many teachers, Deaf studies or its equivalent was not a part of their course requirement for teacher certification. What they have learned is mostly related to the medical and audiological fields, with dabblings in the area of technology and sign language. For example, they know about the etiology of deafness, measurement of hearing loss, and use of assistive listening devices, as well as TTYs, visual alerting systems, and basic signs for the classroom. What they might have not studied is the impact of deafness on people's lives throughout history, the influence of the civil rights movement of African Americans on progress in accessibility issues relating to communication and employment for deaf people, and divergent perspectives on what the future holds for today's deaf children from the sociocultural and medical fields. With such a background in the study of deaf people, teachers may lack the confidence needed to institute this study into their teaching routine.

Following are suggestions to help teachers become comfortable with the notion of teaching about deaf people. As we have done throughout this book, we use the term *deaf* loosely to apply to people with a hearing loss that is significant enough to impact their way of living.

1. *Become familiar with the literature relating to deaf people.* The body of literature about all things related to deaf people and more generally deafness is still meager when compared to what's available for studying other groups of people. Begin your research by identifying various areas of interests, and alongside these areas make note of related literature. You can find a listing of books in several ways. You can do a search of catalogs and publishers that specialize in books about deafness such as Gallaudet University Press, TJ Publishers, and Harris Communications.[3] You can look up any of these publishers or distribution companies on the Internet simply by using the search engine on your Internet program. You can also do a search for books on the Internet by calling up Web sites that sell books. A visit to the library is always an option, and it is a good idea to ask around and find out what people are reading.

Catalogs provide a good start for categorizing areas of interest. A recent issue of the Gallaudet University Press catalog included the following headings American Sign Language, Signed English, Deaf Studies, Deaf History, Deaf Culture, Sociolinguistics in Deaf Communities, Language Skills/ESL, Audiology/Speech, Parenting, and Young Adult Books. The Harris Communications catalog is similar but also has sections on Interpreting, Entertainment, Consumer Education, Religion, and Teaching Resources. The TJ Publishers catalog includes the headings Telecommunications, Sign Language and Linguistics, and Software. To these headings you should add Arts (visual and performing arts) and Sports. Take any or all of these headings, and make a list of books that are available. Order a couple or check them out from the library.

In addition to books, there are a number of newspapers and magazines that contain information about deaf people. These include the following:

- *Deaf Life*: A glossy, monthly magazine that delves into controversial issues. The writing style is blunt but pleasant to read. Regular features are "Deafview" (reader's viewpoint); "For Hearing People Only" where, for example, one issue addressed the question "I've noticed that deaf people stare. Why do they do that? Don't they realize that this makes hearing people uncomfortable?"[4]; and DEAF LIFE Plus, which is a listing of news releases, announcements, upcoming events, and late-breaking news.

The magazine brings to the public lively discussions of newsworthy events such as the one about a hearing interpreter who pulled off a stint in a Saturn car commercial by pretending that she was deaf.[5]

- *DeafNation*: A monthly newspaper that includes informative pieces such as the those relating to sports, the regular sections titled "ASL Corner" and "Deafinitely Our Life!," and stories that investigate difficult issues that gnaw at the soul of the Deaf community. One such article challenged the comments of Dr. David Bruton, North Carolina's Secretary of Health and Human Services, who made a comparison of German deaf children who spoke with their deaf counterparts in North Carolina who signed (Suggs, 1999). In his comparison he argued that for deaf children, learning to speak should be preferred over learning to sign, because then they would be able to communicate with hearing people. This could be an interesting article for debate in a Deaf studies class.

- *Deaf USA*: A bimonthly newspaper that promotes information and marketing opportunities. Given its major focus on business, this newspaper devotes space to stories relating to technology, entertainment, government, and a section on Deaf Power. The business focus brings up discussions about issues that have financial or accessibility implications for deaf people. An example of this was an article that examined the possibility of deaf people being denied social security (SSI) and social security for people with a disability (SSDI).[6]

- *Gallaudet Today*: A quarterly magazine put out by Gallaudet University. Although much of the information contained in it relates to the university, it is still relevant to a study of deaf people. Indeed, Gallaudet University has been called a mecca of the Deaf community, and events that happen there can impact Deaf communities throughout the nation as well as the world. The magazine also carries stories that stem from the academic world such as one about the persecution of deaf people in Europe during World War II.[7] This article and others are oftentimes based on academic conferences sponsored by Gallaudet University, and the information they contain is valuable and timely and abetted by the thorough research of the presenters at the conference.

- *NAD Broadcaster*: The official publication of the National Association of the Deaf. It is distributed monthly and contains regular columns; reports about the NAD; opinion pieces about issues such as interpreting, civil rights, and education; news items; book reviews; and a calendar of national and regional events relating to the Deaf community. It also contains the names and addresses of various regional NAD offices that can be used as resources.

- *Newswaves for Deaf and Hard-of-Hearing People*: A monthly publication with a combined July/August issue. Its regular sections carry a broad focus and include the headings Arts, Life, Work, Sports, and Books. One might think that there would not be much news relating to deaf and hard of hearing people and that all of the newspapers listed in this section would carry the same stories. Not so. There is some overlap but where have you read a story about a deaf woman competing in a deaf modeling competition? Or about a deaf motorist suing a highway patrolman?[8]

- *NTID Focus*: A news magazine aimed primarily at students, staff, faculty, and alumni associated with the National Technical Institute for the Deaf (NTID). It contains fascinating stories about Deaf people, which are especially useful in discussions about Deaf role models and career exploration with deaf school-age students. The newsmagazine contains frequent interviews with NTID graduates that are enlightening because they trace the paths that deaf people with diverse backgrounds have taken to success in their careers.

- *Silent News*: Calls itself the world's most popular newspaper of deaf and hard of hearing people. It is published monthly and like other newspapers it offers a range of reading, including articles with an international flavor. In a section called World Events, one issue, for example, contained two articles entitled "Deaf author's journey during takeover of Hong Kong" and "Deaf Frenchman's struggle for pilot's license."[9] Both of these articles are good examples of the type of information that can be integrated into a social studies unit with the added benefit that they may inspire deaf students to learn more about the topics under discussion. Other regular sections include an extensive covering of education issues along with Sports, Travel, Milestones, People, Health, and book reviews.

- *Volta Voices*: Published bimonthly by the Alexander Graham Bell Association for the Deaf. It reports on issues that are of particular interest to deaf and hard of hearing people who prefer to speak rather than sign. There is even an "Oral Hearing Impaired" section in it, and educational issues are popular.

- *Hearing Loss*: The official journal of the national organization, Self Help for Hard of Hearing People (SHHH). The journal, which covers coping with hearing loss as a common theme, contains information about developments in technologies, research, products, services, and SHHH events as well as profiles of hard of hearing people and articles by professionals in the hearing health care field.

- *ALDA News*: The official newsletter of the Association of Late-Deafened Adults. It regularly contains personal accounts of adults who have lost their hearing. The newsletter serves as part of a support network for adults whose gradual or sudden hearing loss has confronted them with many new challenges in their day-to-day living.

In addition to printed literature, there are numerous video products that are excellent resources for classroom teaching. The most popular ones have to do with ASL or one of the English sign systems such as Signed English and Signing Exact English. Some videos feature books that have been translated to ASL. There are also videos of Deaf adults telling stories in ASL on a variety of topics.

Finally, there is the Internet. We hesitate to name some of the better Web sites that we have found on the Internet because of the changes that many of these sites undergo over a short period of time and the increasing proliferation of new sites. However, with today's Internet search engines it does not take much time to get a comprehensive listing of available and still active Web sites. Moreover, searching and ranking the Web sites relating to a particular aspect of Deaf studies is a good instructional objective for school children.

While you are becoming familiar with the literature and other sources of information about deaf people, you should also be on the lookout for stories that might be of interest to your students. Note also that relatively few deaf people engage in writing for publications, and many stories of interest can only be found through interpersonal interactions with deaf adults and others who have ongoing contact with deaf people in either a professional or personal capacity. The box titled "What's Glamorous About Being Deaf?" illustrates this mingling of information. It also provides an interesting platform for discussing reasons hearing people choose the fields of teaching and interpreting as a career.

2. *Create a Deaf studies resource center.* To teach about deaf people it helps to have good resource materials, and creating your own Deaf studies resource center is one way to do this. You should start with the materials you have gathered in your exploration of the literature relating to deaf people. Some of the materials you will need your school might order for you or you might find them in your school library. The rest of the materials you will have to collect yourself. As you gather resources, organize them. Use filing cards or computer software programs such as Endnotes and FileMaker to keep track of everything you have read or collected. You will likely want to allow your students access to this center, but also let other teachers and parents know about your Deaf studies resource center and encourage them to use it and contribute to it.

You may want to solicit funds for this center from your administrator. If you have indicated on your students' IEP that they are going to learn about deaf people, then your case for getting money should be easier. When purchasing books and videos, remember that this resource center will likely be used by a lot of different people, including your students, their parents, fellow teachers, and other people.

What's Glamorous About Being Deaf?

One of the authors was working at a school for the deaf when a deaf woman accepted a teaching position in the high school department. She was one of the most dedicated teachers anyone at the school had ever met. She worked very long hours, often leaving the school three hours after the final bell of the day. She spent this extra time working in her classroom by herself. The author often tried to coax her into doing some afterschool activities with him but she steadfastly refused. She seldom allowed herself to be coerced into joining the staff for a little get together after school because she always had work to do. She did attend an occasional party, quietly. The story of her deafness was that she got spinal meningitis when she was 13 years old. She learned to sign but everyone marveled at her speechreading and articulation skills. Her speech skills never deteriorated as with most people who lose all of their hearing. About fifteen years after the author left the school, a friend e-mailed him to say "You have probably already heard, but in case you haven't, Mannie [not her real name] got fired for pretending that she was deaf." The author's jaw struck the desk. A short time later, he read in a *DeafLife* magazine about an interpreter in Indiana who pretended she was deaf to get a spot in a Saturn car commercial. She fooled everyone until someone uncovered her ploy. So what's glamorous about being deaf?

3. *Incorporate goals for studying deaf people into the IEP.* Teaching about things related to deaf people should not be incidental or an afterthought once a deaf student's educational program has been signed. The benefits of teaching this subject matter are too great to be left to the whim of the teacher. Figure 5.4 provides examples of how concepts of relevance to the education of deaf students can be broken down into instructional objectives by subject matter and incorporated into a student's IEP.

All of the instructional objectives shown in Figure 5.4 can be taught in a school for the deaf, a self-contained classroom, a resource room, or a general education class. The concepts governing the objectives are applicable to hearing students with either minor

Subject	Concept	Instructional Objective
A. Social Studies	• Not all deaf people think and act alike.	• The student will recognize and respect the similarities and differences in the social behavior of deaf people.
B. Language Arts	• Deaf people in the world of literature; themes in books.	• The student will read a book or an essay written by a deaf person and identify the author's theme.
C. Science	• Etiology of a hearing loss.	• The student will be able to describe at least three different causes of deafness and (if known) identify one of the causes as the reason for the student's hearing loss.
D. Math	• Estimation of the number of deaf people living in different parts of the United States.	• Using the incidence of deafness and population figures, the student will be able to estimate the number deaf people who live in each state.
E. Computer Science	• Impact of computers on the lives of deaf people.	• The student will be able to describe how he or she communicates with friends and others using computer technology and compare his or her manner of communication with how deaf people communicated with their friends in the 1960s or earlier. (Note: This is an excellent opportunity to bring deaf guest speakers to class who can describe how they communicated thirty or more years ago.)
F. Physical Education	• Using community resources to determine options for involvement in sports and recreation with other deaf people.	• The student will demonstrate a self-developed procedure for determining the availability of organized sports and recreation activities for deaf people in his or her area.

FIGURE 5.4. Examples of how instructional objectives can be incorporated into a deaf student's IEP.

modification or none at all. The key is to match concepts with the subject matter curricula used for the deaf student.

The Role of Teachers in the Teaching of Deaf Studies

Teachers of the deaf have many opportunities to incorporate a study of deaf people throughout their teaching of all subject matter. We have described how this can occur in our chapters about how to teach various subject matter to deaf students. For example, discussions of scientists should include the names of deaf people who have made significant contributions to the world of science. In social studies, an analogy can be drawn between the civil rights movement of African Americans in the 1960s and Deaf people's growing awareness of their linguistic and cultural heritage during the 1970s and 1980s. A language arts class can draw some of its literature from stories written by deaf authors and stories about deaf people. Whatever the class is, something about deaf people can be integrated into the curriculum.

We cannot, on the other hand, expect that all general education teachers will have the knowledge to infuse information about deaf people into their teaching. They can be helped by itinerant teachers and resource room teachers of the deaf who are in contact with the deaf students that the general education teachers have in their classes. In this respect, the following guidelines may be of help:

1. The general education teacher and the teacher of the deaf (e.g., itinerant or resource room teacher) should meet on a regular basis to discuss topics and concepts that are being covered in a particular subject. This would allow the teacher of the deaf to make suggestions about infusing information about deaf people into a lesson.
2. The teacher of the deaf should be familiar with the interests of his or her deaf students and from this be able to deduce what areas in the study of deaf people might appeal to them. This interest can then be matched with topics and concepts that are being studied in various subjects by the general education teacher.
3. The teacher of the deaf can provide the general education teacher with a list of resources relating to deaf people including books, magazines, and Web sites.
4. The teacher of the deaf should compile a list of local deaf people who have expertise in certain subject matter or who can speak about being deaf and working in a world dominated by communication in speech and audition. This list should be shared with the general education teacher who might be seeking guest speakers to talk to all students on some topic of interest.

Conclusion

The teaching of Deaf studies was initially spurred by a growing appreciation of the linguistic and cultural value of ASL along with a more general acknowledgment of the uniqueness and importance of all activities associated with the Deaf community. Once this happened, the notion that sign language and cultural events relating to the Deaf community are unique began to work its way into the psyche of the Deaf community. Until recently, Deaf studies has largely been associated with the study of the language and culture of the Deaf community. The time has come to expand the boundaries of who it is we teach about in a study of deaf people.

We need to look at the greater deaf population and include those people who are commonly referred to as Deaf, hard of hearing, or late-deafened. In this way, the scope of a Deaf studies program will reflect a variety of topics and issues relating to people with a range of hearing loss. To some extent, this make up of the deaf population mirrors the makeup of the deaf students we teach.

Finally, a major goal for teaching Deaf studies is to provide deaf students with information and experiences that will help each of them shape his or her own unique identity in whichever community or communities he or she feels most comfortable. Thus, where our teaching leads deaf students once they leave school should be of little concern to us other than the hope that they lead a healthy and well-balanced life and that they are satisfied with whom they have become.

KEY WORDS AND CONCEPTS

Deaf community: The lives and activities of a group of people who have shared experiences relating to deafness and who use American Sign Language as their primary means of communication. Thus, the Deaf community is defined by sociocultural and linguistic parameters rather than by ethnic and/or geographical ones.

Deaf studies: The study of deaf people—the study of all aspects of life relating to people who are deaf. Topics that can found in Deaf studies include the following:

- Linguistics of American Sign Language.
- Influence of ASL on the socialization of people who use it.
- Deaf sport activities that range from the activities of local sport teams that have all deaf players to the events of the Deaf World Games.
- Influence of educational institutions on the lives of deaf people. Examples of such institutions are schools for the deaf and public school programs where deaf students are mainstreamed alongside their hearing peers. Gallaudet University and the National Technical Institute for the Deaf are prominent postsecondary institutions that devote much resources to the education and welfare of deaf people.
- Organizations of the Deaf such as the National Association of the Deaf, Canadian Association of the Deaf, National Fraternal Society of the Deaf, USA Deaf Sports Federation, and the Canadian Deaf Sports Association.
- Literature about deaf people.
- Technological influences in the lives of deaf people stemming from the use of TTYs, closed-captioning, Internet, assistive listening devices, and so forth.
- Federal legislation that have impacted the lives of deaf people such as the Americans with Disabilities Act (ADA) and Individuals with Disabilities Education Act (IDEA).
- And many more topics.

global-interactive approach to Deaf studies: A more eclectic approach to Deaf studies than the traditional approach. In addition to the selection of topics normally covered in a traditional approach, the global-interactive approach encourages teachers to shape the content of a

Deaf studies program to reflect the characteristics and interests of the students in the classroom.

integrated approach to Deaf studies: An approach aimed at deaf and hearing students in the general education classroom. Rather than being taught as a separate course, information related to deafness is infused throughout the curriculum.

late-deafened: The acquisition of hearing loss during the adult years. Presbycusis is one cause of deafness in adults and is especially prevalent in the elderly population.

oral deaf: Someone with a severe or profound hearing loss who uses speech and hearing as the primary means of communication.

traditional approach to Deaf studies: A curriculum that is primarily focused on the people and activities associated with the Deaf community. In most instances this approach relies on a curriculum that is predetermined.

QUESTIONS

1. What are some similarities and differences between Deaf and hard of hearing people? Between Deaf and late-deafened people? And between oral deaf and late-deafened people?

2. What is an important advantage to a global-interactive approach to Deaf studies when compared with a traditional approach?

3. What are the key features of an integrated approach to Deaf studies?

4. What are six premises in the selection of what should be taught in Deaf studies?

5. As a general guideline for teaching Deaf studies, what perspective about deaf people would you pursue and why?

6. Name five different sources of information that should be a part of a Deaf studies program.

7. Name and describe the six strands of the KDES Deaf Studies Curriculum Guide.

8. Why is it important to incorporate goals relating to Deaf studies into the IEP?

ACTIVITIES

1. Create a list of resources that includes organizations, service agencies, journals, newsletters, books, and Web sites relating to each of the following groups of people:

   - Deaf
   - hard of hearing
   - oral deaf
   - late-deafened

2. Marnie has a seventh-grade class of five deaf students, all of whom have been signing since their preschool years. Jackie has a seventh-grade class of five deaf students, two of whom are hard of hearing and three who have cochlear implants. In a unit on "The Development of Self," use a global-interactive perspective to first draw up a list of subtopics that Marnie

and Jackie might discuss with their classes, then compare the two lists. What are the similarities and differences?

3. Design an outline for a social studies lesson for high school students that explores the reasons there are postsecondary institutes (i.e., NTID, Gallaudet University) that primarily serve the educational needs of deaf students. In your outline, consider the pros and cons of deaf students' attending these institutes as well as their attendance at other colleges and universities.

NOTES

1. An order form for the KDES Deaf Studies Curriculum Guide can be obtained from the Gallaudet Bookstore (202-651-5380) or by writing to Laurent Clerc National Deaf Education Center, Kendall Demonstration Elementary School, 800 Florida Avenue, NE, Washington, DC, 20002.

2. We are only able to provide an overview of the KDES Curriculum, and readers are advised to review the original materials.

3. Requests for free catalogs can be made via the distributors respective Web sites or by phone: Gallaudet University Press, 800-621-2736 (v), 800-630-9347 (TTY), 800-621-6476 (fax); TJ Publishers, 800-999-1168 (v & TTY), 301-585-5930 (fax); Harris Communications, 800-825-6759 (v), 800-825-9187 (TTY), 612-906-1099.

4. *Deaf Life* (1997, June), IX(12), 8.

5. See Trudy Suggs' article, "Faking it: How a hearing woman fooled thousands of people into thinking she was Deaf—and how she was unmasked by a Deaf reporter." *Deaf Life*, IX(12), p. 10–12,14, 16,17.

6. See the Therese Shellabarger's article, "SSI: Will Deaf be pushed out?" *Deaf USA* (1999, January/February).

7. See Laura-Jean Gilbert's article, "Deaf people in Hitler's Europe." *Gallaudet Today* (1998, Fall).

8. See *Newswaves for Deaf and Hard-of-Hearing People* (1997, December) for both of these stories.

9. Both articles can be found in *Silent News* (1997, November).

6 Teaching Mathematics

CHAPTER OUTCOMES

After reading this chapter, you should be able to:

1. Describe why prior experiences impact on a student's ability to learn mathematics.
2. Describe at least six different strategies for helping deaf students learn the language of mathematics.
3. Design hands-on activities that will help deaf students think about mathematics using a variety of resources such as newspapers, a gymnasium, and bodies of people.
4. Design a mathematics field trip that encompasses experiences relating to a number of mathematical concepts.
5. Design activities in other subject matter that can be used to help teach and reinforce mathematics.

It's not easy for schools to teach mathematics to children, deaf or hearing. Politicians, academics, parent groups, and others want you to believe that mathematics is essential for going to college, getting a job, and keeping track of your finances. But there are computer programs that track your stock and bond investments to the second. Other programs tell engineers what mathematical operations are appropriate for calculating the strength of steel needed to construct a bridge and how much it will cost to build it. Clerks in a store double-check the cash register to know that they owe you $1.55 in change after you gave them $5.00 for the purchase of a book that cost _____ .

Why teach mathematics at all? First and foremost, knowledge of mathematics opens career options for students. It has been called the queen of the sciences, and numbers and statistics are ubiquitous in society. At a more mundane level, mathematics allows us to calculate numbers in our heads as we look over our grocery list, estimate the amount of sand needed to fill a play area, look for geometric patterns in land forms and architecture, and dream about how we are going to spend our winning lottery prize. Mathematics makes us less dependent upon others when we are making decisions concerning numbers. It also helps children learn other subject matter. How long ago did World War I occur? Were your grandparents alive at that time? How many teaspoons of salt are needed when you triple the ingredients for baking bread? If the climate warms up 1 degree Celsius, how much of the polar ice will melt? Mathematics shows no favors. It is good for all of us.

The Third International Mathematics and Science Study (TIMSS) examined mathematics and science education in dozens of countries by comparing curricula, textbooks, teaching practices, and student achievements. The study found that U.S. schools tend to cover a lot of mathematical topics for short periods of time relative to other countries that cover fewer topics but spend more time on each of them. In addition, general education classes in the United States tend to focus on seatwork and homework activities (Schmidt, McKnight, & Raizen, 1997; Schmidt et al., 1999).

The TIMSS research indirectly indicates how mathematics is likely taught to deaf children because most deaf children are educated in public schools. One implication is that deaf students in general education classes are likely learning mathematics in the same manner as their hearing classmates—they cover a lot of topics briefly. We must ask whether the time allocated to each of the topics covered is sufficient for a deaf student, given the limitations that language imposes on the learning of mathematical concepts, possible difficulty in following all classroom communications, and in the case of a signer, a dependency on an interpreter for communication. Each of these factors may adversely affect the ability of a deaf student to learn the mathematics content being taught and the rate at which it is being taught.

Another concern for teaching mathematics to deaf students is that the instructional strategy used in classrooms should be matched with the learning style of a student. For example, the fact that general education classes tend to focus on seatwork and homework activities during mathematics activities does not necessarily mean that teachers of the deaf should do likewise. The Individualized Educational Plan (IEP) is one way of allowing teachers to match instructional strategies with students' learning needs. Yet, Kluwin and Moores (1985) found in their study of how teachers taught mathematics to deaf students in self-contained classes that teachers tended to have a narrow focus on selected topics and relied on repetitions as their students' primary method of learning the mathematical concepts.

In our discussion of teaching mathematics we are focusing on three of our recurring themes:

- Creating authentic experiences to help deaf students make connections with mathematical principles and real life experiences.
- Integrating vocabulary development to help deaf students overcome the limits that language imposes on learning mathematics.
- Creating opportunities for self-expression by engaging students in talking about mathematics.

How Should We Teach Mathematics?

It is too easy to say that deaf children will have trouble with mathematics because of their lack of proficiency with the English language. Starting from a deficit approach may doom teachers in any area. Nevertheless, language is important and we will talk about teaching the language of mathematics later in this chapter. Beyond language there are things that teachers need to do to effectively teach mathematics to any student regardless of the student's hearing loss. This includes a careful perusal of the standards in mathematics education for all children as well as looking at adapting mathematics teaching to the instructional demands of the situation and to the deaf student's experiential background relative to mathematical concepts.

There are many things that need to be considered when teaching mathematics to deaf students. However, given the large number of mathematical concepts that are taught throughout the school years, it would be impractical for us to make suggestions about how to tackle each of these concepts with deaf students. Rather, teachers of the deaf need to improve their ability to teach mathematics through coursework, workshops, exploring the Internet for teaching ideas, and reading the literature on how mathematics can be taught. Essentially, the principles involved in learning mathematics are the same for deaf children as they are for other children. We will, however, devote some space to a discussion of the following three particular mathematical aspects:

- Numbers and patterns
- Sequencing
- Specialized vocabulary

Learning about numbers and patterns, recognizing sequences, and acquiring a facility with specialized vocabulary is greatly helped by experiences outside the classroom; experiences that some deaf students may be lacking.

The reasons that mathematics is challenging for deaf students are varied and complex, likely ranging from the ability to learn from experiences outside of the classroom to cognitive considerations in the classroom such as the ability to assign meaning and language to mathematical problems. Attempts to delineate these reasons have focused on the language aspect of mathematics. Yet, the recognition of patterns in mathematics along with sequencing is a major concern for many deaf children.

Moreover, if a child—regardless of hearing status—does not spend sufficient time working with and talking about sequences and patterns, then the child may struggle to do well in mathematics. Thus, one key to understanding and enjoying mathematics is to have sufficient real-life experiences that attune a person to the existence of mathematical phenomena.

Patterns are everywhere in life. Highway departments use road signs in special shapes, colors, and symbols. To be a good, safe driver you have to recognize the meaning associated with each shape (i.e., recognize the pattern). Patterns are found in the rhyming schemes of poetry and in the repetition of chords in pop music. Patterns such as rush hour traffic and a swimmer's attendance at an outdoor pool are only visible over a period of time. Some patterns are idiosyncratic, such as the eating habit of a person always on the go or our own notion of how best to organize our day.

Sequencing is also important. Sequencing for many children begins well before schooling starts, and their dialogue with parents plays a role in this process. Children experience sequencing when their parents read to them and talk about the stories. Dr. Seuss's

One Fish, Two Fish, Green Fish, Blue Fish is a good example of this. Children learn about sequencing in the TV programs they watch. They readily come to know what program follows "Lambchops" and "Blues Clues," and parents reinforce their children's learning of sequencing in the things they say:

> MOM: You may watch "Wishbone" and "Sabrina." But after that you will have supper and then we are going to visit your aunt.

Along the way, some children learn self-monitored routines for getting up or going to bed:

> DAD: Please take off your dirty clothes and jump in the bath. After that, put on your pajamas, brush your teeth, and then I will read you a book before you go to sleep.

Think about how many parents would take the time to sign or say a long sentence like this to their deaf children. If they do not, then it is one less opportunity to facilitate language development and one less opportunity to get their children thinking about sequencing.

Sorting laundry, organizing the tools in the garage, and putting different shaped blocks in different shaped holes are part of a lifetime of learning patterns and sequences. Interestingly, national standards in mathematics education emphasize the teaching of mathematics in daily life. In fact, this is backwards—with appropriate experiences, life begins teaching fundamental mathematics skills long before children meet their teachers.

To teach mathematics, teachers and parents have to overteach many of the fundamental elements of mathematics. This means talking about patterns, making children aware of patterns, stressing the importance of order and structure in our daily activities, and so forth. The home and the classroom have to be full of schedules and systems in words and colors that deaf children have to articulate. If order is a part of their thinking, then they will use order as a principle in sorting out mathematical puzzles.

We now come to the problem posed by the vocabulary of mathematics. "Bruz" is the older brother of one of the authors. It is also a chisel with perpendicular cutting edges that is used to clean out the corners of mortises (a hole, groove, or slot through which something fits) during furniture making. This goes to show that mathematics, like furniture making and every other area of human endeavor, has a specialized vocabulary. Mathematics did not invent the arcane, so the claim that the vocabulary of mathematics is a special problem for deaf children distracts from the real issue. Every child, deaf and hearing, has to learn the vocabulary. The issue with deaf children is how they are going to learn it.

To help deaf children learn the vocabulary of mathematics, the teacher has to search for the point of contact that will permit the child to add new information to his or her knowledge base. One sequence for instruction is as follows:

Step 1:   Identify the strengths and interests of the child. Use this information to motivate the student and to ensure that your lessons have accounted for student limits when such limits will affect the student's ability to participate in an activity or comprehend a lesson.

Step 2:   Expand the current knowledge base through broadening experiences.

Step 3: Teach the concept in relation to known information.

Step 4: Teach the vocabulary, which includes some or all of the following: spelling, fingerspelling, sign, and pronunciation.

Step 5: Reinforce the meaning (and multiple meanings) of the vocabulary in other nonmathematical activities.

An example of an activity that combines the teaching of pattern recognition with the introduction of mathematics vocabulary would be to find the perimeter of a rectangular object or area. Think about how you might teach a child to find the distance around a desk, room, and school building. Think also how you might teach the vocabulary words *measure*, *distance*, *length*, *width*, *total*, and *perimeter*. Using the above sequence of steps you might come up with the following:

Step 1: Three weeks prior to a lesson plan about perimeter, engage the students in a series of measurement activities the purpose of which is to have the students get used to measuring things and recording this information. This can occur at any time during the day and should last no longer than five minutes. First, create a chart with three columns in it to represent Week One, Week Two, and Week Three. For the first week, concentrate on single measurements of an object such as the length of their pencil, a book, a room, a bookshelf, and so forth. Use target vocabulary (i.e., measure, length) but do not formally teach them. That is, during this period, the students will be exposed to these words although they might not be able to define them or use them in a sentence themselves. You might want to have the students use the following two types of measurement units: (1) simple ruler, where students measure to the nearest whole number; and (2) steps, where each student uses a normal step to count out a measurement. Have them record all of their measurements during this time period in a single column.

Step 2: During Week Two, expand the activity to include measurements of each side of an object such as a book, room, table, and desk. Have the students record their measurements in a column next to the column created during Week One.

Step 3: During the third week, and before the actual mathematics lesson on measurement, have the students go back and measure the total distance around each of the objects measured in Step 2. They should record each measurement in the third column on the chart so that the same objects are on the same line in each column.

Step 4: This is the actual lesson plan where you will talk about the measurements that they have recorded over the previous three weeks. Begin by asking questions about the relationship between columns. For example:

- What did we do to get the measurements in each of the columns on your charts?
- What similarities do you notice between the Column A and Column B?
- Review what you did to get the measurements for Column B and Column C. What do you notice about the two columns? Prompt until someone says that the total in each column is the same.
- How can we show that the total in Column B is the same as the number in Column C? What patterns can you see in the numbers? Can you write an equation to show this? Prompt until the students come up with suitable equations.

- What names can we give to the numbers in Columns A, B, and C? The following vocabulary words should either be said by the students or formally introduced by the teacher: length, width, distance, total, and perimeter.
- Go back to the equation written earlier and ask the students to rewrite it using the vocabulary words. Move from [l + l + w + w = p] to [2l + 2w = p] for rectangular objects.
- What is another way to get the same information that you have in Column C without measuring all four sides of an object? Prompt until someone says that you only need to measure the length and width of rectangular objects.

Provide a lot of visual representation of what the students are learning in this lesson.

Step 5:   Design activities that will allow the students to demonstrate their knowledge of how to find the perimeter of rectangular objects. Some things that can be measured are an indoor and an outdoor basketball court, a lunchroom table, a floor tile, the biggest book in the library, and the school playground.

In this foregoing activity, students are provided with the experiential background they needed for a formal lesson on finding the perimeter of a rectangle. The three weeks spent measuring objects prepares the students for learning vocabulary words related to finding the perimeter. The students were all exposed to the emergence of patterns in numbers through their measurement activities. Finally, they learned that finding the perimeter is an orderly activity and performing operations in a sequential manner will lead to the answer.

Teaching the Language of Mathematics to Deaf Students

Mathematics has both a common and a specialized set of vocabulary. The common set occurs in everyday speech, examples of which are related to operations (e.g., add, subtract, multiply), comparisons (e.g., greater than, lighter than, equal), shapes (e.g., squares, circles, sphere), measurements (e.g., meters, liters, acres), estimation (e.g., rounding off, about, close to), temperatures (e.g., degrees, conversion), and finances (e.g., interest rate, mortgage, monthly payments). These are terms that many hearing children might learn just through social interactions with family members, watching TV, and listening to the radio. Most of these are terms that repeatedly show up in mathematics workbooks at all grade levels. Many of these terms can also be signed (e.g., FRACTION, INTERSECTION, PERCENT) or are commonly known by their fingerspelt representation (e.g., I-N-C-H for inch, O-D-D for odd number, K-G for kilogram).

Then there are the specialized vocabulary that we usually come across only in a mathematics class. Examples of these are distributive principle (a key concept in estimation: a(b + c) = ab + ac), factorial ($6! = 6 \times 5 \times 4 \times 3 \times 2 \times 1$), trapezoid (an equilateral in which one pair of opposite sides are equal), multiplicand (the number that is multiplied by another number), and googol (a 1 followed by a hundred zeroes). These are the terms that most children are taught as part of a mathematics lesson. Most of these terms do not have a sign equivalent, and their expression is reliant upon saying the word, printing it, and fingerspelling the whole word or its abbreviation. Even in speech, their lack of common usage may make them difficult to pronounce at least initially.

Teachers have a number of techniques at hand to help teach the meaning of both common and specialized mathematics vocabulary:

1. *Incorporate the teaching of the word in a language arts activity such as spelling or writing a story.* Teach and reinforce the language of mathematics in subjects other than mathematics. Include mathematical terms on spelling tests, as words that are to be included in stories, in practices with the dictionary, and in other language arts activities. Also challenge the students to use mathematics words to talk about a nonmathematical situation. Mathematical expressions such as "common denominator" and "square" can be taught whereby a student's understanding of its mathematical reference is used to assist in applying it to a nonmathematical expression. Examples of nonmathematical uses for these two terms are given below:

   What do you think the common denominator is in each athlete's success as a basketball player?

   and

   At the end of the month, the builder needs to square his accounts with his suppliers.

2. *Use mathematical terms in notes that you write to the student.* We know of one principal of a school for the deaf who keeps a stack of blank rectangular greeting cards. She uses this *2-dimensional medium* of print as a *means* for offering *additional* praise for her students. She would write a note to a student and then mail the card. The student is inspired to read the card by the *simple* fact that it came in the mail, something that *seldom* occurs for the *average* student. This might seem an *elliptical* manner for reaching a student, but the reaction of the students never fails to make her *acutely* aware of the *value* of taking just a *fraction* of her time to write the notes in the *first place.*

3. *Write the words on cards and place them on the walls with examples of their meaning.* This is a very common practice at the elementary level but is often ignored at the middle and high school levels. Better still is to attach the words to real world images. For example, the James River Bridge near Richmond, Virginia, is an elegant engineering marvel of a suspension bridge. A photograph of it would convey the concepts of radius, elliptical, curve, circumference, and triangle.

4. *Have the students compile a list of key mathematical words by entering them into a vocabulary book along with a description and an example of their meaning.* This could be done in a book form, or it might be done in large letters on colored papers that are laminated and held together by a ring. The advantage of this latter idea is that students might be more inclined to read what they have written. Both the book or laminated collection of cards should be kept in a desk or close at hand to the student during a mathematics class.

5. *Make a point of using mathematical terms in your own dialogue.* This is a good technique for reinforcing the meaning of words. You might want to set aside a few min-

utes each day for this activity, either as part of your mathematics class or even better, at another time during the day. It can be short, too:

> Class. From now on, the privilege of free time that I give to you as a class will be in inverse relation to the number of incidences of improper behavior. The better you behave the more free time I will give you at the end of the week. The more you misbehave, the less free time I will give to you.

Some teachers might cringe at the thought of using terms such as "inverse relation" in their conversations with deaf children. They should only cringe if they avoid using such terms because their students are deaf.

6. *If your students sign, then make ample use of fingerspelling to clearly indicate which mathematical term you are using.* Even when there is a sign for a term, you may wish to add the fingerspelling. Take the terms "calculate" and "figure out," which are often used interchangeably in mathematics—the sign for both of them can be the same in ASL. If you are concerned about your students' recognizing the word "calculate" in print, then after you sign it, you should fingerspell it. In a dialogue you may wish to switch which word you fingerspell after the sign you make to show that the meaning of both terms can be the same in mathematics. Also, writing the words on the board helps to reinforce the fingerspelling.

7. *Have the students explain the meaning of mathematical terms to the class.* Have the students talk about mathematics and not just in response to a mathematics question. They should be encouraged to describe to others how they arrived at their solutions using examples that will help them illustrate the meaning of new mathematical terms. This technique is a good opportunity for assessing each student's understanding of a particular mathematical term as well as for diagnosing errors in their thinking. It is also an excellent way to get students to use language.

Also talk about the varied meanings of mathematical terms and have the students do likewise. Vince Daniele, a professor of mathematics, proposed that any discussion of language as it relates to mathematics would be incomplete without some mention of the *inappropriateness* of encouraging students to look for one-word clues when solving mathematics problems (personal communication, 1999). He illustrates this notion with the mathematical meaning of the word *more*. Teachers often say to deaf students, The word *more* means to add, which is not always true. Consider the following:

Mike weighs 20 pounds more than his son Eric. If Mike weighs 165 pounds, how much does Eric weigh?

Most of us would solve this problem by subtraction. Indeed, unless a conscious effort to use an algebraic approach was made ($x + 20 = 165$), the problem would not strictly involve addition. So how do we teach the solution of such problems to students? Daniele recommends that teachers stress the meaning of and the relationships between the words involved. A labeled sketch, showing which person weighs

165 and which person is larger, can help. See the box titled "Enhancing the Teaching of Mathematics" for more ideas about mathematics teaching from Dr. Daniele.

Enhancing the Teaching of Mathematics

How deaf students perform in mathematics in college is in large part a result of how well they have been prepared in mathematics during their K–12 school years. Moreover, college instructors know well the strengths and shortcomings of these school years through their work with students in various postsecondary disciplines that require some level of mathematical skills. As university professors, the authors have witnessed much in this respect. We asked Dr. Vincent Daniele, chairperson of the Department of Science and Mathematics at the National Technical Institute for the Deaf (NTID) to draw from his experiences to describe how mathematics teaching can be enhanced for deaf students in their elementary through secondary schooling. Here's what he had to say:

"Teaching mathematics to deaf and hard of hearing students is as much an exercise in advocacy as it is in instruction. Young people with strong mathematics skills and concepts will have access to far more career options than their peers without such strengths. Neither students, teachers, nor parents can be permitted to assume that desirable professional fields will be accessible with inadequate mathematics preparation. Here at NTID, for example, it is not only engineering or computer science majors who are required to study mathematics. Depending upon the degree pursued, business students might be required to study calculus and statistics, and undergraduate social work majors are expected to complete a sequence of statistics and research courses. What do these realities say to teachers of deaf students in the K–12 grades?"

1. *Start early and maintain standards.* Appropriate mathematics education must begin in the early grades and it must be provided daily. The curriculum must be rigorous and it must compare favorably to that which is provided for the general population of all students.

2. *More mathematics in high school.* Deaf students, and particularly those expecting to attend college, should be given the benefit of four full years of mathematics at the high school level. Teachers must resist the temptation to provide "life skills" and "consumer skills" if such instruction deteriorates into nothing more than computation. College students interested in the computer field find they need algebra, geometry, and trigonometry or their career options are severely limited, yet an overwhelming number of them have not had trigonometry before studying it at the college level. That in itself is fine, since we can provide the necessary instruction. What is more disconcerting is the reality that many students are not nearly ready to begin trigonometry until they are in college for quite some time.

3. *Attitudes matter.* Teacher attitudes can and will have an impact on students. While it would be ludicrous to expect teachers to cheerfully admit to "not being much of a reading and writing kind of person," we see that attitude directed toward mathematics with alarming regularity. Teachers and other adults have a responsibility to refrain from using expressions about always hating mathematics or being unable to balance a check-

book. Students must be shown the value of mathematics, and they must be convinced of their ability to do well in mathematics.

4. *Technology helps.* Because scientific and graphing calculators are so readily available in our society, teachers must make use of the power of these instruments in their classrooms. This means teachers are responsible for understanding the workings and applications of such technology, and it means mathematics instruction must encompass far more than simple attention to computational algorithms or algebraic manipulation. Students must learn to apply mathematics and to develop the ability to model given situations with diagrams and equations.

5. *Language is important.* Language that supports mathematical thought needs to be developed, expanded, and practiced throughout the school day. In turn, such attention to language permits teachers to talk about translating from printed English to mathematical symbols and back. In programs in which sign language is used, the potential to elaborate on the way something might be expressed in sign, in English, and in mathematics symbols presents an opportunity to enrich all of these areas concurrently. Programs that make use of speech therapy have an additional component to add to this "reinforcement mix."

6. *Get support.* Mathematics education is a complex endeavor. Teachers and administrators must appreciate the need for inservice training, they need to be aware of the availability of reasonably priced commercially prepared books and manipulative materials, and they should be mindful of the ability of local colleges, teacher associations, and state agencies to provide practical strategies and classroom activities. Seek these resources. Talk to the professionals.

---

8. *Teach deaf students how to talk about learning mathematics.* Daniele (1993) observed that the language of deaf children may lead teachers to:

> assume that students do not know certain material, when in fact the students know more than the students can demonstrate. Conversely, . . . teachers [may] assume incorrectly that understanding exists when students . . . are able to communicate one or two words to the teacher and the teacher assumes the student's understanding is the same as the teacher's. (p. 80)

But a teacher who is alerted to the possibility of misinterpretations is better positioned to consider the language of the student when diagnosing student mathematical knowledge and skills. Thus, deaf students should be encouraged to think aloud—explaining the mathematical relationships and processes that they are observing. As a teacher, model the language that students can use to do this and use whole sentences (in whichever language is used, English or ASL):

> **TEACHER:** Now, let's see. I want to know how many beans I have on my desk. All of the beans are in cups. I have 4 cups on my desk. I added up the number of beans in each cup. Each cup has 5 beans. I can find out how many beans I have all together by adding them up like this (write on the overhead)
>
> $$5 + 5 + 5 + 5 = 20$$
> What's another way of writing this equation? Can someone help me?

STUDENT: Multiply.

TEACHER: That's good thinking. Multiplying could be another way of writing this equation. Can you show me how you can write an equation with multiplication in it?

STUDENT: (Writes $4 \times 5 = 20$ on the board.)

TEACHER: That is correct.

When modeling language, do not look for shortcuts in how you communicate a concept to a student. Use the language of mathematics as you would find it in books. Do not, in the above dialogue for example, ask "What's another way of writing this?" while pointing to the equation. Say the word *equation*. Likewise, in signs, do not use the sign THIS as a replacement for *equation*. Point to the equation and then fingerspell E-Q-U-A-T-I-O-N.

When teaching students to talk about mathematics, teach them to look for relationships with what they have previously learned. Learning mathematics is a sequential activity. Mathematics textbooks are designed so that each chapter or unit contains a series of related lessons covering a specific topic. Do not, however, assume that your students will know the relationship in question simply because of the way a book has laid out the lessons. Have the students explain it to you.

Further Suggestions

The *National Action Plan for Mathematics Education Reform for the Deaf* (Dietz, 1995) attempted to bring the teaching of mathematics to deaf students to the same standards as those brought to hearing students under the standards proposed by the National Council of Teachers of Mathematics. In this section we will focus on how those standards can be met.

In the mathematics content standards, all children from preschool to grade twelve will:

1. Learn to value mathematics.
2. Become confident in their ability to do mathematics.
3. Become mathematical problem solvers.
4. Learn to communicate mathematically.
5. Learn to reason mathematically.

As we show below, these goals can be achieved primarily through activities that are designed to get deaf students to think about mathematics outside of the time they are doing textbook mathematics. Several of the classroom instruction criteria from the report are worth expanding upon because they demonstrate how to implement the goals.

1. Instructional approaches must facilitate students' construction of their own complex knowledge structures. We illustrate the idea of how to move from what students already know to the absorption of new information in a description of a lesson about circumference in geometry for younger students.

Example A: First, have the students make a list of circular items to measure such as a hula-hoop, mouth of a cup, and a lid. Next, have one student stand in the middle of the gymnasium, holding one end of a known length of string. Then walk the other end of the string around to form a circle, placing students evenly on the imaginary circumference.

When finished, you should have your students representing a fairly good circle, with one in the middle. Use the tape measure to find the diameter, using the center student for accuracy in measuring through the circle's center. Then measure the circumference as well.

Then, go back to the classroom and measure the circular things on the list the students had made. Carefully write down all your information using a data recording sheet with columns for the object's name, the diameter, and the circumference. Finally, calculate for pi by dividing the circumference by the diameter.

Example B: Fridricksson and Stewart (1988) designed a system specifically to help deaf students move from the concrete to the abstract. This system is called **Uninterrupted Silent Sustained Mathematics** and is similar to reading programs that encourage more involvement with literacy. For ten minutes each day, students explore mathematical concepts in ungraded activities. The sessions begin with the teacher giving directions and help so the students can explore a particular concept. After that the students are left to themselves. Each student is expected to go through three steps:

- Manipulate concrete materials.
- Conceptualize the mathematical concept in semiabstract ways such as a sentence or verbal rule.
- Conceptualize the principle at the abstract or symbolic level.

An example of how a teacher can move from the concrete to the abstract in thinking about the concept of multiplication is illustrated below:

> The concept of multiplication ties in closely with that of addition. Hence, the initial assignment is to expose the students to repeated addition. Distribute fifteen tiles to each of the students. Have them make different piles so that at least two of the piles contain the same number. An interaction like the following should then commence:
>
> TEACHER: Would someone like to tell the class what addition equation they have created?
>
> STUDENT: I have made a pile of three, another pile of three, a third pile of three, and a pile of six.
>
> TEACHER: Fantastic. Could you show me an arithmetic statement to describe what you have?
>
> STUDENT: (Writes $3 + 3 + 3 + 6$)
>
> TEACHER: How many piles of three did you make?
>
> STUDENT: Three.
>
> TEACHER: I will show you a short way to record that. (Writes $3 \times 3 + 6 = 15$ on the board) and I will put a circle around 3×3. (Fridriksson & Stewart, 1988, p. 54).

Fridriksson and Stewart (1988) reported success with this program with deaf fourth and fifth graders in simple arithmetic operations. In fact, Fridriksson experienced so much success with his deaf students that he later parlayed his effective mathematics teaching skills to work with hearing elementary-age students also. In recognition of his accomplishments he was awarded "Mathematics Teacher of the Year" in the province of British Columbia.

2. Instruction must build on students' prior knowledge and experience. This is true for all types of learning. We will use geometry to show how teachers can construct activities that build upon prior knowledge. Geometry is a particularly good example because it is a difficult subject to grasp if students have no real-world connection. But some cardboard squares in a semidarkened room can move students into thinking geometrically.

Give each student a square and then ask the students if the shadow of a square on a flat floor or wall could ever be non-square. Could it ever be nonrectangular? That is, can the angles in the shadow ever vary from 90 degrees?

After talking about the possibilities for a few moments, turn down the lights and have the students experiment with the squares. Like a shadow puppet, the square is placed between the light source and the floor. Students should start by trying to get a square on the floor and then turning the square different ways, including tilting the square out of the horizontal plane to observe how the shape changes.

Working in teams of two or three, students can draw the outlines of different shapes to look at later and for other students to see. Next, show the students some possible four-sided shapes and ask the question: Which of these shadows could be cast by a square and which could not? Then have the students try to get that shape to appear on the floor or on the wall.

From here you can move to the requirements of a square and the number of degrees required inside all the angles, which is one of the abstract concepts you would like to them to understand.

3. Instruction should require students to actively make use of a variety of tools to construct knowledge, to solve problems, and to communicate ideas. Such tools include manipulative materials, calculators, videotapes, computers, and related technologies. One quick source of mathematics instruction is the newspaper. In a newspaper article consider the report that a model makes a seven-figure income just for having the right face. Do your middle elementary students know what minimum amount she makes? The answer is $1,000,000. Have the students estimate and figure out how high a stack of 1,000,000 one-dollar bills would be; how many rooms they would fill; how many miles they would stretch if placed end to end; and when placed on a balance scale, how many students would be needed to balance the scale.

To collect ideas you may wish to pick up the newspaper and write down five mathematics activities that you can think of given something that you have read. Do not wait until these activities are needed. Compile a list of activities and file them away for later use.

4. Show students how an understanding of mathematics can be applied to the world they live in. Have you ever thought about taking a mathematics field trip? You can start with a short trip around the block and focus on one or more of the following concepts:

- *Measurement*. The distance from the front door of the school to the road. The different pathways from the front door to the parking lot. The distance from one corner of the school playground to another. The perimeter of the school grounds. The number of students who can fit into one parking space. The height of the basketball hoop. The height of the shortest tree in the school yard. The number of cars that pass the school each minute.
- *Estimation*. The number of cars that can be parked along the perimeter of the school ground. The number of students standing side by side that it would take to ring the school. The number of bricks on one face of the school building. The number of cars that will pass the school in one hour; in one day.
- *Graphing*. The number of cars that passed the school during one minute at the end of each period. The color of cars in the parking lot. The percent of cloud coverage in the sky at the end of each period. The number of students who played different types of activities during recess.
- *Geometric shapes*. The shape that is most visible when looking at the back of the school building. The most common shape in the school yard; in the parking lot. Things that can be described as a trapezoid, circle, parallelogram, and so forth.
- *Fractions*. The number of classrooms that would be visible from the street if half of the school building was covered up; if a quarter was covered up. How many parking spaces are available if three-fifths of the parking lot was full.

You can reinforce and combine skills learned during these short field trips when taking the class on a long field trip. See the box titled "The Best Mathematics Trip Ever" for ideas that can make a field trip a venture into mathematics.

5. Integrate mathematics teaching across the curriculum. Many deaf children do not grow up in homes where they have fluent communication with their parents and significant others. Even in those homes where the deaf child does communicate well with the family, we have no basis to think that a higher level of communication will lead to more meaningful discussions about mathematics as it relates to everyday living. The onus is on teachers to pick up the slack in the experiential deficit that their deaf students might have when it comes to knowing about how mathematics is applied in the real world.

Therefore, every teacher should have a "Let's check out the numbers" activity in all of the subjects that they teach to deaf students. This is a relatively easy thing to do. You should be able to find a mathematics activity to do in every lesson you teach. In the following, we have provided examples for you to get started on this.

a. Reading. If your students are reading a book, you might ask them how many pages they have read in a fifteen-minute period. Then ask them to estimate how many pages they could

The Best Mathematics Field Trip Ever

Divide the class up into groups of two. Go to a shopping mall and drop off each pair of students in front of a store. Have the students do an activity relating to each of the following mathematics concept:

1. *Counting/measurement.* Count the number of customers that enter the store over a fifteen-minute period.
2. *Estimation.* Estimate how many customers would probably enter the store in an hour and in a day.
3. *Graphing.* Graph the findings for each store. Do this using a bar graph and a pie graph and then discuss the merits of each type of graph.
4. *Comparisons.* Many different types of comparisons can be made. Derive a total for the number of customers that visited all stores then calculate the percentage of customers that went into each store. Determine the mean number of customers that visited each store.
5. *Problem solving.* Tell the students that they are to divide the stores into low-volume and high-volume stores with respect to the number of customers entering a store. They are to figure out a criterion for determining the volume of customers entering a store.
6. *Patterns/hypothesis.* Look for a pattern that can be used to predict the volume of customers that enter each type of store. Derive a hypothesis that will allow a person to predict the volume of customers entering a certain type of store.
7. *Application/inference.* Plan a second field trip to a different shopping mall. Have the students make predictions about the volume of customers that will enter each store during the day based on the hypothesis that they developed in number 6. If the mall has different types of stores, infer which ones would be low- or high-volume stores based on the nature of the store.
8. *Demonstration of knowledge.* Make a presentation to another class or to a group of parents and other adults about the activities conducted during the two field trips.

As with any field trip, this one is loaded with opportunities to exploit language and communication usage as well as social interaction skills. Students interact in pairs and then as a group. They might also interact with shoppers querying them while they are at the mall. They are forced to use mathematical terms to convey their thoughts to one another. Recording information, identifying patterns, determining hypotheses, making inferences, and then making presentations are just some of the opportunities for developing the language and communication skills of the students.

---

read in thirty minutes, forty-five minutes, and sixty minutes. Have the students estimate how many books, piled one on top of the other, it would take to reach the top of a desk, the ceiling, and the moon.

b. Deaf studies. If you are studying about deaf people, create a chart showing the number of deaf students in your state who are receiving an education in kindergarten through twelfth grade. Create another chart comparing the number of students in schools for the deaf with the number of students in public schools.

c. Social studies. If you are studying the exploration of Spanish and Portuguese sailors in the fourteenth and fifteenth centuries, ask them how long ago this was. Have them find out how long the voyages were and calculate how far the ships traveled on an average day of sailing. Compare this time with traveling by air today or by traveling a similar path by diesel-powered ships.

d. Science. If you are studying about the solar system, have them total up the number of planets rotating the sun and compare this with the number of moons that are rotating all of the planets. Get a book about the solar system published in the 1960s or earlier and have the students compare the number of moons that were thought to be in the solar system at that time with the number we know today. Have them calculate the percentage growth in the number of known moons over the past thirty years; fifty years.

e. Physical education. Let your students calculate the change in their times for running a quarter of a mile over a semester. Let them estimate the number of dribbles they can do with a basketball in two minutes and then let them do it. Have the students estimate how far they can throw a ball, and then calculate the difference between this estimate and the actual distance thrown.

There are abundant opportunities for exploiting the learning of mathematics in other subject matter. This does not have to be an everyday activity in each of the subject matters, but it should be something that is planned and inserted in subject matter teaching at regular intervals so as to continually introduce deaf students to new applications of the mathematics concepts that they have learned.

6. Get the family involved. Many teachers of the deaf are already doing this. You should make a habit of regularly sending suggested activities home in a note and indicate the vocabulary words that the family might use during this activity. For some of these activities, you might ask that the parents sign a paper indicating that they have helped their child do the requested tasks. For other activities, you might merely make a suggestion and give the parents the option of reporting that they completed the tasks with their children.

As important as the activity might be, perhaps the more important point of suggesting mathematics activities in a note home to the parents is that you are regularly reminding them about the importance of communicating with their children.

Teaching Mathematics to Deaf Students in General Education Classes

Much of what we talked about in this chapter is applicable to all situations involving deaf students learning mathematics. Our heavy emphasis on the importance of teaching the language of mathematics and of reinforcing the varied meaning of mathematical terms in other subject areas is of particular concern to teachers of the deaf. However, the ability of deaf students to succeed in a general education class can be enhanced if their teachers in these classes are aware of the implications that language has for deaf students learning mathematics.

The following suggestions can help the general education mathematics teacher who has a deaf student in the class optimize this student's learning:

1. When an interpreter is present in the classroom, learn how you can help facilitate communication with the deaf student. Effective interpreting is not the sole responsibility of the interpreter because all participants (i.e., teacher, deaf student, and interpreter) interact with one another and contribute to the dynamics of the interpreted situation (Stewart et al., 1998). For all types of interpreters, teachers should speak in a clear, easily heard voice and at a rate that allows the interpreter to keep pace. Meet with the deaf student and the interpreter to discuss your delivery of lessons. Normally, interpreters will approach a teacher if they are having difficulty following what is being said or if the pacing is too fast. Deaf students, on the other hand, tend not to take steps to improve their access to instructions (Seal, 1998; Stewart et al., 1998). Therefore, teachers can promote better communication by initiating a dialogue about their teaching style with the deaf students.

It can be helpful if teachers are aware of an interpreter's style of interpreting. They should know, for example, that oral interpreters tend to mouth almost everything that the teacher says with some exceptions. A good oral interpreter will substitute for a word if the word the teacher uses is ambiguous for a speechreader. For sign language interpreters, there are some who essentially transliterate in that they tend to sign almost exactly what a teacher is saying. Other interpreters will translate a teacher's speech to ASL or use their knowledge of ASL to assist in conveying what is being said in English.

Seal (1998) spoke of the challenges that the syntax of mathematics presents to interpreters and noted that ASL's linguistic features can help them illustrate the meaning of word problems. She demonstrated this technique for the problem, "One-third of Ryan's paycheck is spent on rent; another two-sixths is spent on groceries. Do the rent and groceries take up the same amount of his paycheck?" as follows:

> Interpreters who capitalize on their expert knowledge of the language and its grammar are likely to subscribe to the spatial manipulations that belong to ASL in negotiating some of the ambiguities of these problems. Setting up a space for Ryan's "whole check," for example, and representing one-third of that space for rent and another two-sixths of that space for food should add to, not detract from, a sign language interpretation. (p. 91).

2. Use charts, overheads, computers, boards, and other instructional tools to provide visual information. This gives deaf students another medium through which to contemplate and absorb mathematical concepts. Create charts for displaying mathematical terminology, steps to solving problems, and mathematical games. Use the computer to reinforce learning. When a deaf student is paired with a hearing student, the computer can also be used to promote social skills and the development of communication skills.

3. Have the deaf student describe the steps used to solve a mathematics problem. Some deaf students might be reluctant to talk in front of the class. Give these students the opportunity to explain their solutions to you in a one-on-one situation. Take note of the language they use in their explanations. Model appropriate use of mathematical terms directly to the students.

4. Make deaf students feel that they are a part of the class. The difficulty with communicating with classmates and teachers makes some deaf students shy about actively partaking in class activities and discussions. Call upon them for answers. If they show difficulty in providing answers, work with them individually so you know their strengths and weaknesses. Build up their confidence in solving problems by providing them with opportunities to successfully demonstrate their mathematical knowledge to others.

5. Discuss with deaf students their strategies for completing homework assignments. Many deaf students, and especially those who use sign communication, do not communicate effectively with their parents and other family members. This lack of effective communication may lead to situations in which the deaf student receives little or no support for his or her homework. Provide deaf students with support by ensuring that they know how to do their assignments. One of the authors recognized the difficult and complicated foster home situation that one of his deaf students had. He provided the student with a strategy for using school time, including lunch, to complete all homework assignments before going home.

6. Some deaf students may have an itinerant or resource room teacher, or they may be integrated for mathematics classes from their separate classes where they are taught by a teacher of the deaf. Develop a good working relationship with these teachers. Provide them with a list of key mathematical terminology that is being learned in class. If a student if falling behind in class or is experiencing difficulty learning new concepts, share this information with the deaf student's other teacher. Be specific in any requests that you might make for obtaining extra instructions in mathematics for the student. It is not enough to say that a student is having difficulty with multiplying fractions. Instead, use your expertise about this subject to diagnose the reason for the difficulty and provide the other teacher with specific areas to work on. The problem with multiplying fractions, for example, might be related to the student's lack of understanding of the relationship between addition and multiplication.

The foregoing suggestions are aimed at helping deaf students learn, but hearing students can benefit from some of them, too. Some hearing children learn better when information is presented visually. Language presents barriers to learning to hearing children just as it does to deaf students. It can also be a valuable tool for diagnosing a student's understanding or misunderstanding of mathematical concepts. Therefore, having students explain their answers verbally is an instructional strategy that teachers can use with all students.

For the resource room and itinerant teachers, there might be a tendency to use their time with deaf students to mainly address issues and problems relating to language development. This unbalanced perspective fails to account for a deaf student's total educational needs. With respect to mathematics, these teachers should meet regularly with the general education mathematics teacher and do the following:

- Review student progress and link this to the IEP goals. If a student is falling behind and in danger of not achieving goals, devise a plan for helping the student catch up. Do not, however, push for quicker progress if the rate of learning is optimal for this student, because IEP goals can be changed. Conversely, if a student is easily attaining all goals then discuss what can be done to challenge the student. Enrichment activities such as solving mathematical puzzles, group or independent mathematics projects, and computer mathematics programs can be used to create challenges.

- Review specific areas in which the deaf student needs additional instructions or reinforcement that the itinerant or resource room teacher will provide.

- Inquire about resource materials that can be used to supplement learning. The resource room and itinerant teacher should have greater access to funds to make these purchases than does the general education teacher. Certainly, the IEP can be used to justify the purchase of extra materials on the basis of optimizing the student's chance for success in the mainstreamed class.

- Ensure that deaf students have adequate time to complete tests. More time might be needed to allow a deaf student to solve word problems. Although some general education teachers might be reluctant to allow this, it can be argued at an IEP meeting that this is reasonable accommodation in light of the deaf student's language skills.

- Help the general education teacher understand the language level of a deaf student in the class and the implications of this level for learning mathematics.

- Address any concerns that the general education teacher might have about the deaf student, including adjusting to the presence of an interpreter in the class and using techniques for facilitating communication. Such techniques comprise a range of behaviors such as not turning one's back to the class while speaking, speaking at a comfortable rate, repeating or rephrasing what other students in the class have said, and providing positive reinforcements.

Conclusion

Learning mathematics is important for all children. Whether they grow up reliant upon computers and pocket calculators for even the simplest of mathematical operations or whether they become mathematicians and accountants, all children can benefit from a firm grasp of numbers and the manner in which numbers can be manipulated. Historically, mathematics has been viewed as part of a total, or liberal arts, education. Knowledge of mathematics is important for responsible citizenship. It relates, for example, to a thorough understanding of the causes and impact of pollution and helps us keep on top of our own financial affairs as well as to comprehend the discussions of budgetary issues by our government.

As a group, we have not succeeded in eliminating the disparity between the mathematics performance of deaf students and that of hearing students as evidenced by scores of the **Stanford Achievement Test** or **Stanford 9**. Although deaf students achieve at a higher grade level in mathematics than in reading and other language arts skills, the achievement level is still unacceptable.

For deaf students, mathematics poses the same sort of challenges that all school-age students face when learning it as well as some others that are related to their understanding of language and the experiences with mathematical concepts that they bring to the classroom. Thus, what we do differently with deaf students is to provide an additional focus on the language of mathematics not only during mathematics class but throughout the curriculum and incidentally throughout the school day. We must also help deaf students experience the application of mathematics in the world in which they live.

KEY WORDS AND CONCEPTS

Stanford Achievement Test: The most widely administered test given to deaf and hard of hearing students ages 7 through 18 in the United States. It is a norm-referenced test, which means that it produces a score that tells us how a student's performance compares with other students. There are eight different levels of the SAT that range from Primary 1 to Advanced 2. Depending upon the level taken, there are nine to ten subtests, including achievement testing in the areas of reading, language, spelling, science, and social science. The acronym for Stanford Achievement Test is SAT and is the same acronym used for Scholastic Assessment Test, which is used as an admissions test for colleges in the United States. Earlier versions of the Stanford Achievement Test used with deaf students were called the SAT-HI, where HI stood for hearing impaired. This led to the misunderstanding that the SAT-HI was developed specifically for deaf students. It was not. But it does have norms for deaf students just like it has norms for all general education students in grades 1 through 9. To avoid confusion that the acronyms SAT and SAT-HI raise, it is now common practice to refer to the test by its most recent edition. Thus, the current edition, Stanford Achievement Test, 9th Edition, is called the Stanford 9.

Uninterrupted Silent Sustained Mathematics: Proposed by Fridriksson and Stewart (1988), a program with a period of short duration during which time students explore mathematical concepts in ungraded activities.

QUESTIONS

1. The Third International Mathematics and Science Study found that when compared to the United States, other countries that performed better on measures of mathematics tended to devote more time to the teaching of fewer mathematics topics. Why might deaf students benefit from a similar approach to teaching mathematics in the United States?

2. What can a teacher do to gain confidence in his or her ability to teach mathematics to deaf students?

3. What are some benefits of implementing an Uninterrupted Silent Sustained Mathematics program in a classroom for deaf students?

4. Provide some examples of common mathematics vocabulary and specialized mathematics vocabulary.

5. Why is it important to engage students in instructional activities designed to facilitate students' construction of their own complex knowledge structures?

6. What are some of the things that a general education mathematics teacher should know about an interpreter?

7. What are five things that an itinerant teacher or resource room teacher can do to help a deaf student learn mathematics?

ACTIVITIES

1. Design three activities using the idea of a daily period of ten minutes of Uninterrupted Silent Sustained Mathematics that was proposed by Fridriksson and Stewart (1988).

2. Design a field trip to a neighborhood that will involve the following mathematical concepts: counting/measurement, estimation, graphing, comparisons, problem solving, patterns/hypotheses, geometry, applications/inference, and the demonstration of knowledge.

3. Select an article from the newspaper and design mathematics activities based on something that was said in the article. The activities should require students to make use of a variety of tools to construct knowledge, to solve problems, to and communicate ideas.

7 Teaching Physical Education and Extracurriculars

CHAPTER OUTCOMES

After reading this chapter, you should be able to:

1. Provide a rationale for why physical education (PE) in general should be a necessary part of every child's education program plus provide further reasons why it is especially important for deaf students.
2. Explain why deaf children should be tested for overall physical fitness and motor ability from the perspective of IEP planning and from the perspective of lifelong fitness.
3. Describe at least five things that a general education PE teacher can do to help make PE more accessible to deaf students.
4. Give three reasons why deaf people become involved in Deaf sport activities.
5. Describe five ways in which deaf students can benefit from participating in extracurricular activities.
6. Describe two accessibility-related concerns for a deaf student planning to participate in extracurricular activities and state how these concerns can be addressed.

Changes in curriculum over the past twenty to thirty years have been propelled by parents and politicians calling for an increased effort by schools to improve students academic performance and to hold them accountable for doing so. This movement got a boost with the publication of "Nation at Risk" and "The Holmes Report" in the 1980s, and it is being sustained by a media watchdog that now publishes report cards on school achievement scores so that schools can be compared with one another. This places much pressure on schools to make changes in programming in an effort to improve academic scores on statewide achievement tests such as the Michigan Educational Assessment Plan that assesses students on reading, writing, math, science, and social studies beginning at the fourth grade and continuing through high school. With this race to achieve, something has to give in traditional school programs, and PE and art education are often the first to go.

Yet, getting through life is no longer a matter of knowing your math facts and how to read and write. Children must be prepared to know what to do with time on hand. DVDs and the Internet are not the answer. No doubt they are valuable technology and resources but they are also activities conducive to a sedentary lifestyle—one that leads to significant health problems later in life (Biddle & Armstrong, 1992; U.S. Public Health Service, 1991). This is more alarming for deaf children, whom Jansma and French (1992) claimed lead a more sedentary or low activity lifestyle than their hearing peers, which results in lower overall fitness levels.

But exercise is not the only option for whiling away time. Art projects such as painting, crafts, stained glass making, and photography are good stress-relieving activities as are the performing arts such as drama and dancing (Dance away stress, 1998; Landers, 1994). Music too should be found in all children's educational programming if only for its intellectual value—knowing, for example, about the influence of music on cultures. Thus, exercise and intellectual stimulation via the arts and music are options that our deaf children must have. Together, these added educational experiences will help them lead a healthy, well-rounded lifestyle without the burden of undue physical and mental stress and fatigue (Wilmore & Costill, 1994).

Physical education and extracurricular activities should be an integral part of all deaf students' educational plans. They are important in preparing deaf students for a healthy lifestyle and years of fitness-related and leisure-related activities.

Physical Education

We teach PE because exercise is good for the body. A healthy and well-conditioned body leads to fewer medical problems later in life. Being fit physically makes staying fit mentally easier because the mind is accompanied by a body less susceptible to fatigue and better able to handle everyday stress (Siedentop, 1998). We teach PE because we want children to experience the satisfaction that comes with doing physical exercises and playing games and sports. We want them to remain active physically throughout their adult lives.

We teach PE because for some children it enhances their self-esteem. This is a strong incentive for teaching PE to deaf children. Marschark (1997, p. 182) observed that "higher self-esteem and a sense of control better enables children to think for themselves and make good decisions about how to act and who to emulate." Involvement in sports is one way in which many deaf people enhance their self-esteem (Stewart, 1991). Observations of Deaf sport activities in the community and surveys with deaf athletes (Stewart, Robinson, & McCarthy, 1991) and sport directors who are deaf (Stewart, McCarthy, & Robinson, 1988) support this assertion.

How Fit Are Deaf School Children?

Several studies have shown that deaf children do not perform as well as their hearing peers in tests of balance (Brunt & Broadhead, 1982; Lindsey & O'Neal, 1976). This makes sense because the inner ear manages both hearing and balance functions, therefore, there is a close link between balance and sensorineural hearing loss. In fact, it has been estimated that as many as 49 to 95 percent of deaf children have impaired vestibular function (Sherrill, 1993). It has also been suggested that the balance skills of deaf children eventually catch up to their hearing peers by the teen years (Dummer, Haubenstricker, & Stewart, 1996). Yet a study with female deaf and hearing college athletes found that the deaf athletes' performance was significantly lower than that of the hearing athletes in measures of static and dynamic balance as well as cardiovascular endurance (Ellis & Darby, 1993).

All physical games and sports require a person to do at least one of the following **fundamental motor skills**: catching, kicking, bouncing, throwing, running, leaping, hopping, skipping, and striking. Most sports require several of these skills. Butterfield (1986) found that deaf children were delayed in their ability to catch, kick, hop, and jump. But Dummer, Haubenstricker, and Stewart (1996) found that the performance of students at a school for the deaf were not significantly different from norms established for the Test of Gross Motor Development. They did notice delays in deaf children's acquisition of some motor skills (i.e., bouncing, skipping, leaping, throwing, striking, catching, and kicking), but they also found that the same children were actually advanced for their age for the skills of galloping, running, and sliding, although this difference was not significant. The work of Butterfield and Dummer and colleagues, suggests that deaf children experience developmental delays in some fundamental motor skills.

No explanation as to why the delay in fundamental motor skill development occurs was provided by the researchers. Nevertheless, more engagement in physical activity should lessen the nature of the delay if not altogether remove it. In addition, balance is a critical factor in the development of motor skills (Burton & Davis, 1992; Sherrill, 1993), which highlights the need to attend to deaf children's physical education needs.

Simply stated, physical fitness is too important to leave to chance alone. Teachers of the deaf need to be aware of this and insist that educational programming include full participation in a physical education program as well as assessment of balance in young deaf children and, when necessary, physical education goals for improving balance.

Creating a Well-Balanced Child

The key to most techniques that are designed to improve children's balance is to increase their body awareness. Children have to first learn how the positioning of their body or stance affects their balance. They learn this by engaging in many different types of physical activities. They then learn how they can alter their stance to compensate for balance deficits. They also have to learn how to use their vision to maintain equilibrium with their surroundings. Thus, it is critical to engage deaf children in many exercises that will help them explore how each part of their body moves in relation to space as well as in relation to each other body part. In time, they will acquire a sense of what stance gives them maximum equilibrium and hence better balance.

Butterfield (personal communication, 1999) suggested that when planning games and activities relating to balance, it is a good idea to offer activities that require feed-forward (anticipatory) postural adjustments, that is, activities that require deaf students to anticipate where they are going to move next, thus giving them practice in how to plan for these movements. Rhythmic activities, for example, jumping a rope and movement games like hopscotch, are examples of such activities. All sports involve feed-forward postural adjustments but some such as badminton are especially good for playing when class sizes are small.

There are numerous activities, including games and sports, that can be used for helping children become aware of the effects of body movements. These include the following:

Skipping
Jumping rope
Crab walk
Hopscotch
Sack races
Playing on jungle gyms (monkey bars)
Walking/running across rolling bridges
Bouncing balls
Throwing/catching
T-ball
Kickball
Dribbling a soccer ball
Ice skating
In-line skating
Walking on stilts
Cycling
All forms of dance
All forms of gymnastic activities
Oriental exercises such as Tai Chi
Martial arts such as judo, karate, and kung fu

Although it might seem reasonable to select exercises that are appropriate to the physical ability of the students, you must remember that all of the above games are played by children of all ages. Perhaps more important than the actual game or exercise is the fact that children are given many opportunities to engage in physical activities.

Sherrill (1993) suggested that when doing physical activities, deaf children should be coached in what they should be thinking about. That is, they should be consciously questioning themselves as to what their bodies are doing. Two examples of questioning techniques are as follows:

1. Center of gravity. "What is it? How do your movements affect it? In what movements can you keep the center of gravity centered over its supporting base? Can your hands be used as a supporting base? What happens when your center of gravity moves in front of the supporting base? In back of it? To the side of it? What activities lower your center of gravity? Raise it?"

2. Broad base. "How can you adapt different exercises so that the supporting base is larger than normal? In what directions can you enlarge your base—that is, how many stances can you assume? In which direction should you enlarge your base when throwing? Batting? Serving a volleyball? Shooting baskets?" (p. 654).

Creating an Exemplary PE Program

Deaf students can benefit from participating in a PE program that is similar to one in which their hearing peers are engaged. After all, deaf students experience no physical disadvantage because of their hearing loss other than possibly in the area of balance. They are able to participate in any sports without any rule modifications as to how a sport is played. Because of this it has been said that physical education and sports puts deaf people on a level playing field with their hearing peers—something that cannot be said about most other subject matter taught in schools (Stewart, 1991).

It is tempting to say that all deaf students should follow their school's PE curriculum and leave it at that. To do so, however, overlooks the fact that many schools do not follow a curriculum for PE at the elementary level, and many elementary schools no longer employ a teacher who is certified to teach PE (Treanor & Housner, 1999). Moreover, it is not unusual for teachers in self-contained classrooms to assume the role of a PE teacher, and schools for deaf children may or may not have certified PE instructors. Nevertheless, knowledge about the basics of a good PE program is necessary for all teachers of deaf students.

An example of a model PE program was described by Stewart and Ellis (1999) based on the teaching experiences of Ellis at a school for the deaf and designed after the content standards portion of the Michigan Exemplary Physical Education Curriculum program developed at Michigan State University. Their work forms the basis of the following description of an exemplary PE program and should be referred to for further information on this topic.

The key factor of Stewart and Ellis's model is its emphasis on attending to content, performance, and opportunity-to-learn standards. These standards are critical not only for the motor and game skills that they help develop but also because each standard can be modified to fit the limitations caused by smaller class sizes found in both schools for deaf children and self-contained classrooms. Smaller class size imposes limitations on the types of games that can be played and the duration of some games when there are not enough players for substitutions. A description of the standards now follows:

1. Content standards are what it is that students are supposed to learn. Statewide curriculum guidelines or a school district curriculum for PE are intended to address this area. Areas that are typically covered include the following six content areas:

- Body control/management skills (e.g., posture, form, bending, stretching)
- Fundamental motor skills (e.g., balance, throwing, kicking, catching)
- Physical fitness (e.g., cardiovascular capacity, strength, endurance, power, speed)
- Sports, games, and dance skills (e.g., lifelong physical activity, rhythmical skills
- Activity-related cognitive skills (e.g., rules, team strategies)
- Activity-related social skills (e.g., sharing, turn-taking, being a team player)

A class of deaf students might have four to seven students with an age difference of up to four years. In addition, the students are usually working at different grade levels, which makes following a grade-level curriculum difficult. This situation is still manageable in PE as long as teachers attend to the six content areas listed above or whatever major content areas are specified in their state curriculum guidelines.

Moreover, the content areas involve skills that are taught repeatedly over several grades, and a single activity can cover several or all of the content areas. For instance, let's look at how a popular activity such as kickball covers the content areas. With respect to (1) *body control/management*, students learn to position themselves and move within their assigned area, stretch before playing, and demonstrate good posture; (2) *fundamental motor skills*, students learn to kick, catch, throw, and balance themselves when they are about to do any of these actions. They also gain practice in running and agility; (3) *physical fitness*, the game involves running and quick change in directions, which is good for cardiovascular development and kicking and throwing, which develop muscular strength in the legs and arms; (4) *sports, games, and dance skills*, kickball is a game that provides the groundwork for future playing of soccer and baseball; (5) *activity-related cognitive skills*, students learn the rules of the game and to aim their kicks to improve their chances of reaching base, and they learn where to throw the ball when it comes to them; and (6) *activity-related social skills*, students learn to take turns and are encouraged to show good sportsmanship.

Kickball is a popular activity throughout the elementary school years; however, there is a danger in playing this game indiscriminately without regard to students' current level of fundamental motor skill development and the playing of other games that might be more age and developmentally appropriate for the students. The reason for kickball's popularity is easy to understand: Children play it in their streetclothes, it requires a minimum of instructions, and it is quite an easy activity for teachers to supervise.

Every grade has a number of activities like kickball that can be used to cover various content areas of the curriculum. What's critical is for teachers to be cognizant of each activity's relevance to the content areas when planning and not rely upon the convenience of playing an activity as a reason for doing so. In this respect, it is helpful for teachers to know why certain sport, game, or dance skills are being taught or played and to provide a variety of activities over the school year to ensure that requisite curricular skills are taught and are appropriate for the age and physical ability of the students.

One further thought on content standards is the role of the Deaf community in translating a part of the curriculum. In general, content standards should be governed by the values of the community. Look at what activities adults are involved in, then shape the curriculum to lead students up to involvement in this type of activity. We have seen this occur with the inclusion of aerobics in PE classes over the past two decades. But what about the value of the Deaf community in shaping a PE curriculum for deaf students? Stewart (1991) suggested that schools for the deaf should incorporate into their PE curriculum popular sports played in the Deaf community such as slo-pitch, volleyball, and basketball, as well as those sports played in the Deaf World Games (formerly World Games for the Deaf) such as handball, basketball, badminton, and table tennis.

2. Performance standards attest to how well a student can do a certain activity. These standards are used to grade students and to compare their performance with other students. For example, for the performance at the recommended fiftieth percentile, 13-year-old male students are expected to run the mile in less than 7 1/2 minutes, do 41 sit-ups in 30 seconds, and balance on one foot for at least 30 seconds. For 13-year-old female students, the fiftieth percentile expectation is a mile under 9 1/2 minutes, 35 sit-ups in 30 seconds, and balancing on one foot for at least 30 seconds.

Stewart and Ellis (1999) suggested that demonstrating a high skill level should not be the major goal in the measurement of performance standards. Some students because of their physique and natural athletic ability, tend to always do well in most if not all PE-related activities. Other students who do not perform as well should not be penalized. Instead, they should be graded on how much they have improved relative to their performance at the beginning of the school year. Students' participation levels, attitudes towards PE, and cooperation with other students are alternative types of performance that can be used to assess performance in PE classes that are not based on physical ability.

3. Opportunity-to-learn standards are resource-oriented standards. They look at what schools have to offer in the way of staffing, programming, and facilities (Ravitch, 1995). These standards are essentially about a school's commitment to giving students the opportunity they need to access all aspects of the curriculum. Schools for the deaf are usually well equipped in this respect because they typically offer a full-sized gymnasium, soccer and baseball fields, a track, and swimming pool.

Being well-equipped is only part of this standard's goal. The other part is making use of what a school has. If a school uses its track mainly for warm ups during PE, testing for

A Comprehensive Test for Physical Fitness

In the area of physical fitness, what should teachers of deaf students look for before an IEP is drawn up? The following protocol has been used at the Michigan School for the Deaf and was drawn up by Kathleen Ellis, a profoundly deaf Ph.D. student in adapted physical education. The first part of the protocol consists of tests that measure fitness with respect to body strength and endurance. The second part looks at physical skills related to participation in sports and recreation.

Health-related physical fitness (FITNESSGRAM; Hastad & Lacy, 1998)
1. Cardiovascular endurance—timed run/walk for 1 mile
2. Abdominal muscular endurance—sit-ups for 1 minute
3. Upper body muscular endurance—modified pull-ups
4. Muscular strength—grip strength using a hand dynamometer
5. Flexibility—sit and reach toward and past toes

Skill-related physical fitness (adapted from Hastad & Lacy, 1998)
1. Static balance—stork stand with eyes open/closed
2. Dynamic balance—balance beam walk (heel to toe)
3. Speed—50 yard dash
4. Power—standing broad jump
5. Agility—shuttle run

a mile run, and the track team, then it might be missing out on opportunities in the areas of physical conditioning, increasing students' cardiovascular capacity, and exposing students to various athletic events. We have seen some schools for the deaf either not use their swimming pools during PE or use them simply as a fun-time activity. In contrast, other schools for the deaf have implemented a weekly swim schedule that calls for steady increases in the number of laps that each student can do within a single period of PE.

Teachers of deaf students have a role in ensuring that opportunity-to-learn standards are implemented for their deaf students. From our years of involvement in IEPs and from discussions with parents and teachers, it is clear that PE is the subject of choice for pull-outs for speech therapy in public schools. We even observed parents at a school for the deaf pulling their children out of PE for ASL classes. Teachers need to look at the whole child when determining educational goals and keep in mind that PE has a critical role in preparing deaf children for the future. The home environment needs to be considered, too. If deaf children do not have parents who are willing or able to involve them in recreation and competitive sports in the community, then PE becomes crucial to giving these children the chance to acquire fundamental motor skills, conditioning, and experience playing various games and sports. To this end, just as teachers will demand that their deaf students be assessed for speech and signing skills, they should require that their students are also tested for overall physical fitness and motor ability. Only with this information on hand will teachers be able to explore what is required to satisfy the opportunity-to-learn standard.

Ten Tips for the PE Teacher

Most deaf or hard of hearing students receive their education in public schools. Despite this being the case for the past three decades, situations still arise in the general education PE class when these students do not understand what's expected of them until they have watched their classmates do it. Even then they might not pick up on the specific movements that they are expected to do. An interpreter is helpful in these instances, but hard of hearing children typically do not use interpreters.

Even in the presence of an interpreter, PE teachers will be more effective if they adopt instructional techniques such as those that use the visual medium to convey information or actively involve deaf students in the learning process. Some of these techniques might appear to be painfully obvious to anyone who works with deaf children. But teachers in integrated classes also have up to twenty-five or more hearing students to attend to and may forget about basic instructional techniques for their deaf and hard of hearing students. The following tips should be passed on to general education PE teachers by teachers of the deaf in public schools and itinerant teachers:

1. Make sure that deaf students can see you at all times when you are giving directions or performing a demonstration.

2. Explanations are not enough. Always demonstrate the physical movements associated with a skill. If you are unable to demonstrate them, then have a student in the class do the demonstration.

3. Use the buddy system—shoulder tapping—in order to start, stop, and relay information to all deaf and hard of hearing students.

4. Use visual cues such as flags and lights to get everyone's attention when the buddy system cannot be effectively used.

5. Give the deaf students individual attention if it is obvious that they do not understand how to do an activity even after the demonstrations.

6. Ask if rules, skills, and directions are understood by all students, and have several students explain a game or demonstrate how to perform a skill.

7. During assessment allow students at least one trial to ensure that they understand what is expected of them. For example, one difficult assessment activity is walking along a balance beam where a student might not understand that the heel of one foot must touch the toe of the other foot each step of the way.

8. Allow each student to be a "captain" for a day. This will give all students a chance to learn how to interact with the deaf students and enhance their overall social and communication skills.

9. Have students work in small groups. This increases time on task for games and activities. It also allows for more student interactions.

10. Learn to sign. Learning how to sign does more than just introduce people to another medium for communication. It helps them become more comfortable about using natural gestures and incorporating more facial expressions into their communication, which is helpful for many hard of hearing children who do not use signs.

The Potential Sociocultural Benefits of PE

Deaf children grow up with the option of participating in at least two cultures. One of them is the culture to which their parents belong and for most deaf children this means a culture where the majority of people are hearing. The second culture is related to what deaf people do and is most visible in the activities of the Deaf community. **Deaf sport** is a strong institution within the Deaf community and is one in which deaf and hard of hearing people are welcomed to participate regardless of their degree of hearing loss or preferred means of communication (Stewart, 1991). Involvement in Deaf sport activities is an option that all deaf children have.

Stewart (1991) argued that deaf people become involved in Deaf sport activities for essentially social reasons, including the opportunity (1) to meet and associate with other deaf individuals and (2) to take control of a popular societal institution and use it as a vehicle for socializing other deaf people into the world of Deaf sport. He analyzed the social significance of Deaf sport and noted that:

> Deaf sport is attractive to deaf individuals because it provides an environment that is
> protected against society's stigmatization, and its predominant form of communication is

compatible with the needs of its participants. Deaf sport allows for the full involvement of all deaf individuals, unlike sports with hearing persons, where deaf athletes may find it difficult to advance to the level of their athletic ability because of sociocultural differences. (p. 153)

In other words, Deaf sport is popular within the Deaf community because it is a social institution that belongs to them. It is something that all deaf children will eventually have access to, and therefore they should be informed about it and prepared through PE to be an active participant in it.

Deaf sport provides competition in a variety of sports in which deaf athletes compete with one another. All of the sports—from the grassroots level through international competition—are organized by deaf people, and the highest levels of competition are the quadrennial **Deaf World Games** that are held for summer and winter sports (see box titled "Opening Eyes to the World Beyond").

There are several options for becoming involved in Deaf sport activities. The first one is as an athlete. An athlete can play locally in sports sponsored by a Deaf club at both the recreational and competitive levels. Examples of some popular local sports are bowling, slo-pitch, basketball, and volleyball. Each of these sports and several others have regional and national competitions. There are also international competitions in bowling, basketball, volleyball, soccer, tennis, swimming, wrestling, hockey, cycling, shooting, athletics, table tennis, alpine and Nordic skiing, and other sports. Competing at the national and international levels requires a minimum 55-decibel hearing loss in the better ear. This requirement usually does not exist for local and regional competitions as the emphasis at these levels is on participation—getting deaf people involved in a sport activity.

Another option for participating in Deaf sport is to become engaged in its organizational activities, for example, serving on a board of directors for a Deaf sport organization or assisting with the planning and running of a sports event. These are opportunities for involvement that a deaf person seldom finds in other communities because deaf people more readily accommodate the particular communication method that another deaf person might have. And if none of these options appeals to a deaf person then there is always the opportunity to be a spectator.

Information about Deaf sport needs to be incorporated into the curriculum of deaf children. In this section, we introduced you to the role of sport in the lives of deaf people. We only skimmed the surface of this field. Newspapers and newsmagazines such as the *NAD Broadcaster*, *Deaf Nation*, *Silent News*, *Newswaves for Deaf and Hard of Hearing People*, and *Deaf Life* follow the activities of major sporting events in the Deaf community. Several Web sites and contact with Deaf clubs can help teachers gain information about Deaf sport activities. For example, the USA Deaf Sports Federation Web site is a compendium of information relating to the organization. In the box titled "USA Deaf Sports Federation Web site," you will notice that there are seventeen different national sports organizations that are solely for deaf athletes. With this many opportunities, what we cannot do is let deaf children wait until they are adults before exploring the pleasures and opportunities that sports might provide for them. In this regard, PE is an ideal subject for initiating deaf children into the world of sports.

Opening Eyes to the World Beyond

The Deaf World Games, previously called the World Games for the Deaf, are the pinnacle of sport competitions for deaf athletes all over the world. It is a crucial unifying force for Deaf communities all over the world. Regulations require that all athletes have at least a 55 decibel hearing loss in their better ear in order to compete. Over 4,500 athletes from over seventy-five countries compete in the Deaf World Summer Games and about 400 athletes from close to twenty countries compete in the Deaf World Winter Games. This type of information and other information about Deaf sport should be shared with deaf children and can be used as a source of inspiration for young deaf athletes. The following list shows the sites of all Deaf World Games since the inception of the Summer Games in 1924.

Summer		**Winter**	
1924	Paris, France	1949	Seefeld, Austria
1928	Amsterdam, Holland	1953	Oslo, Norway
1931	Nuremberg, West Germany	1955	Oberammergau, West Germany
1935	London, England	1959	Montana-Vermala, Switzerland
1939	Stockholm, Sweden	1963	Are, Sweden
1949	Copenhagen, Denmark	1967	Berchtesgaden, Germany
1953	Brussels, Belgium	1971	Abelboden, Switzerland
1957	Milan, Italy	1975	Lake Placid, New York
1961	Helsinki, Finland	1979	Meribel, France
1965	Washington, DC	1983	Madonna Di Campigilio, Italy
1969	Belgrade, Yugoslavia	1987	Oslo, Norway
1973	Malmo, Sweden	1991	Banff, Canada
1977	Bucharest, Romania	1995	Ylläs, Finland
1981	Cologne, West Germany	1999	Davos, Switzerland
1985	Los Angeles, California	2003	Sundsvall, Sweden
1989	Christchurch, New Zealand		
1993	Sofia, Bulgaria		
1997	Copenhagen, Denmark		
2001	Rome, Italy		
2005	Melbourne, Australia		

What deaf children get out of life will depend to a large part on the type of education that we invest in them. Physical education is a crucial part of deaf children's educational investment portfolio.

Extracurricular Activities

[T]he fundamental goal for participation by deaf and hard of hearing students may differ from that for their hearing peers. However, involvement need not assume a standard

USA Deaf Sports Federation Web Site
http://www.usadsf.org/

One risk in listing Web site addresses and information about the site is that organizations are constantly changing their site addresses and the appearances of their web pages. Still, we are listing that of the USA Deaf Sports Federation because most teachers know very little if anything about Deaf sport activities, and this site provides a wealth of information. Among its content are the following two lists:

Categories	National Sports Organizations
Organization information	Hockey
Summer Games	Softball
Winter Games	Soccer
Retrospective/History	Table tennis
Applications	Swimming/Water polo
Merchandise	Badminton
Sponsors	Bowling
Terminology	Cycling
Contact Us	Golf
Help	Team handball
FAQs	Wrestling
Constitution	Basketball
	Track and field
News Flash	Skiing and snowboarding
	Baseball
Headlines	Flag football
	US Deaf Games

set of outcomes for all participants. Deaf students are unique in their sociocultural and linguistic needs. This uniqueness exists across the deaf population as well as among deaf individuals. On the other hand, hard of hearing students have social needs that reflect their dependence on speech for social interaction purposes. Schools must develop educational and social programs that are based on prior assessment of the needs of each student. In this respect, extracurricular activities can provide a strong support base for implementing socialization strategies. (Stewart & Stinson, 1992, p. 147)

There is not enough time in a school day to give deaf children the type of educational programming they need to prepare for life as an adult. Fulfilling all of the demands of the academic curriculum is a challenge for teachers. The fixed number of minutes that a student spends in school each day is an arbitrary figure, and no research says that this amount of time is sufficient—but one must work with it.

For deaf students, time is important not only because of their lower achievement levels but also because of their lag in social relationships when compared to their hearing peers. Stinson and Whitmire (1992) found that deaf students' involvement in structured social contact (e.g., sports) led to more unstructured social contact. Involvement in

extracurricular activities is one option for helping deaf students further develop their social and academic skills. For those students who are able to remain after school, teachers need to think about their educational program by looking at resources that are available during and after school hours (Kluwin & Stinson, 1993). This can be done by examining the extracurriculars that a school typically offers and then fitting them to the needs and interest of the student. For some deaf students, involvement in sports programs will be their primary interest, but for many other deaf students nonathletic activities such as photography, the school newspaper, and yearbook clubs might be more desirable.

How Extracurricular Activities Got Started

Extracurriculars first appeared on the school scene in the latter half of the nineteenth century. At that time, they were student initiated and student organized (Gutowski, 1988). Students sought activities that emulated those participated in at the college level. Sororities and fraternities were one option, but they were secret societies and frowned upon by administrators who had no control over them. A better bet was sports, which was in the open and provided the greater student body with an outlet for emotions and a chance to socialize with one another. Gutowski (1988) researched the extracurriculars of the Chicago school system at the end of the nineteenth century and found students involved in bands, debating societies, glee clubs (i.e., singing), newspaper clubs, literary societies, and biology clubs. Soon teachers got involved because students had to rely on untrained coaches who were usually just other students, and there were broken game schedules and disorderly behavior among the players, in addition to other factors that worked against the success of these clubs. Control of extracurriculars by the teaching staff has remained to this day.

In schools for the deaf, extracurriculars are especially appealing because they give students something to do while they are on campus. As late as the 1960s, residential students would arrive at school at the beginning of the year and return home for Christmas and Easter and at the end of the school year for summer. Back then most of these schools had large enrollments that made it easier to offer a variety of afterschool activities. Even today, schools for the deaf tend to offer a good selection of extracurricular activities. In sports, they compete against local schools as well as in regional tournaments against schools for the deaf from other states. Outside of sports they might compete against other schools in activities such as Math Pentathlon, Science Olympiad, and Odyssey of the Mind competitions.

The Benefits of Extracurricular Activities

We will start with the obvious: Students participate in extracurricular activities because they are fun. They are doing the activity of their own free will. For some deaf students there might not be many activities that they enjoy in their classes, which accentuates the importance of involving them in extracurricular activities that may interest them.

Stewart and Stinson (1992) reviewed the benefits of deaf students participating in extracurricular activities and concluded that the major aim of "sports and other extracurricular activities is to provide a platform for deaf students to develop a host of skills and personal characteristics that will allow them to capitalize on social, sport, and recreational opportunities found in deaf and hearing communities" (p. 140). They also noted that "extracurriculars provide deaf students with opportunities to enjoy themselves, to experience school in a more relaxed environment divorced from the threat of grades . . . and to interact with others on a common ground and in some instances in a more equitable fashion" (p. 140). The theme of their observation is that the learning environment found during extracurricular activities is markedly different from that of the classroom and should be exploited for the benefits that can be reaped.

More generally, Griffin (1988) identified the following ten skills or attributes that can be developed through extracurricular involvement:

1. Physical fitness,
2. Athletic skills,
3. Effective cooperation skills,
4. Greater self-esteem,
5. Positive self-concept,
6. Leadership skills,
7. Personal recognition for those who do not find it in the classroom,
8. Ability to use leisure time,
9. Improved student and teacher relationships, and
10. Tolerance for differences in others. (taken from Stewart & Stinson, 1992, pp. 138–139)

These benefits are equally applicable to deaf and hearing students, although it would be interesting to know how extracurricular involvement affects deaf students in public schools as opposed to their deaf counterparts in schools for the deaf.

Finally, there is an unheralded benefit associated with extracurricular activities of which all teachers should take note. Being a coach or a sponsor for an extracurricular activity is an excellent way to get to know your students better. From experience, we know that such endeavors lead to teachers having greater respect for the students and vice versa. All students want to perform well and experience a minimum of corrections as they go through their daily activities. Compared with academic classes, extracurriculars is a haven for such experiences. The positive experiences gained from extracurriculars can be transferred to the classroom and especially to those classrooms where the teacher is a coach or a sponsor.

What Can Teachers Do to Help?

In general, this whole area has been neglected in discussions about how to educate deaf students. Therefore, we encourage all teachers to not only take an interest in opportunities for involving their deaf students (and themselves!) in extracurriculars but also talk about it at meetings and conferences and in newsletters and journals. Here is a list of some of the things that teachers can do to facilitate the involvement of deaf students in extracurricular activities.

1. *Introduce deaf students to the potential benefits of extracurricular activities.* Do not take for granted that all students are aware of the afterschool activities that are available to them. Even when students know about clubs and sports programs and have an interest in them, they still might lack confidence in their ability to do the activity. In public schools, deaf students might be shy about getting involved with their hearing peers outside of the classroom. Spend time in the classroom exploring the various extracurriculars that are offered. Students can identify the activities that appeal to them.

Discuss in detail all that is involved once a student agrees to participate and include the amount of time per session, number of days per week, and length of season. Discuss the concept of commitment and the rewards associated with participation. Have the student create a list of questions or concerns that they might have regarding their participation. Arrange for the student to observe the activity and to meet with the coach or sponsor.

Even if a student does not elect to participate in an activity, introducing the student to the activity would still be a good learning experience that involves research, reading, writing, questioning, self-evaluation of interest, and other skills.

2. *Make extracurriculars a topic of discussion at all IEP meetings.* Extracurricular activities can help meet both educational and social goals for deaf students. Parents should be made aware of this and should be encouraged to be active players in helping their children participate in extracurriculars. Once an educational plan for a student is drawn up, teachers should examine what a school has to offer (see earlier discussion of opportunity-to-learn standards) that will help the student achieve these goals. They should then discuss steps that will be taken to monitor implementation of IEP goals related to extracurricular activities. Ensure that all expectations and plans are recorded in the IEP so that there is a record of accountability. This is not an unreasonable demand—extracurriculars are not extraneous to a student's overall educational plan.

3. *Teach communication and language skills associated with a particular extracurricular activity.* Involvement with peers in a nonacademic setting that is less structured than the classroom provides deaf students with an added opportunity to explore communication and language skills. In order to facilitate socialization during extracurriculars, it would be prudent for these teachers to teach the vocabulary associated with a particular activity and to model language structures (in whatever language and modality the student uses).

The following are examples of expressive language goals written for a middle school student with a profound hearing loss:

    a. Will demonstrate the correct use of *wh*-questions when communicating with others.
    b. Will use complex sentences when talking to people.

Both of these goals are critical conversation goals. Students need to be taught how to structure *wh*-questions and how to use various linguistic devices to form complex sentences. They will also need to see mature speakers modeling these grammatical structures in conversations.

All of this can occur in the classroom; however, a good measure of whether a student has internalized the appropriate grammatical concepts is to observe their usage in the student's communication outside of the classroom. Therefore, this should be brought up at an IEP meeting. Discuss what extracurricular activities a student might be interested in and what a teacher might do to prepare the student for asking questions or responding to questions from the coach or sponsor. Note in the IEP specific follow-up protocols: for example, having the student's teacher (or teacher consultant) write a short note to the coach or sponsor explaining the student's expressive language goal and asking for assistance in monitoring achievement of the goal. A visit with the coach or sponsor would help emphasize the importance of cooperation in the student's learning process.

4. *Ensure that extracurriculars are accessible to deaf students.* Some schools refuse to pay for interpreters to accompany a student to all or even some of the extracurricular sessions. That is one reason it is important to incorporate extracurricular involvement into an IEP. Once a goal is identified and agreed upon, the school district is obligated to provide all of the resources necessary to help the student meet that goal. Resources should also be included on the IEP. Sign language and oral interpreters are key resources for some deaf children. Auditory listening devices such as FM systems and directional microphones also provide greater access to communication and, if necessary, should be provided for the students.

5. *Resolve any transportation concerns.* Transportation is an access issue but it is discussed separately because it is a concern found at all types of schools. Also, deaf students in public schools are often transported much further than hearing peers (Kluwin & Stinson, 1993). For those students who are bussed to school, the question is who will drive them home after the game or club activity is finished. If the general student body is responsible for their own transportation, then there is no reason why the deaf student should be treated differently. Or is there? If participation in the extracurricular is linked to the IEP, then the school will have to bear the cost of getting the student home or to school earlier in the event that there is a practice before school starts. If a school has no legal obligation for getting the student home, then the parents should be encouraged to assume this responsibility.

6. *Prepare the coaches and club sponsors for working with a deaf student.* We prepare general education teachers when a deaf student is going to be in their classes and also provide them with a contact person such as a teacher consultant should they need assistance or have questions relating to the deaf student. This is a practice that needs to be instituted with deaf students in extracurricular activities.

Some coaches may feel uncertain about how to communicate with the student, and this needs to be addressed constructively with a teacher of the deaf who can provide tips on how best to communicate with that particular student. To help put coaches and deaf students at ease, arrangements should be made for a visit by a deaf athlete who can talk about his or her involvement in sports and answer questions that others might have. Provide coaches with information about Deaf sport so that they have a better understanding of their potential impact on the future participation of a deaf student in community sports. If coaches are still feeling anxious about the prospect of having a deaf member on their teams, put them in touch with a coach from another school who has had the experience of coaching deaf athletes.

7. *Keep in touch with a deaf student's involvement in an extracurricular activity.* Let the student know that you are proud of his or her involvement in an activity. No matter how well students might perform in a game or how their participation might be viewed by other members of a team or club, the minimal reward that we hope they will receive for their participation is an increase in self-concept and a more positive self-esteem. Let them know that what they are doing is a worthy accomplishment that does not need to be graded and talked about in a report card. Let them know that this type of participation gives them the kind of experiences that will help them both prepare for and enjoy their leisure time once they are adults.

Creating a Well-Fit Child

Physical education classes and extracurricular activities help schools create a well-fit deaf student. But fitness is more than just games, sports, and physical exercises. It's about intelligence, too. About twenty years ago, Gardner (1983) espoused the theory of multiple intelligence, claiming that there are at least seven measurable intelligences: logical-mathematical, verbal-linguistic, spatial-mechanical, musical, bodily-kinesthetic, interpersonal-social, and intrapersonal. Two of these, the logical-mathematical and verbal-linguistic intelligences, are the ones traditionally measured by IQ tests. Although these measures alone tell us little about an individual's knowledge and capacity to do things, they have had a tremendous impact on how we tend to grade children in school and devise educational programs. Schools strive to improve the math and reading skills of all children but essentially ignore the many children whose athletic abilities or drawing skills would soar with a little more attention and guidance from a skilled teacher.

Associated with **multiple intelligence** theories is the now accepted notion that thinking is different in the left and right sides of the brain. In most people, the right hemisphere is the control center for verbal and analytic thinking while the left hemisphere functions mostly in the nonverbal and global mode (Sperry, 1973). In a sense, we have reached the point where educational planning must look at what happens on both sides of the brain and not just at language and numbers. Deaf students will benefit from schools that provide them with as many opportunities as possible to reach their potential in all areas of intelligence.

Children need extra time in school and after school to exercise their multiple intelligences. Deaf children in particular have much to gain from a curriculum that shows that there is more to learning than reading, writing, and arithmetic. Greater self-esteem gained from whatever intellectual, physical, or artistic endeavor deaf children engage in might translate to better overall performance in all of the academic areas. At the very least we need to give them the opportunities to learn using their various intelligences—opportunities that extend beyond the school day and into the eclectic offerings of an extracurricular program. Ultimately, such global programming will lead to well-fit deaf adults better prepared to work and play.

The Role of the Itinerant Teacher and the Resource Room Teacher

It might be a challenge for itinerant teachers and resource room teachers to devote adequate time on issues relating to PE and extracurricular activities. But after the latest amendments, the Individuals with Disabilities Education Act (P.L. 105-17) now recognizes the value of ensuring that all children have access to afterschool activities. Moreover, PE has always been a part of school programming, although the value placed on it varies greatly between school districts. Thus, teachers who have responsibility for the education of deaf children should ensure that these children have access to PE and extracurricular activities.

It is unlikely that many general education teachers and even PE teachers in public schools are aware of the possible discrepancy between the physical fitness of deaf students and their hearing peers. Nor are they likely to be aware of the sociocultural benefits for deaf students who participate in sports—a benefit that includes future participation in community sports programs including Deaf sport events (Stewart, 1991). Thus, it is important for itinerant teachers and resource room teachers to help deaf children and their parents become aware of the benefits of participating in PE and various extracurricular activities. Following is a list of things that these teachers can do.

1. Request that deaf students, and especially those of elementary age, be tested for physical fitness. Include this information when designing an IEP. If a student shows deficiencies, then this needs to be discussed when examining the student's participation in PE. It is also a reason why PE should not automatically be the course of choice for pulling a deaf student out for speech therapy and/or assistance with academic learning.

2. Explain to deaf students the opportunities for involvement in extracurricular activities that a school has to offer. Do not assume that all students already know this information. Also, determine a student's interest in an activity and their willingness to follow through and join an extracurricular activity. Be prepared to encourage participation.

3. Meet with parents of deaf students to explain the physical and sociocultural benefits of participating in sports and extracurricular activities. Talk to the parents about the possibilities for involving their deaf children in community sports programs. Make suggestions as to how the parents might help these programs accommodate communication concerns. In addition, provide parents with ideas about how they can help their children adjust to the socialization circumstances associated with participating in such activities.

4. Meet with the PE teacher to alert him or her to the possibility that a deaf student might need some extra support to develop balance, fundamental motor skills, and physical fitness skills.

5. Compile a list of resources for more information about Deaf sport activities. Share this with deaf students, their PE teachers, homeroom teachers, and their parents.

6. Review communication and transportation issues that might pose a problem for a deaf student participating in extracurricular activities.

7. Monitor a deaf student's involvement in extracurricular activities. If a student enjoys a particular activity, we want to give him or her every opportunity to continue participating. Thus, teachers need to be on the alert for student dissatisfaction that is not related to playing a sport or doing an activity but rather is related to communication and/or socialization concerns, such as a reluctance to talk to others even in the presence of an interpreter.

Conclusion

Physical fitness is good for everyone, yet deaf children do not seem to be as fit as their hearing peers. Why this is the case has yet to be ascertained. What we do know is that for deaf children to get fit means that they have to have opportunities to participate in physical activities—at school and at home. Although teachers cannot be responsible for the amount of physical activity a deaf child is involved with at home, they can be a source of information to the parents on the benefits of their children being active in physical games, sports, and exercises.

At school, teachers can help deaf children take advantage of physical education programs that their schools offer as well as afterschool sports programs. But involvement is not simply a matter of showing up. Communication and socialization issues, for instance, might present barriers to full and equal participation—a concern of which teachers of the deaf must be acutely aware. The concerns related to communication are obvious, yet as simple as some movement activities might look, the importance of verbal instructions must not be ignored. In other words, movement activities and playing sports might seem a perfect match for visual learners such as deaf children, but there might be important verbal instructions that help some children perform a physical task better. Therefore, addressing deaf children's need for access to communication at all times is important in PE and extracurricular sports.

The concerns in the area of socialization relate, in part, to deaf students' willingness to participate in PE and sports. In schools for the deaf, interacting with others is not a major concern because of similarities in communication preference and the fact that deaf children are among others who are just like them. In public schools, where deaf children are integrated with hearing peers, the isolating effect of a hearing loss may discourage some deaf children from fully participating in an activity. By addressing this possibility, teachers might be able to encourage a greater willingness among deaf students to partake in PE and other school activities.

Outside of school, involvement in most leisure activities is a good way to maintain a healthy lifestyle. When they become adults, today's deaf children will be faced with many sports and recreation opportunities in their local community as well as within the Deaf community. Deaf students have to be prepared to take advantage of these opportunities. Thus, involving deaf students in PE and assisting them in their desire to participate in extracurricular activities should be a critical component of their overall education plan.

The role of extracurricular activities cannot be overemphasized. Involvement in sports is a good way to develop physical skills as well as self-esteem. Understanding how a game is played and knowing the movements and skills associated with playing the game is a critical step towards preparing deaf children for a lifetime of participation in physical activities. But not all deaf students enjoy PE, nor do they all want to be involved in an afterschool sports program. Furthermore, even for those who do enjoy sports and strenuous physical activities, there are other activities that can also lead to much enjoyment. Indeed, the benefits of participating in some sort of extracurricular activity is such that all deaf students should be given the opportunity to explore their interests in particular activities. If they express no immediate interest, then their teachers should devise a plan for exposing them to the range of activities their school has to offer, for example, drama, chess, sign language, and recreational skiing.

The key is not to let deaf students' participation in PE and extracurriculars fall by the wayside. These students need to be assessed just as they are for other subject matter. They need to be aware of their opportunities for staying after school and playing sports or joining a club. Some of them might also need encouragement, and certainly many of them who are in public schools might initially, at least, need communication support.

KEY WORDS AND CONCEPTS

content standards: Items listed in a curriculum that describe what it is that students are supposed to learn in a particular subject. Content standards for physical education are typically related to body control/management skills; fundamental motor skills; physical fitness; sports, games, and dance skills; activity-related cognitive skills; and activity-related social skills.

Deaf sport: An institution within the Deaf community that refers to all of the activities related to the organizing, playing, and/or watching of sport events involving deaf athletes. It has been called the strongest institution within the Deaf community because almost all of its activities from the grassroots through international levels are organized by deaf people (Stewart, 1991).

Deaf World Games: A quadrennial event in which deaf athletes from around the world compete in various sporting events. There is a Deaf World Summer Games and a Deaf World Winter Games that are held two years apart from each other. The Deaf World Games began in 1929 and are operated by the Comité Internationale des Sports des Sourds. Until 1999 the Deaf World Games were called the World Games for the Deaf.

extracurricular activities: Any type of school-sponsored activities that occur before or after school hours. These activities are not related to the curriculum, and participation is voluntary. The activities may be sports such as soccer, volleyball, and basketball, or they may be nonsport-related such as a drama club or a sign language club.

fundamental motor skills: The most basic of physical skills used in sports and games requiring gross motor movements. Examples of fundamental motor skills are walking, running, skipping, leaping, hopping, throwing, catching, striking, and kicking. One of the main purposes of physical education is to help children develop fundamental motor skills.

multiple intelligences: A theory that espouses that people have several distinctive types of intelligences that can be nurtured and measured. The measurable intelligences that are most often discussed in the context of schooling are logical-mathematical, verbal-linguistic, spatial-mechanical, musical, bodily-kinesthetic, interpersonal-social, and intrapersonal.

opportunity-to-learn standards: Related to the resources that a school has to offer in the way of staffing, programming, and facilities. Along with content and performance standards, opportunity-to-learn standards are an important consideration in the development of a successful physical education program.

performance standards: In physical education, measurements of how well a student can do a certain activity.

QUESTIONS

1. Jake is a 15-year-old deaf boy who is fully mainstreamed in a public school with the support of an itinerant teacher and an interpreter. He wants to play junior varsity soccer and has requested that an interpreter be present at all practices. What should Jake's itinerant teacher do to ensure that an interpreter is provided?

2. Why might a school for the deaf, or a large center program for deaf students, incorporate into its PE curriculum sports that are popular in the Deaf community?

3. PE is often the subject from which deaf students are pulled for speech therapy. When might PE not be an appropriate subject for pulling deaf students out?

4. What are the Deaf World Games and what is the hearing loss requirement for participation?

5. Describe three different ways in which a deaf person can become involved in Deaf sport activities.

6. How might involvement in extracurricular activities help in the development of a deaf student's social skills?

7. Why are extracurricular activities important for residential schools for the deaf?

8. What are some of the benefits experienced by a teacher of the deaf (or any other teacher) when becoming involved in coaching or sponsoring an extracurricular activities?

9. What might each of the following types of teachers do to introduce deaf students to the benefits of extracurricular activities: general education teacher, teacher of the deaf in a self-contained classroom, itinerant teacher of the deaf, and resource room teacher of the deaf?

10. What can teachers do to make extracurricular activities accessible to deaf students?

11. Suppose you are an itinerant teacher and that you have a deaf tenth grader who has a keen interest in the school's drama club but is too shy to sign up for the club. What could you do to help the student join the club?

ACTIVITIES

1. The purpose of this activity is to compare PE and extracurricular offerings in different school programs. Working in groups of three to four people, first contact each of the following types of programs:

   - residential school for the deaf
   - center program for deaf students at the elementary, middle, and high school levels
   - public school program that has at least one deaf student enrolled in it

   Then record the following information for each program:

   (a) the number of minutes of PE required at each grade level
   (b) the extracurricular programs including sports that the school offers
   (c) the number of deaf students participating in extracurricular activities and the names of each activity
   (d) the accommodations and provision of support services that the school offers for deaf students participating in extracurricular activities

2. Sherrill (1993) recommended that when deaf children are doing an activity they should be instructed on how to think about what they are doing. For each of the following activities, write a list of five to seven questions or statements that you would use with a deaf child:

   ■ skipping a rope
   ■ jumping through a hopscotch pattern
   ■ hitting a tennis ball with a racquet
   ■ shooting a bow and arrow

3. Contact a Deaf sport club in your area (or on a Web site if one is not available locally) and inquire about deaf athletes who have participated in the Deaf World Games and the name of the sport in which they played. Note that many Deaf sport clubs are affiliated with local or statewide associations of deaf people and therefore might not be listed separately in phone books or Web sites.

8 Integrating Technology into Your Teaching

CHAPTER OUTCOMES

When you are finished with this chapter, you will be able to

1. Describe why you use technology in teaching and why your use of technology will enhance the learning experiences of deaf students.
2. Use technology in meaningful contexts that provide deaf students with authentic learning experiences.
3. Use software for the dual purpose of teaching computer literacy and subject matter content.
4. Design effective evaluation strategies for projects that involve the use of technology.
5. Use a procedure for developing a comprehensive lesson plan that incorporates the use of computers.

Technology has been a boon in the lives of deaf people in many ways. It has helped them become more independent as they interact in a society oriented to speech and hearing communication. One wave of technology to benefit deaf people brought us closed-captioning, TTY (teletype), alerting devices, ever improving hearing aids and other assistive listening devices, and fax machines. Another wave brought the Internet and the everyday use of e-mail as well as online conversations, videophones, videoconferencing, highly accurate speech-to-text software, emerging text-to-signs software, and palm-size pagers with keyboards designed specifically to meet the communication needs of deaf people.

From an educator's perspective, the growing need for deaf people to be literate obligated schools to help deaf students gain access to technology as well as the know-how to use it. This posed a challenge to schools because at the turn of the twenty-first century, there were still many teachers whose computer knowledge was limited to the use of e-mail and the Internet. These uses of the computer represent only a fraction of the ways in which technology can be used to enhance instructions in the classroom.

Thus, it must be emphasized that emerging uses of technology is a call for new learning experiences not only for deaf students but also for their teachers.

Technology in the Classroom

There are at least three reasons given or implied in the use of emerging technologies in teaching: entertainment or motivation, improving learning, and future skills.

The first reason, the entertainment or motivation argument, has several variants. Students like to do it. It's fun. Students may have access to even more sophisticated stuff at home. The counterargument is: If they were supposed to have fun, students would not be in school. Obviously, using technology is motivating in many ways; however, it also requires a learning curve. One curve is for the teacher who is often developer, systems administrator, and software training specialist. The other curve is for the students who can range from knowing more than the teacher will ever know to students who don't know where the power switch is. Finally, you have to spend all of your time teaching the students how to use the system, and the system is not used in any other part of their lives, what is the point? From this perspective, the supposed motivational properties of technology are not sufficient to justify using it.

The second reason for using technology in the classroom is that it will improve learning rates. This claim has been made frequently, has a long history, and has been examined carefully and repeatedly. The computer-based argument for drill and practice is that the computer is patient with the student. The argument goes: The computer does not get bored presenting the same material to the student, therefore the student will learn more. Unfortunately, the problem with factual learning is that it is difficult to learn what you cannot connect to. For example, ask a veteran what his or her military service number was, and you will get an accurate answer instantly. You will be told the number even if the veteran had mustered out fifty years ago. Ask almost anyone what their home phone number was when they were a child. Odds are you will get the correct information and very quickly.

The point to be made is that factual information tied to meaningful events or situations is easier to learn and retain. In other words, there is no rote learning, only the memorization of essential data. If the material is not important to the student, it might not be learned no matter how long the student sits at a computer. And putting students at computers for drill and practice reduces the time they could be using for learning more complex ideas.

The third reason for using technology in the classroom is the best argument for integrating technology into teaching: Technology will be a part of your students' futures. What shape that technology will take and how it will change is something we cannot predict; however, in the future, computer-based technology will play an integral role in everyone's lives.

Before the advent of the printing press, learning involved a lot of memorization, and the key to success in school included learning ways to remember information. Educationally, it was the age of the mnemonic device. With the cheap production of books, libraries became the measure of learning. Higher education became a question of knowing what books to look for and how to retrieve them. At Thomas Jefferson's home at Monticello, there is a wonderful device that Jefferson invented that permitted him to have three or four books open at the same time and to turn to the appropriate page by simply turning his book-laden Lazy Susan. Now and into the future, information will be held within computerized systems, and the skill of the future will be the retrieval and comparison of data. From the age of the mnemonic we will move to the age of the heuristic: the intelligent search strategy.

If the goal of education is to prepare the individual to be a functioning member of society, then education in the future has to include instruction not simply with technology but instruction about technology. The challenge for the teacher comes not in designing the lesson with the most bells and whistles, but in designing the lesson that teaches the deaf child the most that the child is able to learn and ultimately use.

Basic Functions of Learning Technologies

Cynthia King of Gallaudet University advocates the use of the term *learning technologies* instead of educational technology because it places the emphasis on the student. We're going to use her term for that same reason. We want you to think of the "machine" as the servant of the learner.

Currently, there are several forms of software that define the basic learning technologies both in the sense of how a teacher will present lessons as well as in the sense of what the students need to know about information-delivery systems for the future:

- Word processing
- Spreadsheets
- Databases
- Electronic communities
- Computer-based publishing

One other important function is image processing, which we will not discuss in this chapter because it is the most specific and probably the most technical of the computer applications; however, if you plan to do any kind of electronic or desktop publishing with your classes, you will need an introduction to image manipulation.

Word Processing

Word processing software can be used to teach about technology. Small-scale communications are an essential part of any organization whether it is a club, a classroom, or a corporation. While there is a movement away from the use of newsletters to Web sites as sources of small-quantity information, the two- to eight-page newsletter probably will not disappear anytime soon. Consequently, developing a classroom newsletter gives you the opportunity to teach English skills and journalism principles and to develop a means for communicating with the children and their parents.

Using the computer for a classroom newsletter entails that the teacher and student have a solid understanding of the various functions of a word processor and know how to manipulate various commands to facilitate the form and production of a newsletter. See the box titled "Frequently Used Functions of a Word Processor" for examples of the many useful applications of a word processor when creating print.

Frequently Used Functions of a Word Processor

- Store documents for later use.
- Erase and insert text with ease.
- Search for specific text and replace it.
- Move or copy text.
- Wrap text around images.
- Easily change text style and appearance.
- Set margin justification quickly or change as desired.
- Insert text from other sources.
- Run spelling checks.
- Use built-in thesaurus for alternate word choices.
- Insert graphics into text.

Many teachers of the deaf now send home class-generated newsletters as a form of communication with parents since it not only highlights the children's work but provides a friendly vehicle for passing on essential information. (See Chapter 14 for more information about the importance of communicating with the families of deaf children.) Topics include the usual announcements, descriptions of long-term assignments that might require parental assistance, class news, information about sign language, strategies for encouraging speech-reading, events in the Deaf community, accessibility issues in society, and even material on child development.

The inclusion of all of these topics and much more can seem like a daunting task for the uninitiated. But for the teacher with minimal computer skills, the word processor makes the task not only easy but easy to do repeatedly throughout the year. The box titled "Word Processing and the Newsletter" lists some of the advantages of doing a newsletter using a word processor.

Getting started doing a newsletter depends on the sophistication of your equipment. You do not need sophisticated software but the ease with which you can do a class newsletter changes with each level of technical sophistication you achieve. The big difference, aside from cost, as you get into newer and more sophisticated systems is that you move from having to do your own formatting to systems that provide you with newsletter templates where you just fill in the blanks.

Consequently, the way to approach the newsletter is to know the parts—that is, focus on communication rather than on the technology. When you develop the newsletter remember that newsletters tend to be repetitious from one issue to the next. For instance, they will have regular columns or features. Certain news will always be reported, such as schedules for parent-teacher meetings and school events, student accomplishments, and notes from the Parent Advisory Council. Word processors typically have a feature for existing templates or a feature that allows you to create your own and by which you can specify a format for a particular heading. Once you have a template you can simply add information relevant to the heading each time the newsletter is printed. The box titled "Reusable Doc-

Word Processing and the Newsletter

Word processing is a must in the production of any class newsletter. Among the many benefits are the following:

1. Saves time
   Revisions of classwork are simpler for teachers.
   Students can compose more quickly.
   Format for one issue of the newsletter can be used for another issue.

2. Better-looking documents
   Easier corrections.
   Easier improvements.
   Can personalize headings.

3. Sharing of documents
   Teachers can swap materials with each other, with students, with parents.
   Newsletter can be easily placed on a Web site.

4. Portfolio assessment
   Students can decide what work they have created for the newsletter should be placed in their portfolios.

uments (Templates)" has examples of templates that can be used in newsletters or to regularly send information to the families of the deaf students.

When developing the newsletter, the essential parts begin with the *nameplate* or *banner*, which is the portion of the newsletter at the top of the front page. The *newsletter title* is the first item in the nameplate. Below the title is usually a horizontal line. The *newsletter subtitle* and the newsletter *volume* and *date* are contained between the *ruling lines* below the title. The text of the newsletter is called the *body copy*.

Once you have mastered using word processing in one context, such as making a class newsletter, you will have both a grasp of the general potential of your word processing software and some familiarity with using word processing in the classroom. The next step is to branch out into other uses in the classroom:

1. Student writing
2. Group activities
3. Cross-curriculum projects

In Chapter 4, we presented the process approach to writing instruction. Word processing is the perfect tool in using this approach for teaching student writing because it allows students to brainstorm lists of ideas, to easily organize the lists into outlines, and to compose and manipulate text.

Reusable Documents (Templates)

Templates are reusable documents that all word processing programs have. The simplest template is a blank document. But virtually any document that you create and save can become a template for future use. Templates can be used for a variety of written materials. The following are some examples of templates that teachers and/or students might wish to create:

- Welcome back information at the start of the year
- Field trip permission letters
- Information routing for resource room students
- Schedules for students who are seen by an itinerant teacher
- List of classroom rules
- Annual event announcements like Back to School Night and the Spring Ice Cream Social
- Student progress reports to parents
- Worksheets that need to be adapted for different student abilities
- Lesson plans
- Lecture notes from mainstream classes
- Subject matter–related signs that parents should use at home
- Best assistive listening devices for the home
- Educational goals and objectives for each student

Group writing is also discussed in Chapter 4 as an activity that can encourage writing by deaf students because one student's strength compensates for another's limitations. Word processing permits individual student contributions to a group process to be readily combined. An example of this is shown in the box titled "Writing Through Webbing for Elementary Students."

At several points in this book, we mentioned cross-curriculum projects such as integrated social studies projects. Word processing makes a readily alterable document that permits the addition of a variety of sources of material, including images of maps, pictures of individuals, and charts of numeric data. It is also a handy device for tracking instructional objectives across several subject areas. Figure 8.1 is an example of how tables can be set up for such tracking purposes. One adaptation of this table would be to structure it so that students can see how the activities are related between different subject matters. This table can also be adapted to show how each objective is linked to a specific IEP goal.

Spreadsheets

As with word processing software, **spreadsheet** software can be used to teach about technology. If you have ever computed a student's grade from the information in a grade book, you were using a spreadsheet. Spreadsheet software is just a carryover from the old days of accounting ledgers. The difference between your grade book and spreadsheet software is that you can program the spreadsheet to do the calculation for you, but spreadsheet software offers more benefits than that. Spreadsheet software can let students ask questions like:

Writing Through Webbing for Elementary Students

Following is a lesson that shows how the process of webbing can be used to help learn writing skills while using a word processor with young elementary age students:

Purpose: Teachers use word processing in a five-step process to help students learn writing skills.

Activity: Very young children may have a lot to say but often have difficulty getting started because they don't have a structure for their thoughts. The procedure listed below can help them overcome this difficulty. The procedure is tied to five concepts:

Think   Draw   Tell   Write   Share

Procedures: 1. At the beginning of the project children *think* about an idea that they would like to write about. Children then bring in photos or cut out pictures of objects related to this idea. They develop a file of these pictures.
2. They *draw* a picture that ties the images together. Their drawings should *tell* a story. In more elaborate creations this can be done with image-processing software with the teacher's help.
3. After they have drawn their picture, they *write* a story about the picture. The pictures and the story are combined and *shared* by being posted or displayed for others to see.
4. The word processor is used at several points to turn their words into text and to illustrate the stories.

This lesson was adapted from C. Etchinson (1995). A powerful web to weave—Developing writing skills for elementary students. *Learning and Leading with Technology, 23* (3) 14–15.

When (Date)	Where (Subject Area)	What (Activity)	Why (Instructional Objectives)	Who (For Which Students)

FIGURE 8.1   Creating a template for planning cross-curriculum, interactive lessons.

1. What if a mouse was as big as a lion?
2. What will happen if the temperature around the world goes up half a degree?
3. How do wind patterns impact weather?

Spreadsheet software offers us the opportunity to play with numerical concepts. If I weigh 100 pounds on earth, what will I weigh on the moon? Or Mars? Or Jupiter? At what point would the weight of my own body flatten it?

Using a simple spreadsheet program, students can enter their weights and print out reports of their different weights on different planets as a graph. More advanced students can be challenged to compute the point at which their spaceship could not leave the planet. If I weigh X and my supplies weigh Y on earth, and it takes Z pounds of fuel to lift one pound of cargo, how much of my fuel will I need for liftoff from the moon? From Jupiter?

A major benefit of any spreadsheet is that it provides a visual representation of numbers or events (see Figure 8.2 for an example of a spreadsheet layout that helps students visually track wind direction over the course of a year). One of the essential skills related to doing science is the ability to make observations. In order to "make" an observation, students need some way to record it. While the idea of writing it down may seem obvious to adults, it is nonetheless a convention that has to be learned. In the spreadsheet shown in the figure, a check mark is made in the box that corresponds to the predominant wind for each day. A quick scan of a completed spreadsheet will then reveal which wind is dominant during each of the seasons, throughout most of the year, a particular month of the year, and so forth. The top row could be used to write the abbreviations for the predominant wind direction for each month. Further computations will convert this data into percentages (which are the bases for constructing the wind rose). This ties the activity to the goals for creating authentic experiences that we discussed in Chapter 6 on teaching mathematics.

One way to create a data entry sheet is to use the *Table* function provided in a word processor. You will need to create a table with enough cells to complete the project. Save a completely blank version of the data entry sheet (this becomes a template). Make a copy of the data entry sheet and enter all of the data yourself. You can then go through and make multiple copies of the complete data entry sheet. It would be helpful for the child to see one entire row that is completely filled in. This approach can be used for any number of projects when compiling information from another source. For example, in social studies students may want to compile information about the U.S. presidents from the encyclopedia.

The possibilities for "what if" questions is unending, offering numerous opportunities for enriched language experiences, thus reinforcing our theme of self-expression. The students start with a simple question such as, How many buffalo can a park ranger keep on ten acres of park land? Then they move on to introducing new conditions: If the rainfall is heavy? If the deer and antelope want to play? If a two-week annual hunting season is allowed? Spreadsheet software can be used to plot the variables associated with each of these questions.

A valuable reason for using spreadsheets is that they help deaf students organize data in an easily managed visual chart. This setup makes it easier for deaf students to visualize possibilities, especially if numbers are involved. It gives them a sequencing device as we discussed in Chapter 6.

Finally, spreadsheet software offers the deaf student the opportunity to explore the world on his or her own terms. It is a convenient means for tracking and thinking about real world issues in a manageable way.

Wind Direction	Jan.	Feb.	March	April	May	June	July	Aug.	Sept.	Oct.	Nov.	Dec.
North												
North by Northeast												
Northeast												
East by Northeast												
East												
East by Southeast												
Southeast												
South by Southeast												
South												
South by Southwest												
Southwest												
West by Southwest												
West												
West by Northwest												
Northwest												
North by Northwest												

FIGURE 8.2 Creating a spreadsheet for a science project.

In sum, using spreadsheet software is an excellent way to explore mathematical relationships and to solve problems relating to changing conditions. Moreover, by establishing a convenient and visual presentation of numbers, teachers can facilitate the integration of mathematics into other subject areas, which in turn can serve as a basis for conceptualizing the applications of various mathematical principles. For example, is a segment of society making or losing money this year? Students could plot the cost of living against salary increases over a particular time frame. Did this segment of society make or loss money? To make this type of activity more meaningful, students can be asked to track fund-raising efforts with which their class or school might be involved. If each student raised 3 percent more funds each week, how much more would the school have at the end of the month?

Plotting expenses related to a field trip is another authentic use of a spreadsheet that can lead to more self-expression on the part of the students as they debate the cost-benefits of visiting different sites. For instance, in a unit plan on marine life, students might debate the relative merits of chartering a bus and visiting an aquarium twenty miles away that charges a $5.00 admission fee versus going eighty miles to a observe a university marine biology laboratory that has no admission fee. Which will provide the most beneficial experience in relation to the science objectives of the unit plan?

Once you become comfortable using spreadsheets you can become more proficient with other instructional applications for them.

Databases

Have you ever tried to find something in someone else's purse or kitchen or desk? If the location to be searched is fairly empty or the object is large relative to the space to be searched or if you have very specific directions, the task is not too hard. In the real world, the drawer is cluttered, the directions are garbled or nonexistent, or what you are looking for is about the size of a needle in a backpack as big as a haystack.

Databases are like big bags or cluttered drawers full of stuff. The difference between an electronic database and someone's purse or desk drawer is that because the database is structured, the database can be searched quickly and efficiently.

If you have tried to book a ticket on an airline or get a book out of the library, you already have had experience with searchable databases. The person behind the counter at any large car parts store or auto dealership can look for a hubcap for your 1968 Mustang using a searchable database. Bought tires recently? Your local tire store has some wonderful searchable databases that cover almost every make of tire available in North America.

Similar to the business world, you can have your deaf students create their own databases. By doing this, the students are given ownership of the database. If the information contained within the database is of immediate relevance to them, then they may be more receptive to the language associated with discussing the database. Relevance and immediacy are always central to the learning process of children. The box "Student-Created Databases" lists examples of databases that students can easily create in the classroom.

Instructional Implications for Learning About Databases.   There are at least three reasons for teaching children about database systems:

Student-Created Databases

Creating databases is a beneficial activity for many reasons, including that it helps organize information, allows for quick analyses of large amounts of information, helps reveal patterns, and more. Whatever the reasons are, database projects should be meaningful to the students, and they should comprise an authentic experience for the students. Here are some examples of databases that can be generated by students:

Information about the U.S. presidents
  Who had the shortest term?
  Who was the youngest? Oldest?

Information about the states
  How many state birds are the same?
  Which has the densest population?
  Which has the most deaf and hard of hearing support agencies?

Any observational data
  Plants around school
  Plant characteristics during different seasons
  Clouds, time of year, temperature, shape

Endangered species
  Where do most of them live?
  What kinds of animals are endangered?

Is the school lunch healthy?
  Calories
  Fat content
  Food group membership

Selecting a college
  Location
  Support services (e.g., interpreters, real-time reporters)
  Cost
  Programs offered

Life of hearing aid batteries
  Which brand lasts the longest?
  Which size lasts the longest?

Information relating to the Americans with Disabilities Act
  Companies that are affected
  Institutions (e.g., schools) that are affected
  Applications of ADA in everyday life, e.g., Does a restaurant have to provide an interpreter for its customers? Do movie theaters have to provide open captions?

Language analysis
  Signs that are formed with the "Y" handshape
  Signs that are made around the head
  Signs that are made in front of the body
  Signs that have two "Y" handshape

1. If a person knows how a system works, he or she can make better use of it in life.
2. Databases are useful for organizing things.
3. The thought processes involved in databasing information force a person to think about the amount and structure of that information.

If a person knows how a system works, he or she can make better use of it in life.   If students know that there are things such as databases that store information in the form of categories, then they can be better prepared to retrieve needed information when necessary. This includes numerous possibilities such as finding books in the library, searching for a university, searching for a job in a particular geographical area, locating an interpreting agency, buying a cheap hearing aid, or getting a better interest rate for a car loan when they become adults.

Databases are useful for organizing things.   Databases help you keep track of things. Suppose your girl's basketball league needs to create balanced teams of girls for league play. You have names, addresses, phone numbers, available practice times, and ratings of the girls' basketball skills. From this information it is a relatively simple matter to find out how many average skilled 11-year-olds are in the pool of girls who can practice on Wednesdays. Closer to the classroom, students can create a database of subject area-specific vocabulary words that they are learning. On this database, they could insert information about each word such as definitions, sentences in which they first saw the word used, availability of a single sign for the word, tips for lipreading the word, and much more.

The thought processes involved in databasing information force a person to think about the amount and structure of that information.   If you have ever done laundry, then you are likely aware of the process of sorting clothes into piles. This sorting activity forces you to think about the characteristics of the clothes. Are they naturals or synthetics? Colors or whites? Iron or permanent press? When you database you need to organize the world into categories. When you ask a student to organize, the student has to think about the attributes of an object and the relationships between categories of objects. For example, if mammals are warm-blooded, give birth to live young, and produce milk, would the platypus fall under this category?

If schools aim to create literate deaf students, then the process of thinking and talking about databasing can contribute to the process of becoming literate because, eventually, much of what is talked about will have to be translated to a category or a description of a category in a database. In fact, some student-generated databases can serve as an example of a student's self-expression. For example, deaf students might be asked to create a database titled "Famous Deaf People." This database forces the students to consider questions and items such as the following:

1. What did this person do to become famous?
2. Where did this person grow up?
3. What type of education did this person have?

4. How did this person come to do what made him or her famous?

5. Is this person famous within both the Deaf community and the greater society?

An example of a database classroom activity for a social studies class is shown in the box titled "Classroom Database Activity."

Any body of information that has component parts that you would want to retrieve and organize in a systematic way is a candidate for a database. For years, an argument has raged over which version of Chaucer's *Prologue* to the *Canterbury Tales* (there are nearly sixty of them) is the closest to Chaucer's original document. The problem was too huge until scholars began to database the material. This intellectual activity forced them to categorize the elements of the *Prologue* but at the same time gave them the opportunity to easily search and compare them, thus resolving tyhe controversy.

Classroom Database Activity

Brainstorming is a good way of getting students to think about what type of information they wish to collect on a particular topic. A teacher who monitors the brainstorming session can provide key vocabulary words and phrases at an opportune time to facilitate discussion among students as well as to expose students to a timely language experience. Following is an example of setting up a classroom database activity.

A. Students will work with a partner or in a group. Each group will be assigned a particular explorer who will be set up in the database. The groups are then required to brainstorm a list of information that will be collected about this explorer. Once the brainstorming is completed, the list is set up in a database with the following information:

1. Name
2. Date of birth
3. Place of birth
4. Socioeconomic status
5. Education
6. Occupation
7. Sponsor country
8. Date of first exploration
9. Date of last exploration
10. Land discovered
11. Date of death

B. Once each group has located the information about its explorer, students in the group will enter it into the database.

C. Each student will individually write an essay about the information in the database. Students can select a single category such as date of birth for a number of explorers and create a time line. Or each student can select more than one category.

Electronic Communities

There are two main ways for creating electronic communities: sending information via e-mail and using the Internet or **World Wide Web** in the classroom.

E-mail.   When e-mail first came to Gallaudet University in the early 1980s, it revolutionized how deaf and hearing people communicated with each other. Likewise, it helped deaf people all over the world attain some level of parity in communicating with hearing people, because other than language-related issues, the requirements for using e-mail are the same for both deaf and hearing people. In other words, deaf people are not disadvantaged by the requirement for using voice and hearing or the added costs of long-distance phone bills when communicating by TTYs. Since then, each improvement to e-mail system has only expanded the uses of e-mail. We have gone from sending and receiving messages to attaching documents, photographs, video, and other images. While separate software has been developed for facilitating online discussion, features of the newer e-mail systems permit users to create their own discussion groups for special topics. "Virtual meetings" are beginning to replace face-to-face meetings with the added advantage that no one has to take notes because the system keeps track of the messages.

Everything from making appointments to doing consumer surveys to writing books at a distance can be done through electronic mail. The spread of e-mail has been so rapid and so ubiquitous that teacher-training textbooks often do not include any mention of it. Yet for working with deaf students, e-mail offers wonderful instructional opportunities. There are at least three things any teacher can work on in regard to e-mail communication:

1. Etiquette
2. Clarity
3. Language development

Etiquette.   Respect for another human being's feelings is not always innate and needs to be taught. Just as a teacher needs to teach and reteach the etiquette of the school and social graces that can be used outside of school, appropriate behavior online is also important. Students should be reminded that profanity, threats, and harassment—which are easy to use online—are inappropriate and can be illegal.

Clarity.   Just as we teach the form of the business letter so too should we teach deaf students how to structure various forms of e-mail messages. In the same vein, presenting information via e-mail must be done in a manner that can be clearly understood by another person. To do this requires some essential language skills. E-mail is more interactive than other forms of print because of the speed at which responses can come back. However, e-mail can be a wonderful form of miscommunication as well. Teaching students how to present a request or how to lay out a description of a process or elaborate upon an argument are skills that can be used in e-mail.

Language Development.   A perusal of back issues of the *American Annals of the Deaf* yields an interesting look at a whole series of experiments with remote and realistic approaches to language development, particularly the early TTY communication experiments in language development. E-mail can provide the same kind of experience for deaf children who need to practice their written English in meaningful ways.

Sites are already available on the web where pen pals can be found. There are also schools for the deaf or other classes within public schools with large populations of deaf students who would be willing to become e-mail pen pals. Regular exchanges between a deaf and hearing peer can be a motivating and effective means for both learning English and developing friendships (Kluwin & Kelly, 1992).

World Wide Web.   Four general strategies can be used effectively to build the web into your teaching:

1. Internet workshop
2. Internet activity
3. Internet project
4. Internet inquiry

Internet Workshop.   The **Internet workshop** itself does not occur on the web, but instead the students meet in small groups or in other forms of classroom presentation to discuss the Internet. They do this by sharing what they have learned about the Internet, asking questions, or seeking information. In order to develop the search heuristics necessary to successfully navigate the net, students (and teachers) need to see examples of successful and unsuccessful strategies. To encourage participation, you can ask students to share their progress on a successful search and to describe a problem they are having. Emphasis needs to be on students describing what they have been doing. The exact form of students' presentations should vary from workshop to workshop to maintain interest as well as to suit your instructional goals.

Internet Activity.   With a little effort, you can locate sites on the Internet that will provide activities for your students such as data sources or virtual tours of museums. The **Internet activity** is a specific task that is assigned to make use of the sites. For example, children during the Holocaust produced various forms of art that have been preserved. An activity in conjunction with a unit on the Holocaust, World Wars, racism, or the like would have students locate these sites and respond about the content and quality of the work, how the work reflects the triumph of the human spirit in the face of great suffering, the outcomes of those young lives, and much more.

Internet Project.   An **Internet project** is a large-scale endeavor that makes use of web publishing and/or video display on web sites to create some other form of document. Students use the Internet as a resource where they gather information to include in a book report, a page in a journal, a short essay, or some other document. The information gathered could be text or video and could span the range of information that is available on the Internet. The Internet project is not just responsive, but creative as well. The goal is to build a web site or to create a presentation using other sites. The teacher defines the creative goal, which might be a web site, speech, term paper, brochure or something else. The student searches the web for materials to be included in the document, taking note that one of the benefits of the web is accessibility to images not found in books. Just as the students have to weigh the value of information from printed primary sources versus printed secondary sources, they need to learn how to evaluate sources on the web.

The American Library Association, the National Council of Teachers of English, and other professional organizations provide both print and web sites that describe criteria for students to use in evaluating web sites.

Internet Inquiry.   **Internet inquiry** focuses on the quality of the information on the web. A topic, such as the rise of the Sioux nation, is selected. Web sites and printed materials— including both primary and secondary sources—are searched. Baseline information is established for judging the material as being more or less accurate. Finally the material on the web is evaluated for its quality. For example, students might research the use of ghost shirts that were a part of the ghost dancing of the Plains Indians. Do written descriptions of witnesses from this time period match or differ from images picked up of the Internet? How representative are the images on the Internet? Generally, only the most unusual or most attractive appear in secondary source books because of the cost of printing, but Web sites often contain harder-to-find images.

Computer-Based Publishing

Computer-based publishing can typically be divided into electronic publishing and desktop publishing. **Electronic publishing** refers to the process of creating a document that will exist only in electronic form. A web site is an example of electronic publishing. **Desktop publishing** is the process of creating a document on a computer then printing a hard copy (i.e., paper copy) of the final document.

With respect to computer-based publishing the first question is what is going to be published? Or maybe more appropriately, why will something be published? The answer should fit in with our recurring themes of self-expression and authentic experience. The same issues and ideas we have presented elsewhere in this book about using realistic situations for writing as a way to motivate deaf students also apply to electronic and desktop publishing, which are more complicated than simple word processing.

Computers can be used to create reports or documents, print media, and web pages. *Reports* or *documents* are the bread-and-butter activities of academia and business. They refer to term papers, annual reports, research reports, and proposals of all kinds. The focus of the publication is to inform a limited audience about a topic in which they are already interested. The emphasis is on transmitting information as clearly as possible. *Print media* include publishing newspapers or magazines as well as advertising media such as flyers or brochures. In these kinds of publications the focus is on visual impact and persuasion as much as on conveying information. Color, visuals, and structure of the material are as important as the content. The print media move us into a world of layouts and images and an entirely new class of software in which both image and text become "objects" that are moved around the page. The old "paste-up" days of newspaper or magazine layouts are reproduced electronically, although the terminology—cut, copy, and paste—has remained the same. **Web pages** are the new form of electronic medium and range from straight information to pages that move and talk or even dance. It is a new and evolving form of communication with most of its concerns focused on technical issues or graphic design.

In essence, computer-based publishing is an idea as revolutionary as the invention of the printing press. Instead of being bound by an entire industry of writers, designers, and printers, a single individual can turn out his or her own publications.

Another important question is, who should publish? Following are some examples:

- English and language arts teachers can use desktop publishing as an opportunity to teach deaf children how to read and understand the various forms of print communication. The child who has made his or her own newspaper or advertisement will have a better appreciation of the forms of written persuasion in our society.

- Social studies teachers can use various forms of desktop publishing such as imaginary newspapers about historical events or brochures advertising the sale of land in the west or recruitment posters for the Crusades not only to teach the information, but to permit students to extend their imaginations and consider the alternatives if history had gone differently.

- Science presentations can be made more interesting and effective through better layouts. Graphs and charts do not have to be simple piles of lines or symbols but can use different forms of counting or include balloons to explain the significance of different parts of a chart.

- In Deaf studies, students can use both electronic and desktop printing as a means for informing others about their lives and various aspects of the Deaf community and the community of hard of hearing people, plus anything else related to deafness. This would be a unique publication that differs greatly from other school publications. It would also be an avenue for self-expression and could be used as a means for enhancing the self-esteem of deaf students.

Getting Started with Computer-Based Publishing.   The class newsletter is a practical starting point because it serves a real need and does not require a lot of writing. Another simple project to do is to have students prepare *family histories* that can include stories, old photos, and even copies of documents such as deeds or birth certificates. With a family history, there is no fixed layout or style requirement, which permits students to create documents that suit their visions of their own families and their histories. The added advantage is that there are lots of web resources for finding additional materials about families, which makes this a good candidate for a web inquiry project.

The *electronic scrapbook* is the same concept as any other scrapbook but, unlike the family history, which is a genealogy project, the scrapbook focuses on the student's current family and ongoing events. Again, there is no layout requirement, so students are free to design and redesign the layout.

The advantages of desktop publishers for these kinds of projects are cost, storage, and flexibility. There is no printing cost until you make a hard copy. No supplies are required beyond the software package. Storage is simple because students can save the entire body of material to a hard drive, a diskette or another medium like a CD or ZIP disk.

Flexibility provides several opportunities: Students can redo their layout or overall appearance of the document at any time. Or, if cousin Maude has the one and only copy of the picture of great uncle Cletus in his Grand Army of the Republic uniform, Maude can have an electronic copy made and share it with your student for inclusion in his or her electronic project.

The important point for you as a teacher is that before you try to do electronic publishing with your students, you need to do it yourself and become comfortable with the process.

General Planning for Using Technology

Morrison, Lowther, and DeMeulle (1999) use a planning model for integrating computers into a teacher's thinking. Figure 8.3 lists examples of database functions that are matched up with various learning tasks that are repeatedly taught throughout the school years.

1. *Decide what you are going to teach.* Your curriculum or a specific lesson objective is a good place to start. Use the computer to support your teaching. Do not bend your objective to fit the machine. With respect to incorporating a particular function of the computer, there are three primary options: word processing, spreadsheets, and databasing.

Learning Task	Database Function
Arrange	Arrange states.
Assemble, produce	Assemble information about your community.
Choose, select, categorize	Categorize a list of animals by their eating habits.
Classify, identify, isolate, list	List nineteenth century artists by type of work or preferred medium.
Collect, gather	Collect daily observations of almost anything in the environment (or of almost anything in the world using the Internet).
Combine, match, sequence	Match agricultural products with regions.
Compare, contrast, differentiate, discriminate, relate	Compare male and female reading preferences in your class.
Report	Report differences in types of environmental protection laws by country.
Solve, determine	Determine which state has the lowest costs of living and lowest crime rate.
Synthesize	Synthesize a list of foods by common elements.

FIGURE 8.3   Examples of matching a database function with a learning task.

In word processing, in which the skill seems to be in entering and manipulating text, you might want to focus on language skills related to language forms. Spreadsheets, on the other hand, are opportunities to explore mathematical relationships. A large part of a database project can take place away from the computer. Designing fields and collecting data might represent large amounts of time in the overall project. The goal could be either directly teaching about databasing or using the database as a way to organize information.

2. *Determine a manageable problem for the students.* A problem's manageability for your students depends on their developmental level, their level of computer literacy, and their access to information and equipment.

Younger children will not be able to look for subtle relationships among abstract ideas but can easily see the value in using a database to keep track of leaf types, endangered animals, or the physical characteristics of the students in the class. High school age students can database fairly complex or abstract information. In either case, the decision should be based on whether the students would understand the problem on paper. The same holds true for a spreadsheet problem.

The child's dexterity and his or her level of language sophistication are limiting factors in the use of word processing. The language factor especially can be a disincentive for deaf children to type. However, some software packages will let even very young children write simple sentences and then add pictures to the sentences to create storybooks. This is very motivating for deaf children.

3. *Determine the most important end product.* One way of determining the end product of a teaching activity is to ask whether you are teaching about the technology or are using the technology as a way to explore an idea.

If your goal is to teach about the concept of the technology such as using spreadsheets to keep track of a class trip's expenses, then your end product should emphasize the range of possible end products of a spreadsheet such as graphs as well as narratives. If your goal is to use the software to give scope to student expression like integrating images with text, then the text itself is more important than the possibilities of image manipulation. For example, using a single photograph as a background for a student-written haiku that will be printed and posted on the board is more appropriate than a more elaborate multimedia display. The greater the elaboration required in the image, the less time a student might have to developing the text.

4. *If necessary, make plans for grouping students.* You will have to decide whether your activity is an individual, paired, or small group project. Some considerations for deaf children will be related to language and communication skills. Other considerations might include the age of the children, the complexity of the topic, and the availability of the equipment and software. Basically, as children get older, the issue of the relationship of the complexity of the topic to the abilities of the children gets simpler. Further, the more access you have to equipment, the more you can move from group to individual projects.

5. *Decide upon an instructional format.* Your instructional goal will help determine the instructional format that you will use. In a database project, the goal might be to have the students compile a volume of information or for the students to understand the structure of the information. If the goal is to have students organize a large volume of data, it is probably simpler and more efficient for the teacher to provide an information structure and to send the students off to collect and record the data using a predesigned information entry form. If the goal is to have students learn about the complex structure of a body of information or to learn how to generate a classification system, then individual or small group work with guided discovery is probably a better approach.

6. *Plan what students will do prior to using the computer.* Experiential background or how much knowledge the students already have about the topic is the key here. With little background information, the students may have to conduct some research first.

In a social studies class students might be creating a database about American presidents. It would be helpful if the students have already learned several facts about a single American president. With this experience, they could brainstorm and create a list of information categories that will be applicable to all presidents. However, if the students were going to work in an entirely new area or in an extension of an already known area, they may require help or even be provided with an initial list of possible categories to use as fields.

Group discussion to brainstorm ideas or categories or resources can also be an essential part of the precomputer part of the process. Individual work with books or other forms of information gathering need to be considered prior to sitting down to work at the computer.

7. *Plan what students will do at the computer.* This is the main part of the instructional activity. According to your planning, students may be working alone, in pairs, or in a small group. Cooperative learning techniques, such as students taking turns entering the information as well as performing other computer tasks on a database project, fit in nicely with many activities using the computer.

Whatever approach is taken, a rough estimate of the amount of work has to be made by the teacher before the students begin. During this phase, the teacher needs to monitor working groups to make sure that the more computer-literate students do not dominate the process.

8. *Plan what the students will do after using the computer.* This is a critical point in your planning. There should be a clear connection among the lesson goal, the post-computer work time, and the project evaluation. It helps to ask questions about this phase and to refer back to previous steps to answer them. For instance, is the draft of an essay the goal? Will students append comments to each other's documents or will they mark up hard copies? At this point, activities such as databasing and creating a spreadsheet have been completed. Thus, the task at hand is to focus on preparation of the final product.

9. *Determine what supporting activities will be conducted by the students.* One type of supporting activity is to engage the students in cross-curriculum work. If, for example, the end product is a poster display related to a social studies objective, then a supporting activity might be strategies for reporting information in chart form as opposed to writing an essay. This is also the time to think about enrichment activities that will allow students the opportunity to go beyond the information that has been collected.

10. *List all resources needed for the activity and make arrangements to obtain them.* Resources will be needed such as appropriate hardware, software, information sources, and other classroom materials required to complete the project. You can use the table-making option in most word processing packages to create a table with those headings.

11. *Determine how the students will be evaluated.* When planning the evaluation, the first question to ask yourself might be: Why did you want the students to do the task in the first place? Tailor the evaluation to meet the objectives of the lesson. For instance, if the goal was to learn to assemble and organize information, then the complexity of the database should be graded. If the goal of the project was to generate information from the database, then the quantity of the information and the quality of the report are what should be evaluated.

In deciding on the evaluation to be used, note whether this is a new activity for the students. If so, then part of what they must learn is how to present their findings. Do not simply ask them to write a report or draw a graph. Students will need some direction as to the length and contents of a report. If they must graph their findings, you will need to provide specific directions on how to prepare the graph. Numerous examples of topically current graphs can be found in newspapers.

Instructional and Management Applications of Technology in the Classroom

The value of computers to the teacher extends beyond their instructional applications. Below we have briefly identified a number of these applications, all of which can be performed using any word processor.

IEP Management

There are at least two ways that computers can be used for managing IEPs. First, some firms offer specific IEP writing software that will permit a teacher to use a menu to select a behavioral goal after entering basic student information. The software then prints out the IEP for the teacher. Another way is to use a word processing program to create one's own IEP maintenance system. Basically, the electronic editing ability of the word processing software permits the teachers to "cut and paste" repetitive information.

Electronic Gradebooks

Like the IEP management software, there are software packages that will do grade books for teachers. In addition, by using spreadsheet, database, or even word processing software, it is possible to construct your own electronic gradebook.

Lesson Plans

Lesson plans can be done to a specific format using a word processor. Word processing formats for lesson plans are especially useful when you must leave a detailed plan for a substitute, when more than one person is involved in the planning of a lesson, or when you have to plan for several separate students within one lesson.

Student Groupings

In situations in which teachers are using cooperative or collaborative projects, database software is a convenient way to keep track of group membership or the completion of activities.

Seating Charts

Graphics packages can be used to create seating charts or room layouts. This would be helpful for those teachers who wish to design a classroom layout that will allow their students to easily move through learning centers or who desire a seating arrangement that allows all students to have eye contact with each other.

Communication with Other Teachers and with Parents

There are two primary forms and a third alternative form of the use of the computer for communicating with other teachers. First, standard communication and response forms can be stored on a word processor and printed out, or reports can be generated from databases. These are then sent around with the student or through the teacher's mailbox. Second, if the school has e-mail or the individual teachers have personal e-mail, an address book in the teacher's own e-mail system can be used for sending reports or inquiries. Third, a web site can be used as a system for posting nonsensitive information.

Mailings

Merging address lists with a body of a letter using a word processing program is probably the most common use of a computer for mailings. In addition, the system can be used to print envelopes.

Web Pages

Web pages can have several goals. One is to teach children about web pages just as we would teach them about reading novels or the newspaper. Another use of a web page is to display student work. In addition, web pages can be used as ways of communicating with parents or other teachers.

Labels and Tags

Word processing software enables teachers to produce name tags or folder labels quickly and easily.

Coupons

Many teachers use some form of token economy as a classroom management tool. Graphics and word processing software permit the making of a variety of rewards. One of the easiest ways is to use the label-making option on a standard sheet of paper. The paper could then be printed and the coupons cut out.

Certificates

Printing of various kinds of certificates is a form of classroom reward. Combined with some of the special papers now available for computer printers, teachers can generate very special rewards for children that can serve as extrinsic motivation for the students to achieve at a higher level. Certificates can also be used as a reward for appropriate behavior.

Conclusion

To end this chapter, we need to go back to the beginning of it and ask ourselves why should we, as teachers of the deaf, and regardless of the situation we might find ourselves in, be interested in teaching with technology. The best answer is that two things can be said about the future. First, whatever technology we use today, it will be different tomorrow. Second, however technology changes, students will have to have some human skills to use it. The forms and situations may be different, but the skills will remain the same.

For these two reasons, we as teachers need to recognize the essential skills that our deaf children will need in the future—such as self-discipline, respect, and clarity in communication—and adapt our teaching so that as those children encounter problems in new situations, they will be able to respond to them. Therefore, we need to focus on the skills that citizens in our society must have and the common and universal characteristics of the technology.

KEY WORDS AND CONCEPTS

database: A collection of related information such as names, dates, and so on that can be sorted and retrieved electronically.

desktop publishing: The process of creating a complete document on a single personal computer that includes writing (word processing), adding graphics (pictures), and printing the final document.

electronic publishing: The process of creating a complete document when the document will exist only in electronic form such as on a web site.

Internet activity: A specific project done by a single student related to a site or a general topic.

Internet project: A large-scale activity whose goal is the electronic publishing of the results of the activity.

Internet inquiry: An individual or small group search into a specific topic.

Internet workshops: When students meet in small groups to plan the search heuristics and other activities related to a web-based project.

spreadsheets: Programs that let you enter and manipulate data arranged in rows and columns like an electronic worksheet.

web pages: Electronic documents stored on a specific computer or server that can be accessed through a browser from any place in the world.

word processing: Software that permits the performance of editing tasks and the saving of revised documents electronically.

World Wide Web: The graphic component of the Internet, that is, a linked series of computers or servers that contain both still and motion pictures that can be accessed through a browser from any place in the world.

QUESTIONS

1. Why should you try to integrate technology into your teaching?

2. What do you think the difference is between "integrating" technology and simply using a computer?

3. What is the difference between teaching about technology and teaching with technology?

4. What are some of the more commonly used types of computer software? Provide examples of how they can be used.

5. Describe how software can be used to teach about using software and how it can be used to support instruction.

6. Describe a general planning process for using technology in the classroom.

7. What is the difference between using technology to teach children and using technology to support teaching? Are the same types of equipment or software used in both situations? If the same software or equipment is used, how are they used differently?

8. Identify some challenges that might occur when using technology to teach in a self-contained classroom or in a resource room or as an itinerant teacher? What strategies can you devise to resolve each challenge?

ACTIVITIES

1. You are responsible for designing a newsletter to be sent out to parents on a monthly basis. Develop a list of regular headings for the newsletter and provide a brief summary of what type of information would be included under each heading. Create an example of this newsletter.

2. Describe different types of information that could be placed in a database that you might create for each of the following categories:

    a. student biodemographic information
    b. student learning characteristics
    c. communication with the parents or families
    d. student achievement

3. Create a spreadsheet that monitors various aspects of the weather, and then fill in the information over a period of two weeks. Describe how this can be used in a unit plan about the weather for deaf students at the lower elementary level.

9

Testing Deaf Children

CHAPTER OUTCOMES

After reading this chapter, you should be able to:

1. Describe the difference between assessment, evaluation, and accountability.
2. Use basic terms related to testing.
3. Differentiate between norm-referenced versus criterion-referenced tests.
4. List the general characteristics of several kinds of tests commonly used in evaluating deaf students.
5. Assign grades that best reflect the learning goals for a deaf student.
6. Write your own tests using criteria that will help you measure performance or achievement that is related to the instructional goals.
7. Incorporate portfolio or performance-based assessment into your evaluation of student progress.

We begin our discussion of testing with a story about a deaf student for whom traditional testing was all wrong.

Why School Failed Jake.   One of the authors was a first-year teacher at a school for the deaf where he had a student in his homeroom period named Jake. Jake was a kind, easy-going kid in the twelfth grade. He had a country boy reputation that the teachers were keen to tell everybody about. For a time, that's what the author knew best about Jake. He was an only child whose parents lived about 500 miles north of the school on a dirt road that wandered deep into the woods. The author had never met Jake's parents, but he marveled at the parents' decision to take the best of what nature had to offer over the faster paced life in a crowded city. But Jake sitting in a concrete school in the city was not something to marvel at. He was an enigma and an all too familiar one at that. He was the deaf student that made you pause to think about what good, if any, that schooling had done for him after more than twelve years in the classroom.

Teachers in this school labeled Jake as being slow and had long given up trying to teach him basic academics. Science to him was filling in the blanks with words he didn't understand. Mathematics was a series of monotonous drills. Social studies was drawing maps. Language was underlining verbs and thumbing through second grade readers.

Then, of course, he was tested so teachers knew he was where he had been for the past five years or so. Neither he nor his teachers cared much about how well he did in school. As much as the author hated to admit it, in that first year he was as guilty as the other teachers, although he felt somewhat protected in that he only had him for homeroom period.

But Jake taught the author about testing. One day in November an older pick-up truck was parked in front of the school during the homeroom period. The author saw two people step out of the truck and start walking down the steps to the school building. Jake saw them too. He stood up and signed in American Sign Language (ASL),

MY MOM DAD. ONE-WEEK HOME ME GO. MOOSE HUNTING.

And off he went, leaving the author standing there with his eyes wide and his jaw hanging low.

He found out later that this was an annual ritual. He stiffened a bit at the thought of the whole week of school that Jake would miss. As if a week of school would make a difference. When Jake returned, the two of them had a long talk about his life in the country, and it turned out that his dad was a trapper. This was when Jake got excited. He rattled off the names of all the different animals he and his dad trapped. Beaver, mink, red squirrel, fox, and more. He dramatically described how they would make the traps and where they would lay them out. How they would skin some of the animals and eat the meat. How much they got for each pelt. He named creeks and hills that you couldn't find on most maps and outlined his passage through them in miles and hours. He talked about the berries they would find and the trout they would catch in the summer. The large extent of his vocabulary and his eloquent description of life as a trapper floored the author. The amount of science he knew about animals, edible foods, meadows, and forests was impressive.

This was the Jake that school ignored. School had never really measured what it was that Jake knew. It only tested what it was that he didn't learn.

Jake was a smart boy and what he needed was something that showed his talent to other people. Now, imagine a teacher who is able to spur Jake's interest by helping him use his real-world knowledge to learn about animal classifications (his knowledge of fur-bearing animals), plant life (his dependency on edible plants and knowledge of the forests for laying traps), and forces of nature (rain, snow, erosion, and other forces of nature that carved the creeks and rivers from which he drank and fished).

Imagine, too, a social studies teacher who uses Jake's experiences to talk about communities (city versus rural life), land development (the exploitation of open space for townships), the life of Native Americans and the pioneering efforts of early settlers (their dependency on the land and animals for subsistence), and the concept of money and trading (earning money to buy things or trading for things).

Let's add the mathematics teacher who uses Jake's experience with income from selling fur to discuss budgets and financial planning. This teacher could also have Jake do a presentation to the school about the cost and benefits of trapping as a means of earning a living. Then there's the language arts teacher who uses videotapes of Jake telling stories in ASL about his experiences as a trapper. The videotapes are then used to teach Jake how to translate these stories to English.

This type of teaching downplays the role of formal testing in favor of portfolio assessment as a means of capturing Jake's knowledge and skills. But even traditional test methods could prove beneficial if they were linked to Jake's expression of his real-life (i.e., authentic) experiences.

Different Types of Testing

There are three basic ways to look at testing as it relates to collecting and reporting information about a student (see Figure 9.1):

- Assessment
- Evaluation
- Accountability

Assessment means collecting information in a systematic way. **Evaluation** incorporates the concept of assessment but has the specific target of measuring progress or a student's rate of success. **Accountability** includes the concept of evaluation but adds the idea of responding to a specific audience or authority such as the students, parents, school board, and taxpayers.

These ideas about testing are nested within each other, and an example of this nesting can be illustrated using the State of Virginia's Standards of Learning or SOL. The SOL was established to define targets that students in Virginia are to meet at certain grades. In this respect, objectives or a set of criteria are formed that are used as the starting point for an assessment system.

The tests that the students take are the assessment component. All students across the state of Virginia are given the same test. For example, all eighth-grade students are tested in English competence while all fifth-grade students are tested in Virginia history. The assessment is the performance of children on the specific tests.

			Objective or standard of performance
		Assessment	Measurement is applied.
	Evaluation		Level of expected performance.
Accountability			Report to an audience.

FIGURE 9.1   Basic purposes for testing.

Evaluation includes the ideas of a standard, an assessment, and a level of expected performance. Schools in Virginia are evaluated on the basis of the number of children scoring a passing grade on each of the tests in each competency area.

Accountability takes the form of the state sending out "report cards" for each school to the parents. Since this is public information, it is also available to the media. The SOL is, in fact, a means of accountability for the teachers too: Are they teaching children what they need to know to pass these tests?

The Virginia SOL is not unique. Almost every state has an equivalent to the SOL or is in the process of developing one albeit using different names. In Michigan, for instance, it's called the Michigan Educational Assessment Program (MEAP).

Why We Test

In addition to evaluation purposes, which we discuss later in this chapter, we test children in educational programs for several reasons, including the following:

- To establish eligibility for services
- To determine appropriate placement in school
- To diagnose a problem
- To provide feedback
- To plan instruction

Eligibility

The first reason we assess children in special education is to determine if they are eligible to receive support services. Obviously, the initial assessment for the deaf child is the hearing test. Depending on input from the parents, medical professional, or other service providers within the school system, the deaf child can be assessed for additional disabilities as well. However, the child is assessed initially to establish eligibility for entrance into a deaf education program.

Placement

Placement means the place where instruction or another form of service to the deaf child will occur. It answers the question: Where will a deaf child be taught? The current interest in full inclusion (i.e., a school district's commitment to educating all children with a disability in a general education classroom with appropriate support) has not removed the issue of placement from the list of reasons for assessing deaf children. Oftentimes, assessment at this level is not simply looking at placement but also at the question of matching the deaf child to the available services. Let's look at a deaf child who is being considered for placement in a resource room setting. He or she will be assessed to determine the degree of support for a specific subject, such as mathematics or reading, that is required to support the child in the general education class.

Diagnosis of Problems

Some deaf children have additional disabilities. These children need to undergo specific testing to determine the nature and extent of their disabilities. The initial assessment is usually conducted at a "macro" level of diagnosis. That is, the assessment seeks to first determine the type of disability that might be present, such as a learning disability, specific visual impairments, or autism. Although this information is important, it is insufficient to help guide instructional planning for a student. Thus, another diagnosis must occur and this time at the "micro" level. At this level, the child might be tested because of a specific weakness in an academic area, such as the processing of algebra word problems or difficulties in reading comprehension.

Providing Feedback

Providing feedback is important because teachers need to know if instruction is successful and parents need to know about the progress of their deaf child. We will look at this issue when we look at grading and grading practices later in this chapter.

Planning Instruction

The Individualized Educational Plan (IEP) determines not only placement but also the details of instruction the deaf child will receive. IEPs are determined largely on the basis of assessment. IEPs in turn guide the development of instruction.

One example of assessment guiding instruction are state-mandated testing programs such as the New York State Regent's exam, the Maryland Functional tests, or the Virginia Standards of Learning tests. In these instances assessment may or may not have been intended to control instruction, but teachers trying to get classes to perform well often end up "teaching to the test."

A more benign use of assessment to guide instruction is to employ a test for diagnostic purposes and identify needed areas of instruction. The simplest form is a test like the ten-item spelling test. Words that students already know are dropped from the required list, and the words students do not know are drilled both as spelling and vocabulary items if necessary. A mathematics test that focuses on basic mathematical functions that need to be learned is another example of using a test to guide instruction.

A Few Words About Test Terminology

It is not our intention to provide a comprehensive overview of all terminology related to testing. As teachers, however, you are obligated to read assessment reports, many of which make use of these terms. We will, however, provide a brief description of the meaning and uses of the terms *validity*, *reliability*, *norm-referenced tests*, and *criterion-referenced* tests.

Validity

In its simplest terms, **validity** means measuring what we say we are trying to measure. Thus, a test is valid if it measures what it purports to measure. It is a flexible rather than an absolute concept in that it looks at the appropriateness of the measure for the situation to which it is applied. There are several types of validity.

Content validity is the "degree to which a sample of test items represent the content that the test is designed to measure" (Borg & Gall, 1989). Content validity is often confused with the term *face validity*, which is a subjective appraisal of what a test appears to be measuring. A person or group of people conducts the subjective appraisal of face validity, while content validity is determined through statistical analysis.

Concurrent validity covers the relationship between a new test we want to know about and similar established tests of the same domain or type of information. In other words, the validity is determined for the new test by comparative performance on a test with established validity. This type of validity gets its name from the fact that the new test and the established test are administered at the same time.

Reliability

Another word for **reliability** in testing is *consistency* or the idea that if you did it once, you can do it at the same level a second time. The reliability of a test tells us the stability of a measuring device over time. Like validity, there are several types of reliability. We can examine each of these types by framing them around the questions that they seek to answer.

Test-retest reliability. If a test is given this week and again next week will the students perform at the same level? This is also known as an estimate of test stability. *Internal consistency.* Will a particular subset of questions unduly influence performance? *Equivalence.* Can Form A of a test be given and get the same result as Form B? Equivalence is important when you have to frequently retest individuals such as on a pre- and posttest in an evaluation. It is also important to know the equivalence of various forms of a test if you are tracking achievement using a standardized test.

The important issue in reliability is the degree of consistency. Measures of consistency or reliability for test-retest purposes are generally given in the form of a correlation. The correlation itself is termed the *correlation coefficient* or the *reliability coefficient*. A test with poor reliability will have a coefficient that is close to zero. A test with high reliability will have a coefficient that is closer to 1.0. A zero obviously means that a test has no reliability at all. A coefficient of 1.0 will mean that a test has perfect reliability (see the box titled "Some Guidelines for Understanding Reliability").

The reason we can offer these general guidelines is that by squaring a correlation coefficient, we get the percentage of cases that are shared between the two data sets. Con-

---

Some Guidelines for Understanding Reliability

1. .85 to .9 and above: Suitable for individual testing, such as for making an individual placement decision.
2. .75 to .85: Suitable for evaluating or comparing groups of people, such as for evaluating the success of a program.
3. Below .75: Suitable only for research purposes.

sequently, a researcher might live with knowing that only half of his cases overlap (i.e., correlation coefficient = .7; percentage overlap = $.7 \times .7 = .49$ or 49%). A teacher making a placement decision, however, will want to know that the test being used will give the same result next week. In this case a coefficient of 0.9 might be acceptable (i.e., $0.9 \times 0.9 = .81$ or 81% of the time that the test is re-administered, the same result will occur).

Norm-Referenced versus Criterion-Referenced Tests

A **norm-referenced** test means that the measure of success is based on the performance of a group of individuals. This group of individuals is called the *norming group*. The norms for most standardized tests are determined from hearing children. Some norms for tests, such as the Stanford Achievement Test, are available for deaf children. Teachers do not develop their own norm-referenced tests. Instead, these tests are available commercially.

A **criterion-referenced** test means that the individual must meet a specific level of performance. This method is set more by the individual teacher and is the focus for evaluating many IEPs. For example, a mathematics teacher might decide that a student must correctly answer 80 percent of all factoring problems on a test before moving on to the next mathematical concept being taught in a sequence. Or a science teacher might require a student to correctly identify eleven out of fifteen indigenous plants in a region.

Norm-referenced versus criterion-referenced measures take on special significance when applied to deaf students. Some behaviors such as using the Internet to research the quality of a product or correctly filling out credit card application forms are necessary for functioning in society as competent adults. These are criterion-referenced measures. Other behaviors are measures of development, for example, a 10-year-old deaf child's knowing a certain number of words or having a certain degree of grammatical complexity in his or her utterances. These are norm-referenced behaviors.

With respect to norm-referenced measures, one challenge for the teacher of the deaf comes with the issue of *who is the norm for the deaf child*. Because of the chronic problem of the late identification of the deaf children's hearing loss, the delayed selection of an intervention program, and the late start of a program relative to the optimal age for language acquisition, deaf children may not meet the language development norms and knowledge domains of hearing children. Indeed, tests that are normed on hearing children might be biased against deaf children, given deaf children's life experiences and their opportunities and ability to talk about such experiences. Most tests, after all, are built on assumptions about the language levels and knowledge bases of the test taker and these may not reflect the true abilities of the deaf child as was the case with Jake.

Testing in Deaf Education

In the education of deaf children, we typically assess hearing, communication, and school achievement. The assessment of communication splits into the assessment of speech or hearing and sign language skills, depending upon the communication modalities that a deaf student is expected to use. We leave a discussion of hearing, speech, and sign language assessment to other texts. In this section, we focus on the assessment of academic achievement.

Academic Achievement: Reading

There are three classic ways to assess reading: multiple choice questions following the reading of a paragraph or a short passage, cloze procedures, and reading performance measures.

An example of multiple choice questions following the reading of a paragraph would be the various versions of the Stanford Achievement Test over the years. Multiple-choice reading tests should have moderate to high content validity because they use a standard measure such as a norm-referenced test. (*Note*: Multiple choice reading tests will have face validity if they are tests that the teacher developed.) They also tend to have good test-retest reliability for hearing populations, although special populations including deaf children will be less reliable in their performance. One of the main advantages of using the multiple choice reading test is its low cost, both in terms of test administration and test scoring. Group testing is possible, and machine scoring is frequently an option, thus significantly reducing costs.

A **cloze procedure** involves the modification of a text of at least 250 words by eliminating every fifth word and replacing it with a blank of a standard length. Deletions can occur less frequently, but they do not occur more frequently than every fifth word. The test subject then has to supply the missing word without any prompt. Cloze procedures emphasize prediction of content rather than comprehension. The original purpose for the cloze test was to measure the difficulty or reading level of different pieces of text. Since its introduction, the method has been expanded to include both measuring the reading comprehension of first language users and the language proficiency of second language learners. The cloze procedure offers classroom teachers a quick and simple assessment of the match between reading materials and student abilities.

There are two ways to score the cloze procedure. One type is verbatim scoring or the requirement that the exact word be supplied. The other is "acceptable alternate" scoring in which a word is accepted if it makes sense, given the grammar and the context of the word. Both methods yield nearly identical results in their ability to rank texts. Since the verbatim method is easier to score and reduces the problem of subjective scoring bias, it is preferred for hearing subjects; however, verbatim scoring may be too severe a standard for second language users. Cloze scores correlate with scores on multiple choice reading tests. In general, if a subject has a cloze score in the 44 to 57 percent range, then he or she is generally considered to have understood the text.

Cloze tests are easy for teachers to construct, quick to score, and represent a range of the skills required to interpret a passage. However, they do not necessarily measure constructs associated with reading comprehension such as questions that ask for things like picking out the main idea, recalling factual information, stating the author's purpose, or paraphrasing the content. One consideration is that the degree of match seen in hearing students between readability indices and performance on the cloze is not as stable among deaf subjects. In other words, cloze tests are less reliable measures with deaf students. Another problem for deaf students is that the 44 to 57 percent range for acceptable responses does not correlate with their multiple choice responding, but the reasons for this are difficult to interpret.

There are two kinds of *reading performance measures*. The first is the oral reading tests in which a child is given a passage and asked to read it aloud. Scoring is based on exact readings of the text. Repeatedly, these kinds of measures have been shown to present problems to users of nonstandard English. The usual problem is that a user of nonstandard English will substitute a dialect phrase for the exact wording of the text. The scorer is generally left with the decision to score the dialect phrase as wrong or to allow it as a substitution. If the dialect phrase is scored as wrong, the validity of the test for that group of speakers is called into question because the substitution may in fact reflect an understanding of the content and the grammar of the passage for that dialect user. If the scorer allows the substitution then the scoring reliability of these tests can suffer.

The obvious problem for the deaf child is that such a test can rapidly become a test of speech intelligibility, thus reducing the test's validity for this population. A solution to this problem has been in the form of story retellings. Story retelling is a form of performance measure in which the child reads a passage and then tells an adult viewer what was in the passage. Martha French's (1999) book *Starting with Assessment: A Developmental Approach to Deaf Children's Literacy* discusses the benefits of story retellings and provides an example of a checklist that teachers can use to grade a retelling. One benefit of story retelling is described by French in the following passage:

> Because the assessment of retelling has the children explain what they know in conversational language, it eliminates the possibility that competencies in writing, including motor skills, might influence the results. . . . Also, the procedure allows teachers to probe for more information and clarification. (p. 74)

Story retelling has moderate face validity as a measure of text comprehension but suffers from scoring reliability problems. Like the other kinds of performance measures, it requires an "on the fly" scoring that involves considerable training and practice to achieve reliable scoring. An alternative is to videotape the child's performance and to score the tapes at a later date. This adds considerably to the cost and time involved in scoring, thus making it a generally inappropriate classroom measure. A further difficulty is the general absence of test materials. Story retellings tend to be developed locally with local scoring protocols, thus there are no norms for comparing behavior with other groups.

Academic Achievement: Writing

There are three popular ways to assess writing skills: *surrogate skills*, *editing skills* or *grammar correction*, and *holistic* or *impressionistic scoring*.

Surrogate skills are the use of substitute measures that are components of writing skills such as spelling or vocabulary tests. There is a reasonably strong correlation between these kinds of tests and general composition skill. In other words, a child who does well in tests of spelling and vocabulary will typically be a good writer. Therefore, for a long time spelling and vocabulary tests were used in lieu of direct measures of writing. *Editing skills* or the ability to correct grammar (e.g., where a subject is asked to select the "right" form from among four options) has also been used because it reflects a skill in editing prose that also correlates with general composition skill. More recently, the Educational Testing Service as well as researchers at National Technical Institute for the Deaf and Gallaudet University have developed *holistic* or *impressionistic measures* of writing skills that have good validity and scoring reliability.

Surrogate Skills.   **Surrogate skills** tests have poor face validity because they are not direct measures of composition, but involve such subskills as spelling or vocabulary choice. They tend to have good test-retest reliability as well as good internal consistency because they can be developed from a large volume of material. This type of testing is becoming less popular as educators and researchers move to using impressionistic scoring of writing samples.

There are specific validity issues in the use of multiple choice surrogate skill tests with deaf children. Specifically, test development is often based on large samples of hearing children who tend to share similar vocabularies if they are users of standard English. Deaf children often have highly variable vocabularies because of their diverse language learning experiences. Consequently, the necessary linear correlations between vocabulary size or spelling knowledge and writing skills that are assumed in the development of these tests may not apply in the case of deaf children.

Editing Skills or Grammar Correction.   The Test of Syntactic Abilities (TSA) developed by Stephen Quigley and his associates at the University of Illinois is an example of an editing skills or grammar correction approach for measuring writing skills. In these kinds of tests, the child is presented with four choices and asked to select the grammatically appropriate option. These types of tests have low to moderate face validity in that children see examples of writing, but these are in essence editing tasks that are a subset of a larger set of skills involved in composing. Their appeal should lie in their lower cost due to ease of administration and scoring; however, in order to get test-retest reliability and internal consistency, it is necessary to have large numbers of items and multiple tests. Machine scoring is possible but testing is time-consuming for the children.

Impressionistic or Holistic Scoring.   The heart of the process of **impressionistic** or **holistic scoring** is the writing prompt or a scenario that states a problem or issue to be addressed, a likely audience to read the composition, and some parameters for the test taker to consider while writing. For example, sixth-grade students could be asked to write a letter to a teen magazine asking for a free poster of a music group. The use of prompts gives this kind of a test relatively high face validity. Internal consistency is not an issue because there is only a single "item": the writing prompt. Test-retest reliability is fairly good because of the constraints imposed by the prompt.

Test administration is as easy as any multiple choice test because the prompts can be given in large group settings; however, test scoring is an issue in general and for deaf students in particular. Scoring protocols or **rubrics** have been developed for these tests that, when used by trained scorers, produce reasonably consistent results. For the most part, scoring time is equivalent to reading time, making this type of testing less efficient than machine scoring but economically feasible. The problem lies in maintaining the reliability of the scorer and the consistency of the scoring from one scoring team or scoring session to another. Considerable scorer training is required.

The issue in the use of these procedures for deaf children is the familiar issue of norms. As performance tests, these procedures do not have norms per se; however, the scoring rubrics are built on assumptions about the writing skills of users of standard English at a certain age and developmental level. The practical problem in their use with deaf students is that deaf students tend to fall toward the bottom of the scoring rubrics that generally have four or five levels. Score differentiation for deaf students is very difficult with these kinds of procedures. Kluwin and Kelly (1992) reported that it is possible to modify these scoring rubrics in order to allow greater variation and to respond to the writing problems of deaf children.

Stanford Achievement Test

The most frequently used norm-referenced measure of deaf students' achievement in school is the Stanford Achievement Test. This test is typically administered only to students who are at least 8 years of age. The current version is the ninth edition and is referred to as the Stanford 9. It measures the abilities and skills of students in such areas as reading, language, spelling, mathematics, science, and social science. The test reflects the curriculum content commonly taught in grades one through nine throughout the United States. The Stanford 9 is available in eight difficulty levels that measure content considered appropriate for hearing students in specific grades in school. A screening test is available to determine placement of a student at a specific level of the test.

The Stanford 9 used with deaf students is identical to the Stanford Achievement Test used with hearing students in that test items and questions are exactly the same for both deaf and hearing students—a fact that many teachers, professionals in the field of deaf education, and parents do not know. However, the Stanford 9, in addition to having norms based on the performance of the students in the general population, also was normed on a sample of deaf students by the Gallaudet Research Institute, thus allowing performance of deaf students to be compared with achievement levels of deaf students as a group.

The subtests that are most commonly used with deaf students are Word Reading/Reading Vocabulary, Reading Comprehension, Mathematics: Problem Solving, Mathematics: Procedures, Spelling, and Language. The Stanford 9 provides various kinds of scores: raw scores, grade equivalent scores, scaled scores, and age-based percentile rankings.

Because of reading differences among deaf students at the same age, assigning the proper level of the Stanford 9 on the basis of age or grade in school is not a viable testing strategy. Instead, appropriate test levels for the Stanford 9 are selected through screening tests. The Gallaudet Research Institute has developed a booklet on the appropriate use of screening tests.

A serious limitation to the use of the Stanford 9 is that the test was designed to measure curriculum appropriate for hearing students in specific grades in school. Thus, there may be a question as to whether the content material was covered in the deaf student's curriculum. A further consideration is that some students may "top out." This will occur when a student is placed at a level that is below his or her capabilities. In this instance, the student should be retested at a higher Stanford 9 level. Also, some students are already performing at an academic level that is beyond the highest level measured by the Stanford 9, and therefore they should not be tested on it. A final limitation comes from the use of the same question forms that are in the test developed for hearing students. This may produce specific items or groups of items that may be biased against deaf students, thus giving them lower scores.

What States Are Asking for in Assessment Programs

There are two fundamental issues that impact deaf education in the face of state mandated testing: (1) the goals of the state testing system, and (2) how deaf students can be accommodated within that system.

State-based testing is not a new phenomenon because state-level testing has been around in some form for a long time (Airasian, 1987) with the classic example being the New York State Regent's Examinations. In the past, the emphasis on statewide testing was to gather comparative information about schools.

In recent years, with a greater call for accountability in public schools, states have entered into very active programs of requiring high school graduates and more recently, of specific grades, to achieve state-mandated levels of performance. Nearly all states have some form of mandatory testing in place or are setting up programs. This is a fundamental shift in U.S. public education in that previously states would develop curricula that would be used as models for local school programs to emulate; however, many states are now requiring student performance at a specific level—that is, they are creating a mandatory state-level curriculum.

These state testing systems tend to be criterion-based tests developed by state level committees based on objectives or standards of the statewide curriculum. Participation in these state-level committees can range from a heavy emphasis on the state educational bureaucracy working in conjunction with local teachers as test writers to a committee consisting of a large component of individuals from outside the usual school community.

State testing systems often show greater variety in test items than commercial tests because of the different goals of the testing programs. Whereas most commercial standardized tests are primarily multiple choice, most state-based tests will include essay and open-ended questions. Some state testing programs require performance assessments such as oral reading or problem solving.

Goals for state testing can take many forms and be administered at different grade levels in the core subject areas of mathematics, language arts, social studies, and science. Whatever form a test might take, results, along with information about pupil attendance and retention, are used in a reward and sanction system for school districts. Some forms of statewide testing are based on specific learning outcomes for high school graduation. Failure to achieve at a particular level can result in a school losing accreditation and being taken over by the state.

All of these systems are driven by a similar set of concerns: the perceived or actual failure of schools to produce students who are competitive in a global economy or the failure to produce moral and educated citizens. Somewhere in the middle of all of this are school professionals who would like to see better schools and are looking for mechanisms to achieve school reform.

Where does the education of deaf students fit into this overall picture? The answer to that question will be very specific to an individual deaf student. For example, in Virginia, deaf students in general education classes must take and pass the state-mandated tests with their hearing peers. The responsibility for performance falls not only on the individual child but on the school as well. On the other hand, deaf students in special schools or in separate programs do not have to participate. The program is still new and once it is fully in place only students passing the high school level tests—Standards of Learning—will be given a diploma. Thus, deaf students in all types of educational placements will eventually have to pass the tests, or they will not receive high school diplomas.

Accommodations for Students in State-Mandated Testing

Elliot, Kratochwill, and Schulte (1998) identified eight possible accommodations to state testing formats for students with disabilities. Using these categories, we have developed the following list of accommodations that are specific for deaf children.

1. *Clarification of purpose.* Explain to the student why he or she is taking the test. For all students, deaf and hearing alike, these kinds of tests are a source of confusion and misunderstanding. Understanding what a test is about may make the student feel more comfortable about taking the test. A desire to do well will produce better results than fear.

2. *Assistance prior to testing.* Communicate not only the belief that the student will succeed but any additional test-taking skills as well. Explain what parts of the test will be similar to experiences the student already has and teach him or her any new forms of test taking.

3. *Scheduling.* Setting up a sequence or timing of the tests outside of the regular schedule may be necessary when dealing with deaf students with multiple disabilities. For other deaf students, it may be necessary to schedule longer or simply open-ended time frames because of the necessity to respond to individual problems during testing.

4. *Setting.* For deaf students, this accommodation will generally involve the assurance of the presence and coordination of interpreting or real-time captioning services. Also, because of language considerations, the interpreter needs to work with the testing staff prior to the event so that he or she can present the material to the student in a manner both appropriate to the student's abilities and to the original intent of the test.

5. *Directions.* This is a balancing act between communicating the original intent of the test and giving away an answer. If the written directions are unusually elaborate or new, deaf students may need the directions interpreted for them. For the most part, this can be dealt with by careful preparation of the student before administering the test.

6. *Assistance during testing.* If examination of the test items is not possible prior to the testing situation, it may be necessary to provide assistance for particular questions during testing. Because of the smaller sample pools available for development of state-level testing, there will be a greater potential for biasing items. Assisting deaf students during testing periods may be the only solution. A quick check in this situation is to ask a student to explain what a question means to him or her.

7. *Support services during the testing.* This typically takes the form of a providing a deaf student with a trained and, preferably, certified interpreter.

8. *Format and content changes.* The common problem to be encountered is that a test-writing bias will show up in the test. The quick solution is to try to rephrase the item for the student; however, that may not be possible without altering the intent of the question. Requesting practice or example items prior to testing will assist the deaf education specialist in supporting the deaf student during testing.

Grading

Evaluation or testing to see how well a student is learning is an inescapable fact of teaching. We give tests and grade papers because they give us a score on how well students are progressing, which is, in part, a reflection of how well we have taught a subject. We measure in the *cognitive* domain looking for mastery of concepts and facts, rules, and principles; in the *psychomotor* domain for motor skills relating to the ability to conduct experiments and to make measurements; and in the *affective* domain for students' attention to lessons, their beliefs about science, and their attitudes towards it.

We assign percentages and letter grades based on our evaluation and write a few words about a student's overall performance in a subject on their report cards. But what a "B" on a report card really tells a student or a parent is a question that you as a teacher must constantly ask yourself. For our purpose, we are content to state that tests and their accompanying grades are just one part of the total assessment of a student's performance.

We use grades in the classroom to monitor a student's progress, to motivate students, to provide guidance to the student, and for administrative purposes.

- *Monitor progress.* Everyone wants to know how well students are doing in school. The first purpose for grades is to provide information to the student and to the student's parents about the student's progress in learning.
- *Motivate students.* Grades typically carry intrinsic rewards (e.g., good grades give students a sense of accomplishment) and extrinsic rewards (e.g., free cheeseburger, TV privileges). Both sets of rewards can motivate students to do well or to try harder.
- *Provide guidance.* Effective grading systems can give direction to the efforts of the student. If he or she is doing well in one subject and not in another, or if a subject that was under control at one point is slipping now, the student and his or her parents have the opportunity to adjust the direction and level of effort.
- *Administrative purposes.* One obvious administrative purpose is to determine who should move on and who should continue to receive more instruction in an area. Who is working up to his or her potential and who is falling behind and needs additional attention? What do you need to cover in more depth and what do the children seem to understand? Just as grades give the individual student an opportunity to monitor individual progress, grades can give the teacher the opportunity to monitor the progress of a class as a whole. For example, if too many students are getting a "D" or below on a quiz or an assignment then this might suggest that material needs to be retaught, that the teacher needs to reevaluate his or her instruction, or that some form of motivation needs to be added to the learning process.

Grading is difficult, time-consuming, and requires considerable mental and emotional effort. It is difficult because of the need for justice, the inherent subjectivity of grading, and the absence of uniform standards. Teaching, like parenting, offers conflicting challenges. The teacher wants to nurture but also has to discipline. When it comes to giving a grade, a teacher will want to reward any effort but must honestly reflect what has occurred. Teachers need to encourage but at the same time they have to rein in errors. If this does not occur, then the teacher is in danger of not giving the student the feedback he or she needs to improve and to learn.

Most grades are calculated using objective criteria. However, eventually individual teacher decisions will enter into the grading process. This is the inherent subjectivity of a grade. Many subjects involve making decisions about multifaceted assignments. The English teacher who reads the beautiful description written in battered grammar. The social studies teacher who sees a flight of intellect and perceptiveness across a page totally unsupported by facts. The mathematics teacher seeing the carefully worked out problem that misses the right answer by a simple computational error. The teacher has to make the call and assign a grade that will reward the effort shown and encourage better work in the future.

For deaf students who are in a general education class, grading becomes more complicated if these students are unable to maintain either the pace or the quality of the work of their peers. For these students, special adjustments to the grading policy in the class are necessary if the efforts of the rest of the class are to be respected while giving the deaf student a chance to compete. The teacher has several options in which to do this:

- *Contract grading.* Like the name suggests, the student and the teacher agree upon what will be graded. The contract specifies the type, quantity, and quality of the work to be done. Each student has a separate contract with unique terms.
- *IEP grading.* The IEP itself sets the standard for the grade. A grade is assigned based on the percentage of completion of the IEP goals. This is a form of criterion-based grading.
- *Multiple grading.* The grading unit is divided into various components such as effort, participation, achievement, and progress. The student is graded separately on each part. Thus a student who only learns a portion of the material might get a "C" for progress but a "B" for effort and participation. Such an approach permits a more detailed description of a student's progress.
- *Level grading.* There are two parts to level grading. The first part is a letter grade (i.e., A, B, C, etc.) that indicates the student's progress or achievement on a portion of the curriculum. The second part of the grade is typically numerical (i.e., 1, 2, 3, etc.) that indicates the difficulty level of the work done.
- *Narrative grading.* The teacher does not assign a numerical or letter grade but writes a substantial description of what the child has accomplished, including the child's weaknesses or strengths based on the teacher's observations.

Grading Issues in Different Situations

Although most teachers face the same issues when grading, there are some issues that are of particular importance in relation to a specific setting. Examples of some of the grading issues as they relate to various educational settings are provided in Figure 9.2. Note that for the itinerant teacher or teacher consultant, grades will generally not be an issue because this

	Self-Contained	**Resource Room**	**Team Teaching**
Monitor Progress	• Effectiveness of instruction • Inform parents	• Effectiveness of instruction • Inform parents	• Negotiated process
Provide Guidance	• Criterion-based	• Criterion-based • Norm-referenced	• Criterion-based • Norm-referenced
Administrative Purposes	• Promotion • Curriculum coverage	• Promotion • Placement	• Promotion • Program evaluation • Curriculum coverage

FIGURE 9.2   **Examples of grading issues in different educational settings.**

type of teacher usually has a consulting role in relation to the student and the general education teacher and not one of direct instruction. Consequently, she or he is not likely to assign grades for work.

When it comes to monitoring student progress, both the resource room teacher and the self-contained teacher (including teachers of the deaf who teach in a school for the deaf) will want to evaluate the effectiveness of their instruction as well as inform parents of the children's progress. For the team teachers, the challenge is grading for a class of deaf and hearing students, and grades will typically be a negotiated process. One consideration will be the pace at which a deaf student is progressing through the curriculum. A second consideration will be the standards that will be applied to each group of students. The general education teacher will want to keep everyone moving along at the pace required by the school district or by state goals. The teacher of the deaf will have to negotiate either a reduced set of expectations for the deaf students or will have to negotiate a more flexible system for grading.

In the resource room and the team-teaching situation, there are always two possible baselines to use for computing grades: a baseline derived from the standards of the general education students or a baseline applicable to the deaf students. Consequently, in these situations the application of a mix of criteria can be expected.

Sometimes specific performance criteria will be needed to be applied as in the case of preparing all students to take state competency tests. This type of consideration will likely become more critical as states move progressively toward not only mandating that all students take state competency examinations but also toward using performance on these examinations to award high school diplomas. Will special education students be held to the same standard?

At other times, normative criteria might be applied. For example, if the decision is to be made to continue the placement of a deaf student in a particular educational setting, then the deaf student's behavior vis-à-vis the hearing peers should be considered.

	Self-Contained	Resource Room	Team Teaching
Contract Grading	Motivate deaf students who lack interest or discipline under conventional means		
IEP Grading		Address specific needs of deaf student	
Multiple Grading			Respond to curriculum pace
Level Grading			Respond to curriculum content
Narrative Grading		As a consultant who works one-on-one with deaf students	

FIGURE 9.3   Examples of strategies for grading deaf students in different educational settings.

Student promotion is a concern when it comes to grading regardless of the placement situation. For the self-contained class and the team-teaching situation, rate of curriculum coverage determines success not only of each individual student but of the success of the teacher as well. In team-teaching situations, student progress is an important consideration in continuing the practice of team-teaching itself.

We earlier listed several alternatives to conventional grading systems. Figure 9.3 contains suggestions as to where each type of grading system might fit.

Portfolio Assessment

Portfolios are a form of performance assessment, and there can be some confusion in the use of the term *performance assessment* because in practice there are at least three meanings of performance:

1. Motor demonstration
2. Product manufacture
3. Action with an authentic performance

Motor demonstration means that a person shows how to do something and is typically the way we test in physical education. Examples of motor performance measures are walking a balance beam, throwing a ball, catching, and so forth. An example of how motor performance can be used in the evaluation of students' fitness levels is found in Chapter 7. *Product manufacture* can range from writing an essay to carving wood. When we look at creative writing, there is a tendency to focus more on the product, although the process can be assessed as well.

The third use of the term, or the "authentic" performance, is one in which the emphasis is on producing in school or through a school activity something that has a value or place in the real world. The freshman essay has little use outside of the classroom but a letter of inquiry to the telephone company does. To use a letter of inquiry in an assessment would be an example of an authentic performance. For most situations in which a student can engage in authentic performance, we can generate a school product. It is this overlap that has produced some of the confusion in school use of portfolios as collections of performance.

Figure 9.4 illustrates various types of performance measurements and the level of intellectual engagement each requires. There is a tendency for the nature of the response to control the level of intellectual engagement. Simple selections tend to generate only knowledge-level responses while authentic performances reach into the area of synthesis. Assessments that require the student only to supply information tend to be only comprehension- or application-level responses. Asking the student to generate a product can span from an application to a synthesis level activity depending on the complexity of the action.

Another way to think about portfolios is to look at them as being road markers, mirrors, and repositories. As *road markers*, portfolios permit students, parents, and teachers the opportunity to track the student's progress throughout the year by giving the student a clear set of reference points. The portfolio gives the student the opportunity to look back and reflect not only on the development of his or her work but on the nature of what is a good performance. As a *mirror*, the portfolio gives the student a chance to reflect on his or her work, thus involving the student in his or her own learning. As a *repository*, the portfolio contains the work of the student. In a classroom in which paper goes in, comes out, and is discarded, it is more difficult for the student to see how what he or she has done relates to his or her learning. Also, as a repository, the portfolio is a concrete example of student progress or lack thereof, thus providing an excellent starting place for a parent conference.

A portfolio contains more than random assignments or collections of paper; it also contains specific examples of selected pieces of work along the lines of the artist's portfolio. A portfolio will show not only the student's best work but typical work as well. Products of group activities and works in progress such as drafts can also be included. A successful portfolio will contain materials selected with the usual rules for good assessment: a clear purpose, appropriate performance criteria, suitable setting, and the scoring protocol.

Determining the purpose of the portfolio occurs in advance of the selection of materials. Things will go into the portfolio narrowly because the goal is to address one aspect of learning, such as following the progress in written drafts of an essay, or it will have a variety of materials drawn at wide spaces during the year because the goal is to show overall

	Simple Selections	Supplying Information	Generating A Product	Authentic Performance
Synthesis			Write a business letter.	Send a letter of inquiry.
Analysis			A speech (videotaped for inclusion in a portfolio).	Engage in a debate.
Application		Short answers	Create an exhibit (e.g., science).	Conduct an experiment.
Comprehension		Labeling		Explain to a another group of students a concept or a topic that was learned in class (e.g., growth of industries and urban areas).
Knowledge	Multiple choice test True/false test Matching items			Answering questions during an exhibit or class presentation.

FIGURE 9.4   Examples of different types of performance measurements for various types of intellectual engagement.

improvement. At the same time, it is important to have some latitude for student selection of materials to increase the student's sense of ownership of the portfolio.

To avoid "mystic" grading, specific criteria for success need to be specified in advance. Part of the process of learning for the student is not simply to learn the material but to learn how to successfully complete the material. As teachers, we want the child also to be able to transfer the learning in one area into another. If the student does not have a clear idea about how he or she has succeeded, then the learning of the overall heuristic and the ability to transfer the learning to another situation is lost. Finally, it is simply not fair to not tell the student what needs to be done to be successful. In our discussion of science in

Chapter 2, we provide a detailed description of how portfolio assessment can be applied to a science unit about "How plants grow."

Conclusion

What makes testing difficult for many teachers is that it deals with numbers and technical concepts while seeming so impersonal. It has the aura of "science" about it. Further complicating the problem is the frequent use of testing to evaluate teachers or programs when the tests do not seem to match the goals of the teacher. This chapter can help you as a teacher if you start with simple questions and work toward more complex ones, asking yourself, for instance, questions like:

- What am I trying to accomplish?
- What do I need to know about my students?
- Does this test fairly measure what my students know?
- How can I communicate to the students and their parents important information like what needs to be worked on and what is succeeding?

If you start at that level, technical concepts like validity become simply the match between what you are trying to teach and what the test measures. For example, writing behavioral objectives is now a well-established tradition in special education, but it was a new idea when one of the authors started teaching. Fitting his lofty goals for his classes into the seeming straitjacket of the objectives was an awkward burden. However, he found that the process also imposed a great deal of discipline on his thinking about what to teach and why he was teaching it. Responding to the demands placed on your teaching by testing programs need not be a threat. Therefore, look at what is being asked of your students, make reasonable accommodations, and try your best to get as many to succeed as you can.

At the same time, think about grading as not a process of sorting out the winners from the losers but as a way to communicate information about progress and to define new goals. Doing a good job at grading is never easy even for experienced teachers, but it gets better the more you work at it. More importantly, it gets better the more you think about what you are trying to accomplish.

KEY WORDS AND CONCEPTS

accountability: Conducting an evaluation and reporting it to a specific audience.

assessment: Generally, to collect information in a systematic way.

cloze procedure: A method of testing reading skills. It involves the modification of a text of at least 250 words by eliminating every fifth word and replacing it with a blank of a standard length.

criterion-referenced: A test whereby the individual must perform a specific set of actions. This type of test is the one that teachers tend to create.

evaluation: Incorporation of the concept of assessment but with the specific target of measuring progress or a student's rate of success.

impressionistic scoring: Also referred to as **holistic scoring**, an assessment of writing skills and generally involves giving the student a prompt (e.g., a scenario to write about) to stimulate the writing and an audience to whom the student is to write.

norm-referenced: A measure of success based on the performance of a group of individuals called the *norming group*. Norm-referenced tests are typically developed by a company or a educational research institute because of the high costs involved in testing a large number of students representing the norming group.

reliability: A concept related to the notion of consistency in testing. There are different types of reliability such as test-retest reliability, internal reliability, and equivalence.

rubrics: Another name for scoring protocols. These are scoring procedures for controlling scores during impressionistic scoring.

surrogate skills: A method of assessing writing skills. It uses substitute measures that are components of writing skills such as spelling or vocabulary tests as a means of assessing a person's overall writing skills.

validity: A concept related to the appropriateness of a test for the situation to which it is applied. For example, when we say that a test is valid we are saying that the test measures what it is supposed to measure. There are different types of validity including content validity, concurrent validity, and face validity.

QUESTIONS

1. Describe the meaning of the terms *assessment*, *evaluation*, and *accountability*.

2. Give an example of how a teacher of the deaf might use assessment and evaluation techniques in her or his class.

3. What do the terms *validity* and *reliability* mean? Describe why teachers should know about the meaning of these terms.

4. What are the differences between norm-referenced and criterion-referenced tests?

5. What are three ways by which reading can be assessed?

6. What are three ways by which writing can be assessed?

7. What are some of the advantages for using the Stanford Achievement Test with deaf students?

8. How can you assist a deaf student who has to take a state-mandated proficiency test?

9. What are some considerations when assigning grades for students' work?

10. What does portfolio assessment mean?

11. What are some reasons that portfolio assessment might be good to use with deaf students?

ACTIVITIES

1. If your state has state competency examinations for school age students, contact three local school districts and one school for the deaf and ask about the following:

   a. Whether the examinations are mandatory for deaf and more generally, special education students
   b. The criteria for exemption from taking the test
   c. The accommodations, if any, that can be made for deaf students taking the examinations

2. Contact several self-contained programs for deaf students, including schools for the deaf and ask what types of achievement tests are regularly administered to deaf students at the elementary, middle, and high school levels. If available, obtain a list of criteria by which a deaf student can be exempted from taking one of these tests.

3. Contact a teacher of the deaf whose students take the Stanford Achievement Test and inquire about the following:

   a. How are deaf students placed at a particular test level?
   b. Who administers and scores the Stanford Achievement Test?
   c. Do students' Stanford Achievement Test scores have any influence on instruction and if so, what is the influence?

4. Through discussions with preservice teachers of the deaf, teachers of the deaf, parents, and/or special education administrators, make a list of the merits and disadvantages of having deaf students take statewide mandated achievement tests.

10 Transition

CHAPTER OUTCOMES

After reading this chapter, you should be able to:

1. Use the IEP process to design a plan that takes into account the unique transition needs of a deaf student.
2. Incorporate employment-related activities into a transition plan.
3. Devise a plan for actively involving the deaf student in the transition planning process.
4. Involve the state rehabilitation counselor in the planning and implementation of a student transition plan and use this counselor as a resource person.
5. Make appropriate preparations for transition planning before, during, and after an IEP.
6. Make use of a variety of resources to assist in the planning and implementation of a transition plan.

This is a true story about Roy, and it is one that needs to be told over and over so that teachers realize that **transition** can and does work.

Roy was a 16-year-old deaf student going to a school for the deaf. He had a first-grade reading level, his math skills were at the basic addition and subtraction level, and he was just breaking ground with carryovers and borrowing. He had been in ten different foster homes since he was 4 years old. Everyone knew Roy, and everyone had a story to tell about him. Teachers and teacher aides, deaf and hearing people. And none of the stories were flattering—most were downright amazing for the suffering and injustices that the school had inflicted upon him. Yet few people had empathy for him and the staff's greatest wish was that he would leave school early. Roy did not endear himself to anyone either. So each year at school was more of the same ol', same ol' for Roy.

Roy was one of the school's best success stories. Except for one teacher in his turn-around year (i.e., the year a transition program was established for him), and perhaps a couple of other people, no one had held out any hope for him. But Roy was a success because of a decision to implement a transition program for him at a time when transitional planning was just trying to gain legitimacy in schools. After having Roy for one year when he was

16 years old, a teacher decided that the school spent too much time on academics and did little to prepare Roy for life when he left school.

The teacher started talking to Roy about school and work. Roy had no idea what he wanted to do or even what was available for him to do. They talked about the difference between welfare and earning a living, and even then Roy had a hard time seeing the benefits of working when money was there for the asking. But he did say that he would rather be doing something like work rather than going to school every day. He didn't see the point of school now that only a couple of years of schooling were left for him.

The teacher met with the school counselor, and it was decided that next year Roy would be placed in a work experience program. The counselor found a place near the airport that packaged meals for a large passenger airline. He took Roy to see the place and Roy agreed to give it a try. Every morning, Roy would pack a lunch and catch a bus to this workplace. There he would put in a half-day's work before catching another bus to take him to school. After a while, he started getting a small amount of money as a token for the work he did. This gave him encouragement to continue. When he left school at the age of 18 years, he went straight to this food service company to work.

At the beginning of the work experience, the school counselor served as Roy's job coach and interpreter. As part of his job coaching responsibility he agreed to take the bus with Roy for the first week. At the end of this week, the counselor reduced the amount of time he spent with Roy to just once a week for about thirty minutes. He got to know Roy's supervisor, who was also the person responsible for approving the initial placement. When it became obvious that Roy was having a positive work experience, the counselor struck a verbal agreement with the supervisor to bring other deaf students for work experiences. This relationship between the school and the company packaging meals for an airline continued for several years, coming to an end only after the counselor left his job and moved to a different school for the deaf.

Eight years later the teacher met Roy at a deaf softball tournament. Roy kept it simple. He said the money was good, and he hardly ever missed a day's work. The teacher did some mental calculation and figured out that no one else from Roy's graduating class had been able to stay employed for this long. For that matter, about two-thirds of the group had spent the better part of their eight years following graduation out of work. They were young and healthy but aimless as they strode through their early years of adulthood. None of the others had been involved in a work experience program. None of them had had a transition plan while in school. So the boy who was not meant to succeed did, while many of his fellow students who had far more emotional stability in their lives and had achieved higher academic levels struggled to become gainfully employed.

Now think of a few high school deaf students you know. Think about their present path through the corridors of their education program. Are they being well prepared for life after school? If so, what is the school doing to make you think this? If not, what changes would you make to better transit these students from school to work?

Transition and the Deaf Student

At the turn of the nineteenth century, schools for the deaf prepared their students to get a job. Perhaps a few students went on to college but the vast majority graduated fully expecting to walk into a workplace and start earning a paycheck. Consider the following survey results:

> In 1893 the Ohio School for the Deaf reported that 62 of its graduates were type compositors, 152 were farmers, 31 were shoemakers, 29 laborers, 27 shoe factory workers, 25 teachers, 3 principals, and 17 bookbinders. The list also included 5 professional baseball players, a card writer, a coal dealer, a deputy recorder, 3 editors, 2 grocers, and a horse dealer. Five were listed as peddlers, probably salesmen. One was a postmaster, 2 were portrait painters, 1 was a railroad foreman, 1 a saloon-keeper, and another was a ship builder. (Gannon, 1981, p. 82)

Note how many of these graduates were working in print shops. This was not unusual because most schools for the deaf had a print shop as part of their vocational education program. Indeed, it would not be surprising to learn that nearly every school for the deaf had a linotype printing machine in their shop until the early 1970s.

These schools also taught farming, shoe repair, carpentry, sewing, barbering, metal work, welding, automotive repair, and many other types of manual labor jobs. They tended to teach skills that matched the jobs that were available. For example, the Michigan School for the Deaf (MSD) is only a stone's throw away from a large General Motors car manufacturing plant. For years it had a tool and dye shop that gave its graduates an advantage over students graduating from public schools. The public school students had to attend a vocational school after graduation to learn about the tool and dye trade before they could take a job in an automobile factory. The MSD graduates, diploma in hand, simply walked the half-mile down the road to the GM employment office and began work. At least until recently. (See Box titled "Transition: A Nostalgic Trip" for further insight about how schools for the deaf used to prepare students for the workforce.)

Today's labor market has been shaped by significant technological changes that have occurred over the past thirty years. The market is highly diversified, and it's virtually

Transition: A Nostalgic Trip

The superintendent's house at the Michigan School for the Deaf is a beautiful historic site. The intricately carved banister is breathtaking when one considers that such work today would cost a small fortune and only if you were lucky enough to find someone with the skills to do it. The wall and hall cabinets are works of art. Time, skill, sweat, and care went into each and every piece of handmade furniture in this house. There is a wooden floor throughout the house as well as on the stairwell to the second floor. In each room the pattern of the wood is different. Nothing is in disrepair. You leave the house marveling at its quality and speechless at the thought that no power tools were used to build any component of the house. You see, power tools were not around at that time. You might even leave depressed at the thought of walking back into your house, which was built with all of today's electrical conveniences but none of yesterday's craftsmanship. The superintendent's house was built in the 1890s by the deaf students enrolled in the school. The skills these students learned building this house prepared them for a vocation once they left school. At graduation they were ready to become carpenters, wood craftsmen, cabinet makers, furniture makers, wood floor layers, house builders, construction workers, and roofers. This was how transition planning took place back then.

impossible for a school to prepare students with the skills needed to immediately obtain employment in the way they used to do it. The nature of jobs is changing, too, as computers are displacing workers in many industries, and the service industry has become one of the fastest-growing industries, offering many different types of career opportunities. Another trend is that more and more jobs require education and training beyond high school. The days of when a grade-ten education would get a person into the police force are gone. Some police officers now study criminal science in universities. Clearly, a high school diploma is no longer a ticket to a well-paying job.

The face of the workforce undergoes changes rapidly, requiring workers to get additional education and more training as they progress through their careers. This is one of the reasons why schools should be preparing students for lifelong learning. Even professionals in the field of law, medicine, teaching, and audiology who are assured of a good future are faced with going back to school at some point in their careers in order to keep abreast of changes in their field that directly affect their ability to perform their jobs. Plumbers, electricians, mechanics, and hair stylists all require intense in-school training and apprenticeships. Hair stylists, too? Think about allergies to shampoo and dye colors and all of the chemicals that go into the hundreds of hair products on the market. Think, too, of the alert consumer and litigation. Just cutting hair no longer cuts it any more.

So what have schools been doing about the changes in the world of work? Schools for the deaf were among the first educational institutions to offer vocational education programs (Gannon, 1981). Then through the early and middle part of the twentieth century, vocational education became a standard part of programming in public schools. Now, with the rapid changes in career opportunities, schools tend to send their students to skills centers or centralized vocational centers run by a Local Education Agency (LEA). This centralization forces LEAs to keep up with changes in job demands and to offer a wide selection of career opportunities. In the meantime, it has not been financially feasible nor practical for schools for the deaf to provide a comprehensive vocational education program. Therefore, they too now tend to send their students to a LEA-controlled skills centers.

To adapt to these changes, deaf education programs have to focus on getting their students ready for postsecondary education and training rather than for a job per se. For deaf students this is important because deaf people experience higher unemployment and underemployment than their hearing counterparts (Christiansen & Barnartt, 1987). This is the case for all people with disabilities. This is why the federal government enacted such laws as the Individuals with Disabilities Education Act and the Americans with Disabilities Act to ensure that students with disabilities have access to a quality education and to the job market.

Getting a job requires a lot of time and effort. Transition planning is now a critical component of a student's education. Furthermore, transition planning must not be mistaken as a way of finding work only for low-functioning deaf students or deaf students with severe disabilities. Transition is just as important for deaf students planning to go on to a college.

What Is Transition?

The Individuals with Disabilities Education Act (IDEA) defined transition services as "a coordinated set of activities for a student, designed within an outcome-oriented process, which promotes movement from school to postschool activities" (Section 626, P.L. 101-476). The intent of the law is for schools to be knowledgeable of the opportunities available for a student entering adulthood and to have the students either sample some of these opportunities while they are in school or be prepared to take advantage of them once they are out of school. Examples of postsecondary activities stated in IDEA are the following:

- Postsecondary education
- Vocational training
- Integrated employment (including supported employment)
- Continuing education
- Adult services
- Independent living
- Community participation

All schools are familiar with this list of postsecondary activities and most schools for the deaf and large public school deaf education programs have long been active to some degree in at least informing their students about what employment, education, and living opportunities are available to them once they leave school. The challenge to schools today goes beyond the provision of information per se to the active engagement of deaf students in meaningful, goal-oriented outcomes-based activities. To do this schools must devise a transition plan that is:

> based upon the individual student's needs, taking into account the student's preferences and interests, and shall include instruction, community experiences, the development of employment and other post school adult living objectives, and when appropriate, acquisition of daily living skills and functional evaluation. (Section 626, P.L. 101-476)

In other words, a lot of legwork is required before successful transition can occur.

Critical to the process of transition is the ubiquitous fact that deaf students do not think and act alike no matter how similar they might be with respect to academic levels, communication style, family environment, degree of hearing loss, and other biodemographic characteristics. Whatever success a school might have with one deaf student, the school should be cognizant of the fact that the transition planning needs of another student with similar biodemographic characteristics might require a completely different program.

Transition planning requires a mentality that differs from traditional educational and even vocational planning. In our education programs, we want students to do certain math operations, write fluently, read at a high level, study U.S. civics, pass the state examination in science, and so forth. In some schools, the presence of a long-standing vocational program might extend this list to include some in-school experience with, for example, furniture making and cooking. For the most part, all of these activities are basically the same for all students in the school. But they are not planned for an individual with specific work experiences in mind—they are generic in nature. They satisfy only a small component of a total school-to-work package.

This is what teachers must come to understand: Transition planning today is a complex process that requires intensive evaluation of each deaf student, coordination of an array of educational and employment experiences, and assessment of the value of these experiences to the student's entrance to postsecondary life.

The IEP and Transition

The IEP has a crucial role in ensuring that transition plans are meaningful to the students. This is true for the role of the IEP in all aspects of a deaf student's education. But role and practice are two different matters, and it is in the practice of writing effective annual goals and short-term objectives that teachers initiate their influence on their student's success. Figure 10.1 outlines some of the steps necessary to assure that a deaf student's educational and postsecondary needs are carefully considered in the IEP.

Before the IEP Meeting

⇒ Teach the student how to be an active participant in the development of her or his IEP.

⇒ Talk to the student about his or her interests and preferences related to work and future employment and living goals. Relate these to the transition process.

⇒ Talk to the student about the need for postsecondary education (e.g., colleges and universities) or vocational education to attain certain careers.

⇒ Guide the student in a self-evaluation of his or her emotional readiness to work alongside hearing coworkers.

⇒ Help the student reflect upon his or her range of communication skills and ability to adapt to various communication situations.

⇒ Talk to the parents about their thoughts about career options and employment for their child.

⇒ Develop a list of people to invite to the IEP and call them up beforehand.

⇒ Send invitations to all IEP team members (at least two weeks prior to meeting) required or requested to attend.

⇒ Compile and share assessment information on the student's present level of performance.

⇒ Identify possible work experience places.

⇒ Identify student needs, resources, programs, service, support, and school/community options in the context of adult life roles.

(Continued)

FIGURE 10.1   Flow chart of the processes involved in writing, implementing, and evaluating a transition IEP for deaf students. All asterisked (*) statements are required by IDEA.

Adapted from "Addressing transition services in the IEP" in Statewide Transition Project. (1995). *Fundamentals of transition*. Lansing, MI: Michigan Department of Education, Office of Special Education.

⇒ Compile a list of possible accommodation, considerations such as job coaching, inter-preting, medical needs on the job, and special transportation requirements for work experience.

During the IEP Meeting

⇒ Introduce participants; encourage active participation by all participants.

⇒ Define and provide the purpose of addressing transition services.

⇒ Ask the student about his or her interest and preference relating to careers and postsec-ondary education or training.

⇒ Develop outcomes that include a statement of transition services.

⇒ Review student's present level of performance and determine if discrepancies exist with long-range goals.

⇒ Write annual goals.*

⇒ Write short-term objectives that will increase opportunities or reduce barriers for student to achieve long-range goals.*

⇒ Identify resources, programs, services, and supports that student will need to achieve long-range and annual goals and short-term objectives.

⇒ Determine communication skills needed for work experience and if necessary write goals and short-term objectives to help students attain these skills.

⇒ Determine behavioral and social goals that must be achieved to enhance the student's opportunity to succeed in a work environment.

⇒ Determine how the education program can be used to prepare student for work experi-ence and other transition activities (e.g., vocabulary learning in a language arts class). Share these with the responsible academic teachers.

⇒ Determine who will be responsible for monitoring actions taken to achieve plan.

⇒ Establish time lines (initiation, duration, annual review).*

⇒ Share copies with all participants.

⇒ Determine which work experience option best meets the interests and needs of the student.

⇒ Share copies of IEP with all participants.

FIGURE 10.1   Continued

Following the IEP Meeting

⇒ Conduct regular checks of the IEP to ensure that short-term objectives are being met and that the student's program is on track to meet annual goals.

⇒ Periodically review the IEP with the student. Watch for changing thoughts about post-secondary education and training and about career interests. Teach the student how to reflect upon these thoughts.

⇒ Formally review student's IEP annually.*

⇒ Identify and determine if alternative strategies are needed to meet goals and objectives in the IEP.*

⇒ If student is on a work experience project, determine if the student's social interaction skills and communication skills with co-workers is adequate.

⇒ If student is on a work experience project, then discuss with her or him concerns about interacting in a workplace that is predominantly a hearing and speaking environment.

⇒ Maintain communication with the IEP team members.

⇒ Record and report the status of the student in relation to the progress achieved in each IEP domain.

⇒ Evaluate the role of each IEP member in facilitating the transition process and determine their effectiveness.

FIGURE 10.1   Continued

The processes shown in this figure are similar, in many respects, to those involved in writing goals and objectives for subject matter learning such as math and science. One major difference is the preparation and involvement of the student in the entire transition process. As we will show later, IDEA states that students must be involved in transition planning. At this point, we want to emphasize that thinking and deciding about career possibilities is a tall order for any teenager. It is a difficult enough task for adults who are faced with one, two, or more career changes as they work their way through adulthood. And unlike academic subjects, we can't say to deaf students, "Okay, let's see. Your career and postsecondary options in our program are X, Y, and Z." We do not know what their options are until we have actively involved the students in thinking about them. In Figure 10.1, active student participation in the transition process is emphasized at all three levels—before, during, and after the IEP is written.

Once the IEP is written, implementing it and achieving its goals and objectives will, of course, be the biggest task that teachers face—well-thought-out and beautifully written IEPs are fruitless in the hands of ineffective teachers. This raises another point about transition and IEPs. Students need to be actively involved in the *evaluation* of the success of the transition program. This is an intellectual skill that students must be taught. As described below, a student's reflection about transition is one area in which he or she can offer an evaluation of different parts of the transition process.

Associated with involvement in the IEP planning process is exposing deaf students to role models who can talk about the many aspects of work and the preparation for it. There are at least two types of role models. First, there are deaf people who are much like the students with respect to degree of hearing loss, communication and social preferences, educational background, and so forth. Also, there are other people, deaf and hearing, who are models of the type of employment that the students might be interested in pursuing. Involving the students in the IEP process and introducing them to role models will help prepare them for the real life in which no one else will be doing the thinking for them.

There are three phases to a student's involvement in transition planning:

1. *Exploration*: This first step encompasses all of the experiences and knowledge that a student has about working. Exploration actually starts at a very young age as there are many times when schools and the family are exposing deaf children to experiences relating to work—beginning with the jobs held by members of a household and the job of a teacher. Although these early childhood experiences are not planned for the benefit of career exploration, teachers should use them to begin talking to children about the concept of working or having a job. With respect to transition, exploration for high school students takes on a more serious meaning as we want students to develop a sound understanding of why people work, how they get jobs, what they do with the money they earn, what they do to advance in a job (e.g., continuing education), and their career hopes. It is here that they should be thinking about the types of work that are and are not of interest to them and explore reasons why this is the case.

2. *Determination*: During the IEP, some decisions will be made. Whether they are about academic issues relating to pursuing postsecondary education, or vocational issues relating to work experiences in school, the student must be apprised of his or her role in these decisions and encouraged to be actively involved not only in making the decisions but in following up on them.

3. *Reflection*: Once the transition plan is enacted, the student must know that he or she is partly responsible for its success and certainly responsible for evaluating this success. Transition is not just about students being able to do something well but also about how students feel about what they are doing. It is during this aspect of the IEP that students can contribute towards evaluating the effectiveness of the transition by providing feedback on the value of employment experiences including the preparation for these experiences (e.g., job coaching, interpreting, transportation), their knowledge of career possibilities, their overall level of readiness to leave school, their anticipation of lifestyles, their relationship with people involved in their transition plan, and so forth.

Once you are confident about the involvement of the student, you can then proceed with the writing of the IEP.

What's Special About Transition in the IEP?

First of all, it should be noted that in some school districts transition planning is recognized as the Individualized Transition Plan (ITP). The ITP is still an integral part of the IEP, and those involved in transition planning should be aware of a deaf student's overall education plan. Decisions made with respect to transition planning (i.e., the ITP) could mean making adjustments in the academic courses that a student takes. Effective education planning (i.e., the IEP) could mean offering work experiences that are related to academic subjects that a student is taking. An example of how transition and education planning are intertwined is seen in the case of Janet, a 17-year-old deaf student who wants to become a veterinarian. Her interest in this area led to a change in her academic science program that had her dropping a physics course in order to take a course in advanced biology. Arrangements were made to have her visit a veterinarian, partially to provide her with more exposure to the nature of this job but also to provide her with an incentive to pursue her academic studies more diligently.

Writing about transition in IEPs requires a mind-set that differs from the task of writing goals and objectives for academic subjects. The difference lies in the context in which the transition goals and objectives are developed. Teachers are typically trained to use the curriculum for guidance in developing IEPs for various subject matters. But transition lies outside of the curriculum. In fact, its context lies in the student's future. A good teacher will attempt to envision the future to help figure out what the student needs to do in her or his remaining school years to prepare for the next phase of life after high school. That is, the teacher will consider a student's interest in future career or education opportunities and use this interest to guide transition planning.

Thus, when a deaf student is 16 years old (or younger if necessary), the IEP takes on a new dimension that includes some reality checks on the student's education. Let's see how this plays out with Janine, who is an average 16-year-old profoundly deaf girl. At an IEP meeting, it is noted that she is reading at a grade 2.9 level. Curriculum-based IEPs tend to be sequential and progressive. Therefore, teachers are inclined to write global goals that are easily measured. These goals might be to raise a student's reading level one grade point in one year, complete an Algebra I textbook, or explore the concept of communities in the context of a social studies class. For Janine, a one-grade jump in reading level would be a good goal but perhaps an unrealistic one unless there is a drastic departure in the manner in which she is taught reading. After all, she has already been in school for eleven or more years. Whatever the reading goal that is decided upon at the IEP, it will be tied in some manner to the curriculum and will reflect Janine's current reading level.

In transition, however, the reading level is viewed in relation to what it implies for the future. If Janine were to be considered for enrollment in a vocational education program, then it is possible that the specific program in which she wishes to enroll will require a certain reading level. For example, at one LEA Skills Center, the reading level requirement for enrollment in a beautician program is grade nine. Is Janine a suitable candidate for this program? She might still be if, for example, it can shown at the IEP conference that Janine will be given sufficient outside support such as the assistance of a teacher consultant to help her learn the written materials and an interpreter to help her access the in-class communication.

Transition planning goes beyond just looking at a student's present academic levels and his or her vocational and career interests. There is much that a teacher or a transition team needs to know before an appropriate transition plan can be drawn up for a deaf student.

What You Need to Know Before You Write the IEP

There are many factors affecting a student's path upon leaving school. Although we tend to think that the higher achieving students will pursue further education, this is not always the case. All we can say about this type of student is that upon graduation they will have a greater range of educational opportunities awaiting them then those with lesser academic abilities. To know more about the activities that deaf students might pursue you will have to do some exploring first. Following are some of the things that a teacher should do.

1. *Talk to the students to determine their interests in and understanding of work.* Students might not know what's best for them, and we should not expect them to at their age. But they do have an idea of the type of work that they might like. Teachers need to find out what type of work students envision for themselves. How knowledgeable are they about career opportunities? Do they understand the education and skill requirements of the various careers that they might have selected? Are their expectations realistic? Are the students ready for a work experience placement? Age might not be a factor but maturity and motivation most certainly will. Teachers should not wait until a student is at the transition planning age before starting to talk about work and jobs. As stated earlier, an exploration of the concept of work and jobs should begin while students are in elementary schools.

2. *Talk to the students' parents.* Parents are great resources for information about their children. They may have some idea about their deaf children's interest in various types of career or employment skills. Ask them about their children's fascination with numbers, computers, manual labor, outdoor activities, and other generic types of working conditions and tasks. While you are at it, find out if the parents can offer an opportunity for work experience at their workplace.

3. *Look at the students' communication and social skills.* Students must be given the chance to succeed. Determine if your students are comfortable interacting with hearing people. Have they been exposed to situations at school or in the community that have helped them learn how to behave socially among strangers? Can they initiate a request for help if they come across a difficult task on the job?

4. *Assess the accommodation needs of the students.* Does a student have a physical or medical condition that will affect his or her performance on a job? Are there special services or accommodations that the student needs in order to meet the demands of a job? Does the student have the communication skills needed to perform the essential functions of a job? Assess all aspects of communication, such as reading, writing, interpersonal communication, signing, speaking, and so forth. Can the student use an interpreter or a job coach effectively? How long will an interpreter be needed before the student can use his or her own communication skills to interact with fellow employees? Can the student use public transportation to get to work everyday? What other support services might be needed to help the student adjust to the demands of the job? The list of questions might appear endless but you must probe until you are satisfied that you have all of the information you need to place a student.

5. *Determine if a student is willing and ready to take an entry level examination.* For those students considering the option of going on for postsecondary education, consideration must be given for entrance examinations that might be required for entry to a postsecondary educational or technical institution. Likewise, vocational testing might be required for a career option that a student might be interested in. If testing is required, does the student know how to go about obtaining necessary accommodations when taking the test?

6. *Explore the financial implications of pursuing academic or technical education.* When students graduate will they have the financial means to continue their schooling? Will they need to work part-time while going to a college or technical institute? One source of financial support is the government rehabilitation agencies available in each state. Do your students know how to get in touch with such agencies?

7. *Investigate the availability of work experience opportunities in the school and community.* What work experience opportunities are compatible with a student's interest? Is the community workplace sensitive to the communication needs of a deaf person? Do businesses in the community have experience placing deaf students in their workplaces? Are workplaces willing to make accommodations for deaf employees such as installing TTYs, providing them with pagers, or providing interpreters for meetings?

All of the above information should be shared with the students and their parents. It may be that a student will feel strongly about a particular career. If so, then you must find a way to inform this student of all that is involved in preparing for this career, including such information as the skills and training that might be needed, income prospects, and turnover rates in the field. If it is obvious that this career might not a good choice for a student, then it is your job as a teacher to inform the student about the pros and cons of this career choice—in a manner that is sensitive to the student's thoughts about the career field in question.

A fair percentage of deaf students will receive supplemental income in the form of a welfare check, at least at some point in their lives. Therefore, a discussion about welfare should be part of a student's transition plan. See box titled "It's a Sticky Subject But You've Got to Address It" for further rationale for discussing issues relating to welfare with deaf students.

We dare to be redundant and state again that the involvement of the deaf student is an important aspect of transition planning. IDEA clearly states that the transition program designed for a student "must be based upon the individual student's needs, taking into account the student's preferences and interests" (IDEA, 34 CFR §300.18(1)). In other words, unlike the curriculum and grade-appropriate textbooks already on the shelf, schools cannot force students to engage in work experiences if the students have no interest in doing so. Therefore, get the students involved early in the transition planning process so that

It's a Sticky Subject But You've Got to Address It

Here's an interesting fact shared by a deaf director of a state division on deafness. Some deaf adults refuse to work because the benefits they receive on welfare outweigh the advantage of taking on a job that pays slightly more than minimum wage. Factored into this calculation is the cost of medical and dental coverage that adults would have to pay if they were working and that would be covered by the government Medicaid program if they were not working. It's no wonder that a mother of a 17-year-deaf boy approached a teacher at a school for the deaf and asked if the teacher would teach her son how to apply for welfare. The teacher replied that her job was to teach English and that the mother should take the matter up with the school counselor or social worker.

This mother is not alone in her thinking about deaf adults and welfare or, more generally, about people with disabilities and the welfare system. We have encountered many deaf students who say that they will apply for welfare as soon as they reach the age of 18. Like Mt. Everest, it's there. So why not go for it? And for some deaf students and especially for those with severe physical and mental disabilities, Supplemental Security Income is a necessity. But is it a must for all deaf adults?

Attitudes about welfare need to be addressed before a deaf student leaves school. It should be a part of the overall transition plan. It could be addressed in a career education class, in a social studies class, during a special assembly for high school deaf students, by an invited deaf adult speaking about the benefits of the workplace, during a reading assignment in a language arts class, and in other ways that you should be able to identify. Take this matter seriously and put it down in the IEP as a component of a deaf student's transition plan.

transition decisions are more likely to appeal to the students. Ideally, student involvement will begin indirectly as early the elementary grades.

Interface with the Rehabilitation Counselor

One of the first steps to exploring transition opportunities is to contact a rehabilitation service (RS) counselor at a local state rehabilitation services agency. These counselors are trained to provide vocational and career counseling services. They are up-to-date with information about the labor market and of job trends in general or for a particular area of the state. They know about training requirements for jobs and where to go to obtain the training. They are often one of the first professional people deaf students will encounter once they leave high school. In fact, many deaf students attending a postsecondary educational or technical institution receive some financial support from a state rehabilitation agency. It is the RS counselor who determines their eligibility and who can point them in other directions for further support.

Also important is the fact that an RS counselor can serve as a consultant at an IEP meeting and throughout the transition program. Indeed, IDEA stipulates that procedures must be in place that facilitate the interactions of state agencies such as rehabilitation services with schools:

> Each state plan must set forth policies and procedures for developing and implementing interagency agreements between 1) the SEA (State Educational Agency); and, 2) all other State and local agencies that provide or pay for services required under this part for children with disabilities. (34 CFR §300.152)

So how can an RS counselor help you? The role of the RS counselor is broad and it is essentially to help a student prepare for the workforce. This could mean providing information about work opportunities, training programs, financial support, disability support groups, and much more. Consider the following example of roles for a counselor:

> [T]he counselor can help develop cash-match or other service agreements between local schools and (State Rehabilitation Services). The counselor can also make presentations to school staff, student groups, or families on subjects including disability awareness, reasonable accommodations, the ADA, and other disability-related topics. . . . [the] counselor can assist students in developing empowerment and self-advocacy skills and provide information to school staff on labor market trends. (Statewide Transition Project, 1995, p. 26)

Further examples of the type of services that an RS counselor can provide have been delineated as follows:

- Provide resource information on services outside of school,
- Assist with students' long-range planning,
- Provide inservice training to schools relative to [Rehabilitation Services] . . . the labor market, post-secondary vocational training options, disability awareness, accommodations, empowerment, and other topics, and
- Consult with school personnel to identify and serve non-special education students with disabilities. (Statewide Transition Project, 1995, p. 27)

This is a lot of support that should be tapped by school personnel. Add to this the fact that RS counselors typically work on transition plans for students from a range of disabilities and with a large number of schools. They have a wealth of experience to contribute to the transition process.

The RS counselor should be invited to be a part of a student's IEP team once that student turns 16 years of age. But the RS counselor can work with anyone connected to a student's transition process, including the classroom teacher, teacher consultant, resource room teacher, vocational teacher, principal, school counselor, social worker, school psychologist, health personnel, community health personnel if they are involved with a student, and, for residential schools, the dormitory liaison with the school's education program. The counselor can also work with a deaf student's family providing counseling services, information about school-to-work transition, and information about other community services and programs that are available for deaf students and their families.

Convene the Transition Team

There is an IEP team, and there is a **transition IEP** team. Astute administrators will make arrangements so that both teams are the same or at the very least that many of the participants are on both teams. IDEA (34 §300.344(1)) left nothing to chance as to who these people are. The regulations identified individuals who *must be present* as being:

- The student's teacher
- A representative of the public agency qualified to provide or supervise the special education services
- The regular education teacher if the student is enrolled in a regular education classroom

IDEA also stipulated who *must be invited* to the transition IEP meeting. These people are:

- The student
- Parent/guardian
- A member of the multidisciplinary team
- A school representative
- A representative of any other agency that is likely to be responsible for providing or paying for transition services

The transition team can be expanded to include individuals not mentioned above. A good choice would be to include an RS counselor and possibly the social worker if one is assigned to the student. Others who might be invited are school-to-work consultants, the vocational teacher, the school career counselor, a representative from the business community, an advocate for the student, and other individuals whom the student or parents might wish to come. Obviously, a team that has too many members becomes unwieldy. It would be wise for the IEP transition team administrator to get to know all of the potential participants before putting the team together.

Know Your Market for Work Experience Programs

We place students in work experience programs because we want them to sample what it is like to work on a regular basis as well as to find out what types of work they enjoy doing. In locating suitable workplaces for students you need to consider first the type of employment that a deaf student might eventually seek or be qualified to pursue. There are three types of employment situations identified by the federal government:

Competitive Employment.   **Competitive employment** consists of jobs we normally think of when we think about work. They are in the open labor market and are either full-time or part-time. The jobs offer competitive wages, and workers have varying degrees of responsibilities. These are also the type of jobs that most deaf students will one day have. They are found in all communities and are open to any healthy, qualified individual.

The type of jobs available are numerous and range from minimum skill and minimum wages to high expertise and high salaries. They include maintenance workers, retail clerks, warehouse workers, parking lot attendants, teachers, doctors, insurance sales people, investment consultants, computer technicians, engineers, sign language instructors, teacher aides, dormitory supervisors, printers, truck drivers, dancers, construction workers, commercial photographers, audiologists, and many other types of jobs.

Some competitive jobs require training of some sort either at a vocational institute, a community college, a university, or some other postsecondary educational institute. Others can be learned online on the Internet or through correspondence courses (e.g., hearing-aid dealers, realtors). Still others require on-the-job training.

What all competitive employment jobs have in common is that the worker maintains the job with no outside support. During a transition program, however, some level of support might be needed, for example, job coaches and interpreters. Interpreters might be required for the occasional meeting once a deaf person assumes a full-time position with a company, and the Americans with Disabilities Act requires companies to provide them. This is the case at many large factories such as automotive assembly plants where it is not uncommon to find several full-time deaf workers.

Supported Employment.   **Supported employment** is competitive work that occurs in integrated settings where ongoing support is provided for the person with a disability. The support begins with training and is maintained for the duration of the time that the person with a disability remains on the job. This type of employment was designed for those individuals with severe physical or mental disabilities. Deaf students with multiple disabilities are candidates for supported employment.

There are different models for implementing and maintaining supported employment (Wehman et al., 1988). There is the individual model in which a single person is placed in a workplace, given training, usually with the assistance of a job coach, and with heavy supervision at the beginning that is gradually reduced. The enclave model is one in which several individuals work in a single business. The mobile crew model has several individuals who move from one business to another providing work as needed by a company. The benchwork model has a larger group of individuals with severe disabilities who do contractual work for companies such as electronics or technology firms.

Supported employment situations have in common the provision of intensive training and continuous supervision. Furthermore, one of the goals of this type of work is to allow the individuals with severe disabilities to work alongside nondisabled workers. Wages are dictated by the type of work provided, which includes maintenance, assembly of parts, groundskeeping, cleanup of land and buildings, and more.

Sheltered Employment.   **Sheltered employment** is also designed for individuals with severe physical or mental disabilities. This type of employment differs from supported employment in two main respects. First, there is no integration with nondisabled workers. Second, the individuals must progress from training in daily living, social, and recreational skills to working in a sheltered workshop. The work they do is typically performed on a piecework basis and can include assembling, packaging, collating, and other manual work that is repetitive and simple.

Many sheltered workshops are supported by state and/or federal funds. They tend to work closely with special education agencies and schools for the deaf, and this is one way for them to recruit employees for future work. They generally have programs that evaluate the potential skills of students and then offer them training while they are still attending school. Evaluation is varied but the main purposes are to see (1) if the students are mature enough to handle a half-day or a full-day of work, and (2) if they are able to perform a manual task such as folding boxes at a certain minimum rate (e.g., two boxes per minute). Information about sheltered workshops in your area can be obtained from your state rehabilitation agency.

Once you know what type of employment your deaf students are seeking and/or are eligible for, you can then begin searching for suitable places for the student to gain experience working. There are many ways you can approach this task, including the following:

1. Check with the special education office at the Local Education Agency for a listing of businesses that are receptive to giving students work experience.

2. Contact the chamber of commerce in your area for suggestions. Most, if not all, chambers have a regular newsletter. Ask if you can place a request in the newsletter for a particular type of work experience placement or make a general request for businesses to contact you if they are interested in participating in your transition program. You could even volunteer to write a short article about the benefits to businesses when they contribute to a work experience project for deaf students.

3. Many larger communities have a network of businesses that are already collaborating with schools in the transition process. These are businesses that regularly accept students for experiences that include working in banks, insurance companies, retail stores, restaurants, golf courses, health care clinics, hospitals, and many more. If there is such a program then you should be able to get this information from the chamber of commerce or your LEA special education office.

4. Contact clubs and business associations. Clubs such as the Rotary Club, Lions Club, Elks Lodge, and Masonic Temple have regular meetings that are attended by business people. They aim to make their communities a better place to live, and they are conspicuous for their benevolent activities. You can also try business associations such as merchants groups, small business associations, and trade organizations. All of these can be found in a phone book under Business and Trade Organizations, Clubs, and Fraternal Organizations or on the Internet. Call them up and drop by in person to show your interest in having them find work experience programs for your deaf students. One of the authors was invited to a Rotary Club luncheon to speak about the education of deaf students. The presentation was limited to just fifteen minutes but think of all that can be said in that time. If you only recruited one business to help in your transition then the presentation was well worth it. Get yourself invited to one these luncheons.

5. Contact transition coordinators working at other schools. This is your don't-reinvent-the-wheel tactic. You are not the first and only person involved in transition planning. Contact high schools in the area and ask for the names of their transition coordinators. Share information with them and seek out suggestions of what they might consider best practices in transition. Use the Internet to contact transition coordinators at schools for the deaf and public school programs.

6. Tap into your personal network of people. Parents, teachers, and neighbors are valuable resources for information about work.

At all times keep track of who you have contacted and the results of such contact. Transition is complex enough without having to deal with misplaced phone numbers and the lack of remembered names.

The Internet

The value of the Internet as a resource is growing exponentially. But gleaning useful information from the Internet is still a challenge. Much time can be wasted in a search for a topic that yields something of value to you. The Internet, however, contains some valuable government documents relating to transition that touch upon such topics as IEPs, transition planning, and vocational assessment. Each of these documents provide information about books and other publications that address transition issues and provide guidance in the planning and writing of IEPs.

One such web site is maintained by the National Information Center for Children and Youth with Disabilities.[1] This web site contains linkage to many recent developments relating to the education of children with disabilities. The U.S. Office of Special Education Programs is another good resource.[2] It provides the latest information about changes in regulations relating to the education of children with disabilities as well as current research findings on best practices. You can also contact your State Office of Special Education for information. Some states have regulations relating to transition that are in addition to those mandated by the federal government in IDEA. Another useful web site is operated by the National Transition Alliance for Youth with Disabilities.[3] Finally, numerous other web sites related to transition but involving a lot more than transition planning and service provision can be found for those state agencies responsible for funding and monitoring transition and school-to-work programming.

What IDEA Expects You to Do

IDEA is a powerful and valuable set of regulations, yet many schools fail to effectively implement the processes it defines (Grigal, Test, Beattie, & Wood, 1997). It is not that these schools do not want transition but rather that transition planning is a relatively new mandate and most school personnel have not been trained in the legal implications of the law, the roles and responsibilities of participants including the various government agencies, and the importance of involving students in the planning process (Grigal et al., 1997). Indeed, the very act of implementing the transition component of IDEA is a first and yet challenging step toward successful school-to-work planning (Furney, Hasazi, & Destefano, 1997). And it must be done. The responsibility for school programs and other agencies is clearly stated in IDEA regulations (see box titled "What IDEA Has to Say About Responsibilities").

What IDEA Has to Say About Responsibilities

Read what IDEA has to say about a school's responsibility for providing a transition program for students with disabilities:

> If a participating agency fails to provide agreed-upon transition services contained in the IEP of a student with a disability, the public agency responsible for the student's education shall, as soon as possible, initiate a meeting for the purpose of identifying alternative strategies to meet the transition service objectives and, if necessary, revise the student's IEP.
>
> Nothing in this part relieves any participating agency, including the State vocational rehabilitation agency, of the responsibility to provide or pay for any transition service that the agency would otherwise provide to students with disabilities who meet the eligibility criteria of that agency. (34 CFR §300.347 (a)(b))

There is no two ways about it—If a deaf student is 16 years old, schools must have a transition plan in that student's IEP. Furthermore, if a transition plan is not implemented properly or some aspect of the plan does not take place, then the transition team may have to reconvene to discuss alternatives.

But even with the best of transition plans, teachers must be on the alert for things that might go wrong once implementation of the plan takes effect. A plan can be meticulously put together with full support from all of the parties involved and still not work. Employers agree to take on a student for a period of time, but they are not obligated to do so even after the IEP is completed. They make decisions that are in the best interest of their business. Anything can happen to make them change their minds about taking on a deaf student. There could be a change in ownership, a downturn in the market, layoffs in a plant, or an unfavorable experience with a different deaf student.

Many other problems can arise. A student might suddenly get cold feet about going to work. Once the work is started, the student and employer might sense that the chemistry for a good working relationship is not present. The student might find out that he or she is not emotionally ready for the rigors of a workplace. The logistics of transportation might be too difficult to surmount. Communication incompatibility between the deaf student and hearing co-workers might lead to stress for the involved workers. Ask any experienced transition teacher and she or he could probably add more reasons why a hoped-for transition plan can fail to be implemented. But whatever the reason for a change in plans, the student's transition team must be reconvened to find an alternative work site or to revise the stated transition goals and objectives.

Begin the Dialogue About Rights

There are laws that protect all people against discrimination on the basis of a disability. **Section 504, Title V of the Rehabilitation Act of 1973** forbids discrimination in the services and employment provided by businesses or individuals who receive federal funds. The **Americans with Disabilities Act** (ADA) is a far-reaching law that prohibits discrimination in a wide range of settings that includes those that do not receive federal monetary support. The ADA does not allow discrimination in employment against a qualified individual with a disability. It prohibits discrimination in state and local government services, public accommodations, transportation, and telecommunications, and it applies to private employers, state and local governments, employment agencies, labor organizations, and labor-management committees. ADA is a powerful law that deaf students need to know about.

A key concept in the ADA is the notion of "reasonable accommodation," which is defined as:

> any change or adjustment to a job or work environment that permits a qualified applicant or employee with a disability to participate in the job application process, to perform the essential functions of a job, or to enjoy benefits and privileges of employment equal to those enjoyed by employees without disabilities. (U.S. Equal Employment Opportunity Commission, 1991, p. 3)

Obviously, it is impossible to spell out exactly what a reasonable accommodation will entail for the thousands of jobs that are available to a deaf person. Some examples of accommodations are the following:

- Modifying equipment or devices so that they are accessible to a deaf person. This could mean adding a flashing light or some other device that alerts a deaf person to the sound of a doorbell, fire alarm, a ringing phone, or some other source of sound.
- Providing interpreters or real-time captioners for meetings.
- Modifying the format and procedures associated with an examination so that a deaf person could take it in sign language.
- Lengthening the time of a training session.

The ADA does not make it easier for a deaf person to be hired before a hearing person is hired. It does, however, attempt to level the playing field so that deaf people (or any other person with a disability) will have a fair chance to get a job provided that they meet the job requirements, which might include specific education experiences, a special certification or license (e.g., a electrician's license), and certain skills. Even then a deaf person must be able to perform the essential functions of a job with or without reasonable accommodations. Thus, the ADA tries to ensure that a qualified deaf person will not be excluded from consideration for a job solely on the basis of a hearing loss.

Does discrimination against deaf people take place in the workplace? It does. Perhaps much of it is unintentional but it happens nevertheless. It might start at the hiring stage with employers who are reluctant to hire a deaf worker. It might concern a deaf employee at a large corporation who is unable to have an interpreter for departmental meetings because the employer does not want to pay for services. It might be something that is seemingly innocuous such as measures not taken to ensure that a deaf worker will always be informed about messages that are spoken to all employees through a public address system.

Whatever the cause of discrimination, deaf students must be taught to recognize discrimination when it occurs, to assess the need to file a complaint about the discrimination, and to report it to the correct government agency, which is the Equal Employment Opportunity Commission.[4]

Foster (1992) interviewed supervisors of deaf employees and the deaf workers themselves to explore the relationship between these two groups of people. Although she did not directly tackle the issue of discrimination, she did discover that communication was a major point of contention between the two groups of people. Moreover, she identified the difficulty of communication as having a detrimental effect on the deaf employee's opportunities for advancement:

> [T]he constraints imposed by communication differences, and the impact of these constraints on the ability of deaf employees to access and participate in informal social networks in the workplace, cannot be underestimated. Since most relationships are dependent on frequent and casual conversations, a deaf person who has difficulty communicating with hearing colleagues is at a great disadvantage. (p. 122)

Foster suggested that career mobility may be contingent upon deaf people's accessing the social network of a workplace—a point that should be heeded by teachers, school counselors, and VR consultants developing transition plans for deaf students.

The Role of the Teacher in the Transition Process

We have found that some classroom teachers think that transition is the sole prerogative of school counselors and vocational education teachers. Yet, all teachers have a role in transition, and this role begins as early as the preschool years during a class visit to the fire station. There is much that can be gained from this field trip in preparation for the student's future. Consider the following questions: Who are the firefighters? Are there ever women firefighters? What is the job of a firefighter? How did firefighters learn to do this job? Did they have to go to school? Do they have to know how to read and do arithmetic? How do they know where a fire is? Can a deaf person be a firefighter?

Even at the preschool level and certainly no later than the early elementary grades, an astute teacher will begin the process of introducing deaf students to the vocabulary of the workplace by talking about what parents do for a living and more generally, what people do once they leave school. They should weave thoughts about work and schooling across all subjects. Take for example, a discussion about early pioneers crossing the nation to settle in the prairies and west of the Rockies. In addition to the usual discussions about routes, hardships, buffaloes, Native Americans, and land claims, consider the following topics for discussions:

- A comparison of transportation via wagon trains with today's trucks. Bring in a trucker to talk about the long hours of driving and the various destinations driven to. Discuss the legal battles that deaf people have had in order to earn the right to drive a commercial semitrailer. Include a discussion about the fact that for many years, deaf people were unable to get a driver's license in nearly all states.
- What sort of jobs were available 150 years ago? What jobs did deaf people likely do? What type of jobs are still around today and which of them would the students like to do?

- How were people trained to do various jobs? Did they go to school? Could the same sort of training take place today?

Another role for teachers in preparing students for transition is to expose their students to role models from the workplace. All schools can benefit from involvement of the community and parents in their programs. Whether as guest speakers or as regular classroom volunteers, these nonschool personnel bring to the students new vocabulary and stories of their experiences as adults. We watched a carpenter talk to a group of second graders about his work, and he also showed them his box of tools. He named each one of his tools, some of which are commonly known and some that are not: hammer, ballpeen hammer, screwdriver, Phillips screwdriver, chisel, handsaw, hacksaw, crescent wrench, nail puller, tape measure, level, awl, plane, square, drill bits, plumb bob, chalkline, and more. You might ask about the value of this much vocabulary if nearly all of the names will be forgotten unless the student has an opportunity to work with the tools. For starters, this experience is not about vocabulary per se but rather about a unique linguistic experience for the students. It also entails any or all of the following activities: listening to someone talk about his or her job; learning that tools have names and knowing these names are a part of a carpenter's job; that building things involves many different skills and that training is needed to learn them; and learning about what this particular carpenter had to do before being hired full-time. The carpenter even talked about hobbies (building sailboats, reading books about nature) and other things that he does outside of his job.

Finally, transition is a staple of the education of individuals with disabilities. General education teachers might not be aware of the importance of transition for deaf students, therefore an effort is needed to make them aware and be apprised of the ways in which they can contribute to the process. This is something that an itinerant or resource room teacher can do. The itinerant or resource room teacher might accomplish this by talking to the general education teachers individually or by planning a workshop about a school's responsibility in the transition process and the particular needs of deaf students.

Given their expertise, itinerant and resource room teachers and teachers of the deaf in separate classrooms have a major responsibility in transitional planning for deaf students. Some of their contributions to the process are as follows:

- Serving as an expert on matters relating to the education of their deaf students such as communication methodologies, language considerations, and their future employability. Transition brings deaf students in contact with employers and business people who likely lack knowledge about these matters or who might harbor reservations about the ability of deaf people to do certain jobs. Teachers of the deaf should consciously work toward portraying deaf people as being a positive asset in the workplace whose limitations in performing a job are no different than that of hearing people.
- Making the transition team aware of on-the-job accommodations that might be needed for a student to participate in a work experience program, particularly with respect to communication.
- Helping to select a qualified job coach if one is needed. There may be situations in which an itinerant teacher might be the job coach if his or her scheduling allows for this.

- Teaching or reinforcing some of the job-related vocabulary in class. For some students, learning specialized vocabulary associated with a work experience may be as important as learning subject matter-related words. In fact, learning the specialized vocabulary may influence a student's long-term interest in a particular job.
- Including the students in the evaluation of a transition plan. This process is crucial not only for the deaf students involved in transition but also for improving transition planning for other students.

Further Thoughts About Transition

Along with longitudinal planning in transition and involving key individuals in the planning process there is a need to evaluate the effectiveness of such planning. Effective administrators take action to make this happen. The following are aspects of planning that might be evaluated:

- The roles and responsibilities of the people involved in the planning.
- The effort made to involve the student in planning and the type of involvement that actually occurred.
- The effectiveness of community liaisons such as that of rehabilitation counselors and business people.
- The relationship with workplaces used for placement of students.
- Students' employment outcomes or their enrollment in postsecondary education institutions upon leaving school.

A time line for this evaluation might be established to ensure that they occur at least annually and that the information obtained by the evaluation can be used for guiding changes in a school's transitional planning process.

Conclusion

Perhaps the key to successful transition planning is to get an early start. Tap into all subject matter to teach deaf students how to reflect upon what they are doing and the directions that they are taking in their schoolwork, social life, and their thoughts about life as an adult. Do not just have your fourth graders plod through their math books. Talk to them about why they are learning math and provide real-life examples of its applications. Teach them early on in their schooling how to think about what they are learning. If all teachers did this, then deaf students will be better positioned to make a valuable contribution to their own transition planning.

At all times, do not compromise transition services with a graduation date. **State rehabilitation services** are there to help in this matter. IDEA is also a strong tool for ensuring that students are well prepared before leaving school. IDEA allows schools to provide services to individuals with disabilities until they are 21 years old. If a student is not ready to graduate at age 18, then use the IEP to offer more schooling and more transition preparation.

Finally, many schools for the deaf and other school programs assign a teacher to coordinate transition planning for deaf students. The nature of this job is complex, and transition teachers are responsible for establishing an intricate network of personnel and agencies with whom they are in contact when devising and implementing a student's transition plan. At one school for the deaf, the transition teacher retired leaving nothing behind for the next teacher. It took two full years for the new teacher to learn the names of key community people and state government agencies; to find new businesses willing to take deaf students and learn about the intermediate school districts skills center; to find job coaches who were also skilled as interpreters; and to learn how to write realistic and meaningful annual goals and objectives. When asked about the most difficult aspect of her position, she responded that it was locating businesses willing to provide deaf students with work experiences. She had learned after a while that there are many people who are willing to provide help in this direction.

Make transition a valuable part of your school program rather than just something for students who require independent living skills and are likely slated for supported or sheltered employment. Transition is also for students aiming for university and a professional career. And besides, IDEA requires that you have a transition plan for them.

KEY WORDS AND CONCEPTS

Americans with Disabilities Act: Enacted in 1990, a law forbidding discrimination against people with disabilities in a wide range of settings, including those that do not receive federal monetary support. As long as the person with a disability is qualified for a particular job then the workplace cannot discriminate against him or her. ADA applies to a wide range of workplaces including state and local government services, public accommodations, transportation, and telecommunications. It applies to private employers, state and local governments, employment agencies, labor organizations, and labor management committees.

competitive employment: Jobs in the open labor market that are either full- or part-time.

Section 504, Title V of the Rehabilitation Act of 1973: A federal law that prohibits discrimination in the services and employment provided by businesses or individuals who receive federal funds.

sheltered employment: Work for individuals with severe physical or mental disabilities. These individuals work in an environment with no integration with people without disabilities. The work tends to be subsidized by state and/or federal funds.

state rehabilitation services: State-run agencies that are primarily devoted to helping people with disabilities obtain and/or maintain employment. Rehabilitation counselors are valuable resources for transition planning.

supported employment: Competitive work that occurs in integrated settings where ongoing support is provided for the person with a disability, usually for someone who has a severe physical or mental disability. The support lasts for the duration of time that a person with a disability remains on the job.

transition: A process for preparing students for postschool activities through a set of carefully planned activities. Included among the postschool activities are all types of postsecondary education, vocational training, continuing education, integrated employment, adult services, independent living, and participation in the community.

transition IEP: A planning document that determines what activities will be enacted during the school years to prepare a student for postschool activities. Transition planning requires evaluation of each deaf student, coordination of educational and employment experiences, and assessment of the value of these experiences to the student's life as an adult. Examples of activities are work experiences, career exploration, volunteer community work, and meeting with adult role models.

QUESTIONS

1. What historical changes in the workforce occurred in the twentieth century that made it more difficult for schools to prepare students for employment immediately upon graduation?

2. What are four main areas of transition that should be considered when planning for postschool activities?

3. Who is responsible for the implementation of transition services?

4. Why is it important to help deaf students become familiar with the programs and services offered by rehabilitation services?

5. How can rehabilitation services help in transition planning for a deaf student?

6. What federal law states that procedures must be in place that facilitate the interactions of state agencies such as rehabilitation services with schools?

7. How can a school get rehabilitation services involved in a deaf student's transition planning?

8. For an IEP meeting, who must be present and who must be invited but do not have to be present?

9. What does it mean to actively involve a deaf student in transition planning? Provide at least three examples.

10. Name and describe the three phases of a student's involvement in transition planning.

11. Name and describe three different types of employment for people with disabilities. What are the implications of each for transition planning?

12. Identify five different sources of information about employment places in the community that can be used for work experiences for deaf students.

ACTIVITIES

1. Interview a deaf high school student about his or her career aspirations. In your interview include the following areas: understanding of the concept of why people work and the value of a career; work experience during school years; ideas about what will happen following graduation; and knowledge of resources to obtain assistance in postsecondary activities.

2. Develop a plan for a half-day workshop for parents that will describe the components of successful transition planning for deaf students and what parents can do to help in the process. In your plan, include the titles of people who will contribute to the presentation.

3. Develop a resource guide for parents, teachers, and others that lists publications, agencies, and web sites that provide useful information related to transition including the following:

   ■ career options
   ■ businesses that accept students for work experience projects
   ■ information about federal laws pertaining to transition
   ■ possible accommodations that workplaces can make for deaf employees

NOTES

1. The National Information Center for Children and Youth with Disabilities can be reached by phone: 1-800-695-0285 (voice/tty) or 202-884-8200 (voice/tty); by e-mail: nichcy@aed.org; or by post: P.O. Box 1492, Washington, DC 20013. Their current URL is: http://www.nichcy.org.

2. The web site for the U.S. Office of Special Education Programs is http://www.ed.gov/offices/osers.

3. The web site for the National Transition Alliance for Youth with Disabilities is http://www.dssc.org /nta/.

4. The Equal Employment Opportunity Commission can be reached by tty at (800) 800-3302, by voice phone at (202) 663-4900.

CHAPTER

11 Other Teaching Situations

CHAPTER OUTCOMES

After reading this chapter, you should be able to:

1. Describe the responsibilities of resource room, itinerant (teacher consultant), and team teachers.
2. Plan for instructions in a resource room.
3. Consult with professional peers in a supporting role as a resource room teacher or an itinerant teacher.
4. Cooperate with a peer to teach a class of deaf and hearing students.

To illustrate some teaching situations other than those in a self-contained or separate classroom, we introduce you to three teachers of the deaf, Dinah, Kris, and Nan.

Dinah is a **resource room** teacher in a large city high school. When she started working as a teacher of the deaf, she had twelve deaf students that she saw throughout the week, ranging from one to three periods a day. The fewest she ever had in the classroom at any one time were two and once a day she would have all twelve students. All but two of the students were hard of hearing and relied on speech as their primary mode of communication. The other two students were profoundly deaf and both relied on signing for communication. During her first year teaching in this high school, she spent her time tutoring students in subject areas in which they needed help and had most of her students working on a special reading program to help them with vocabulary growth and comprehension. She also played the role of counselor and liaison with the general education teacher. But by the time her second year came along she had realized that if she was going to help her students in school then she would have to do more than just tutor. Although she continued to assist students with their core subjects, she selected current events as an area to engage the students in learning more about their lives and the world they live in. She used newspaper and magazine stories to help students develop literacy skills. She continued to do this even as the number of students grew to nineteen and another resource room teacher was added. She said that the current affairs literacy program had the most influence on increasing her students' self esteem, and it was her students' favorite subject of the day.

Kris was an **itinerant teacher** in a rural area at the foot of the Rocky Mountains. For five years, she had a caseload of five to seven students from the elementary through high school levels. Some she would see three times a week while one or two of them she would only see once a month. All of her students were hard of hearing and used speech. None of them could sign although Kris was a good signer. She would average about three hours a day on the road adding 120 to 150 miles to her odometer daily. She spent her time with the students immersed in intense one-on-one instructions. Instruction was aimed at helping the students with their schoolwork in the regular classroom. Students would either make specific requests for help, or their teachers would forward requests for assistance to be given in specific areas. She felt that she had a fair impact on her student's academic work but nevertheless left the job because of the driving.

Nan was a teacher of the deaf in an inner-city elementary school, where she team taught with Kathy, a general education teacher. Nan had taught in a self-contained classroom for over ten years when the switch to team teaching occurred. The switch was a result of the school district's commitment to inclusive education (i.e., the education of all children with disabilities in a regular classroom). There were six deaf students who used a mixture of signs and speech (the program subscribed to a total communication philosophy) and nineteen hearing students. The class was a multiage classroom with students from six to nine years of age. The two teachers engaged in **team teaching** for two years, after which the team was disbanded because Nan began teaching part-time. Both teachers enjoyed their team teaching arrangement. Each had responsibility for taking control of certain subject areas. At various times during the day Nan would pull some deaf students to a special place in the room where she would work on language arts activities. When asked about what they thought was the key to the team's success, the two teachers mentioned four things in particular. First, when they agreed to team teach, they convinced the school principal to give them the largest classroom in the building, which was actually a former art room. The extra space allowed them to create activity centers, have pull-out sessions within the classroom, and allowed them both to have their own space for planning. Second, they had complementary personalities. Nan was a disciplinarian and a skilled reading teacher. Kathy was a good hands-on mathematics teacher and incorporated art activities throughout the week that made the class a fun place to learn for all students, deaf and hearing. Third, among the general education students there were several students who were identified as having learning disabilities. Kathy found the instructional methods that Nan used with her deaf students to be helpful with her learning disabled students. The teachers felt that the deaf students benefited from seeing other hearing students learning in the same way that they were learning. The fourth was the teaching of fingerspelling and signs to the entire class. Instructions were done either during the first period in the morning or at the end of the day. None of the hearing students gained fluency but several of them picked up enough signs to feel comfortable conversing with their deaf classmates.

Each of these teachers is a real person, and the situations described above are true portrayals of their teaching situations and quite possibly will be yours one day. If you do not teach in a self-contained or separate classroom, then you will likely end up teaching in one of the following three teaching situations:

- Teaching in a resource room.
- Teaching as an itinerant teacher or teacher consultant.
- Teaching in a team teaching situation.

Teaching in a Resource Room

What a Resource Room Teacher Is Expected to Do

By looking at what teachers report both as the real and the ideal in what is expected of them, we can get some idea of what is expected of the resource room teacher (Glomb & Morgan, 1991; Voltz & Elliot, 1990). In general, there are three major roles: consultation and collaboration, resource room teaching, and general education classroom support. Specific tasks correspond with each of these roles follows:

Consultation and Collaboration

- Respond to mainstream teacher's requests for assistance with a student.
- Develop academic, social, or behavioral goals for student with mainstream teacher.
- Develop and coordinate instructional plans.
- Suggest effective materials or strategies.
- Confer with mainstream teacher to establish classroom expectations for student.
- Share diagnostic testing information.
- Provide assistance in interpretation of test results.
- Conduct joint parent conferences.
- Participate in joint problem solving.

Resource Room Teaching

- Use a variety of examples when teaching a new skill.
- Teach students study skills.
- Give several examples of and require several variations of a response.
- Use general education curriculum materials.
- Use a variety of locations or teaching situations in the resource room.
- Plan for transfer of skills learned.
- Preteach and postteach mainstream lessons.

General Education Classroom Support

- Modify general education classroom materials for use by students.
- Supply specialized learning materials.
- Tutor students in the mainstream classroom.
- Provide input to grades and promotion decisions.

The Experience of Resource Room Teaching

A few years ago, the authors conducted an extensive study of teachers of the deaf in resource rooms in local public schools (Kluwin, Stewart, & Sammons, 1994). Figure 11.1

	Physical Situation	Administrative Support	General Education Involvement
Fort Apache	Included	Unsupportive	None
Guerrilla	Isolated	Unsupportive	Involved
Happy Camper	Included	Supportive	Involved
Lone Wolf	Isolated	Unsupportive	None
Wallflower	Included	Supportive	None

From Kluwin, Stewart, & Sammons (1994).

FIGURE 11.1   Teaching situations associated with resource room teachers.

shows the five types of resource room teachers that emerged from the interviews: Fort Apache, Guerrilla, Happy Camper, Lone Wolf, and Wallflower.

Fort Apache teachers were found in rooms that were physically part of the instructional flow of the school, but the building principals ranged from unsupportive to actively hostile toward the deaf education program. Fort Apache teachers were found in superdistricts that had been created as a way to efficiently provide service to a low-incidence population. However, this arrangement had created an administrative environment or professional separateness that prevented these teachers from productively dealing with the building principal in their day-to-day activities. They considered themselves as "just renting space."

Guerrilla teachers were physically or administratively isolated from the rest of the school but were socially integrated. As such they were often very effective advocates for their children. What made them unique was that they saw their role as one of advancing the needs of their students through informally providing inservice to other teachers and defending the rights of the children by finessing rather than confronting the system. For example, a regular complaint of all teachers was that deaf children were ignored in seating for the auditorium programs. The Guerrilla teacher's approach would be to elicit the cooperation of the school secretary in order to ensure an appropriate situation.

Happy Campers were physically, administratively, and socially integrated into the general education program. They had better physical situations, active general education administrative support, and more homogeneous classes.

Lone Wolves were the opposites of Happy Campers. Lone Wolves were in poor physical circumstances, dealt with social isolation from other professionals, and had a negative outlook on their own situation. The typical Lone Wolf teacher worked in a small room that had been converted from a storage room or had been used for some other purpose such as a projection booth in the school auditorium. Unlike the Guerrilla teacher, the Lone Wolf coped with the situation rather than trying to triumph over it.

Wallflowers were teachers who were physically and administratively integrated but would not make an effort toward social integration. These were primarily teachers of high school age students who were often new to the school and had little or no contact with general education classes, either as interpreters or as teachers.

These five types of resource room teachers are not exhaustive of all the possible situations, nor can any percentages be provided about how many of each type there are out there. However, these types of teachers are the product of how the school district structures resource room teaching, the physical resources available to the teachers, and the teacher's own personal response to the situation. Guerrilla teachers were wonderful people to interview because, in spite of difficult situations, they reported personal successes. Wallflowers were not pleasant to interview because although they had excellent situations they wanted something different, often a vague "ideal." It was clear from the interviews that personal attitude is a large part of the key to success in resource room teaching.

Duties of a Resource Room Teacher

The difference in planning for the resource room teacher is the shift from planning for one goal to planning for several goals. We should add that there are many resource room teachers who have students with disabilities other than deafness as part of their responsibilities, thus the resource room is the place for extra help and the model of instruction should be individualized instruction. The shift in thinking is from establishing a goal for a child to figuring out what goal another teacher has established and moving a child toward that goal.

A lesson chart (an example of which is depicted in Figure 11.2), rather than a lesson plan, is one way to approach this situation. It is the responsibility of the general education teacher to set the instructional goals for deaf students. Materials that the resource room teacher will use will often consist of the materials that the general education teacher has assigned. Whether the student needs help organizing and planning, or needs to be taught or retaught the material, it is likely that additional materials will be needed. The methods used to teach will be set by the instructional goals. Evaluation should be in terms of what the resource room teacher and the student can reasonably expect to accomplish. Feedback both to the student and to the general education teacher is an essential part of this arrangement.

The next step is to complete the chart for the other deaf students who will come in during the same time period. When all students' activities have been listed, then more efficient planning of the time frame can take place. For example, one student might require a ten-minute brainstorming session at the start of a lesson, a quick check mid-hour, and a check at the end on how much progress was made. Other students might be able to start independently. The goal for the resource room teacher in this kind of planning is to have as efficient a classroom as possible, so that students do not waste time or, more seriously, miss an opportunity to get needed help. The alternative and all too frequent solution is to pass out vaguely related worksheets, which serves to shortchange students' learning. With experience, the elaborateness or even the necessity of this kind of plan should diminish.

In general, younger students will not be served in a resource room model for language arts. If, however, a younger deaf student is supported with literacy instruction in a resource room, the role of the resource room teacher will typically not be to teach material to the deaf student but to assist the deaf student in learning what the general education teacher is presenting. Some methods that can be used to support these children include:

- Semantic maps
- Preteaching important vocabulary and concepts

Student Name	Instructional Goal	Materials	Method	Evaluation	Student Feedback	Teacher Feedback
Alfred Brown	Five-paragraph essay	Assigned work and organizers	Brain-storming	First draft completed	As needed	Possible modifications to scoring

FIGURE 11.2   Example of a class lesson chart for resource room teachers.

- Providing study guides
- Other supporting activities
- Addressing specific language concerns

Semantic Maps.   One of the frequent tasks for the resource room teacher is to prepare the deaf student to write an essay or a report. Obviously, the resource room teacher does not want to write the paper for the student, nor does the resource room teacher want to diverge too far from the general education teacher's work, so he or she needs a generic response that will help the student complete the assignment.

Semantic maps are a useful device in these situations because they can be used by one student, a pair, or even be worked on in small groups. Since the approach is basically a planning strategy prior to writing, it is compatible with several different approaches to the language arts.

For individual or even small group work, self-stick notes are a good way to start. Ask the child to simply list words related to the topic. For example, if the child has to write an essay about slavery, ask him or her to brainstorm all of the ideas that he or she can remember from class, readings, and so forth. Each word or phrase should be written down on a self-stick note or a scrap of paper.

When the student has generated a list of a dozen or more related words or phrases, she or he then tries to organize the pile. Since the essay is about slavery, stick that piece in the center of the table. Next, ask the student to put the most important or closely related idea next to it, such as "owning people." Perhaps something like "no freedom" will fit in next to slavery or form a triangle with slavery and owning people. Go through the pile of self-stick notes or paper scraps until all the words have been looked at and placed near related ideas.

The next step is to connect the related ideas so that you can begin to establish a hierarchy of ideas. If the self-stick notes are placed on a large sheet of paper, then the student can draw lines between related groups of words. As the student is doing this, have him or her explain why each connection is being made.

The second to last step is to have the student combine related groups of words into sentences. Finally, sentences can be grouped into paragraphs. Obviously, if at some point the student begins to write freely, the map can be ignored because it has done its work.

Some students will find mapping easy and clear while others will struggle to comprehend its usefulness. The goals of semantic mapping are to stimulate thinking about a topic, provide an initial organizing tool, and support writing. The focus should be on the number of ideas generated and the rough structure for writing that was created.

Preteaching Important Vocabulary and Concepts.   Obtain from the general education teacher a list of important vocabulary and concepts that will be taught, then preteach these to the deaf student. Even a rough outline of the pages to be covered will give you a sense of what material needs to be taught. If you introduce key concepts or vocabulary in advance of their presentation in a general education class, you will give the deaf student an extra edge in understanding what is happening in class. It will also give you a point of departure for reteaching and review: "Remember two weeks ago when I showed you . . .?" You can preteach signs as well as introduce mnemonic devices. Sometimes you may come up with an image or a mnemonic that the general education teacher will find helpful for his or her students, thus contributing to the sense of collegiality in the relationship between the resource room teacher and the general education teacher.

Providing Study Guides.   All students can benefit from a study guide. Teachers can use a word processor to quickly create a study guide of the key concepts, questions, vocabulary, and facts for new material.

Other Supporting Activities.   There are numerous other supporting activities. Luckner and Denzin (1998) delineated the following:

- Provide a copy of the general education teacher's notes.
- Highlight key words or concepts in printed material.
- Use games for drill and practice.
- Use concise statements or simplified vocabulary.
- Demonstrate directions to clarify what needs to be undertaken.
- Check for understanding by having the student restate the directions.
- Break long-range projects into short-term assignments.
- Increase the number of practice examples of a rule, concept, or strategy prior to seatwork or homework.
- Provide duplicate sets of materials for family use and review.
- Have students summarize at the end of the lesson.
- Supplement lessons with visual materials (e.g., objects, pictures, photographs, charts, videos).
- Use graphic organizers to present material.
- Write short summaries of the lesson or of the chapters of the textbook.
- Teach organizational skills and assist students to generalize these skills.

- Teach student reading comprehension strategies (e.g., textbook structures such as headings, subheadings, tables, graphs, summaries).

Addressing Specific Language Concerns. Reed (1987) offers a classic sequence for addressing specific language-related concerns that resource room teachers might find useful when working with deaf students whom they might only see two to four times a week.

1. *Assess language needs and identify the target structure.* This might involve correcting an error or expanding the student's language repertoire. As this is inherently a corrective rather than a developmental procedure, keep in mind the relative value of the structure to be changed. For example, plurals and possessives are more important to correct than third-person indicative active voice, all of which involve the addition of "s" to a base form. Inappropriate use of plurals and possessives can alter the basic understanding of the communication while the third person typically reflects social or educational differences.

2. *Analyze target structure grammar.* Because the deaf student may be operating in more than one language, that is, English and ASL or some other combination of languages, the source of the error might be an overgeneralization from an English form or may be interference from a second language. Overgeneralization of an English form can be addressed through a series of contrasting examples showing the general rule versus the particular exception. Second language interference may require a more elaborate approach that addresses the "logic" of the difference in the two languages.

3. *Analyze target structure for language sense.* Human beings generally communicate for a reason, therefore, do not simply correct errors, but consider what is being communicated by asking the student to explain what he or she is trying to say. Sometimes the mistake is the use of an acceptable form in a new but unacceptable context. In this case, expansion will be more rewarding than correction.

4. *Design and implement activities.* Along with our general support of realistic language settings, we would urge that instructional activities aim at meaningful practice. Worksheets that use disconnected sentences or strings of unrelated words are easy to produce but may not be as effective as examples embedded in continuous pieces of language or drawn from real writing. Recall how our resource room teacher, Dinah, used current affairs as a focus for literacy instruction. Finding examples of the structure or form in a sports report or a movie review can also be effective.

5. *Reinforce the target structure.* In special education, reinforcement is often equated with material rewards or praise, but the student's ability to recognize the appropriate usage is reinforcing in itself. Presenting the target in a series of situations in which the student can be easily successful at first is also a way to establish recognition of the target form.

6. *Assess student progress.* Formal or informal assessment of grammar can be used. One thing to note is the total disappearance of a target grammatical form, correct or incorrect, from the student's writing. This might mean that the student has learned that something is wrong but has not integrated the correct form.

7. *Generalize target structure to other areas.* In educational psychology, this step is also called teaching for transfer. This is not a process of telling the student: "You did it this way here, now do the same thing here." To make the transfer, the student must know why two situations are alike. Before you can generalize, you need to establish with the student how the new situation is like the old situation. What are the characteristics of the new situation that allow for the use of the same form?

Teaching as an Itinerant Teacher or Teacher Consultant

Three-quarters of the students taught by itinerant teachers (or teacher consultants) are served on a pull-out basis; about 15 percent of the time, teachers work with students in the general education class; and only about 5 percent do they team teach. Luckner and Miller (1993) summed up the itinerant teacher as someone who does the following:

- Spends so much time in the car they can't remember why they came to this school today.
- Needs more time to get materials out of the car than to change a flat tire.
- Eats while driving.
- Knows the names of more school secretaries and custodians than the district personnel director.
- Can teach anywhere in a building.

These points might sound like an exaggeration but they in fact are an accurate reflection of reality of teaching for many itinerant teachers.

Swenson (1995) characterized her job as an itinerant teacher in one word: variety. The itinerant sees many students in one day whose ages can range from 2 through 21 years, have a wide range of abilities, and varying degrees of hearing loss. No two days in a week are ever alike for the itinerant. Affolter (1985) says that the hardest part of being an itinerant teacher of the deaf is working with classroom teachers because so few teachers understand the implications of a child's disability.

The most important job requirements for the itinerant teacher are to provide direct service to students and to consult with other professionals and parents. In addition, the itinerant teacher engages in monitoring students in general education classes, adapting classroom materials, conducting student assessment, conducting in-service programs, and attending staffings for students. The greatest barrier to providing services is the time constraints on the general education teacher.

Swenson (1995) described several other problems related to scheduling. Because itinerant teachers are often visiting several schools in one day, they do not have the time to focus on one student. Scheduling with other itinerant service providers such as occupational therapists, speech clinicians, audiologists, sign language instructors, and so on can make for a complex schedule.

Some other problems that an itinerant teacher might face include the failure of the classroom teacher to follow through on recommendations, a lack of administrative support, and the number of students on the caseload. We hesitate to say much about the caseload of an itinerant teacher because it varies from one state to another. However, a 25:1 student to teacher ratio is a fairly common example of a caseload.

A typical student served by an itinerant teacher of the deaf is an orally educated hard of hearing student without any additional disabilities who has a moderate hearing loss. Often, the student wears a hearing aid, has intelligible speech, and gets along well with others. The primary IEP goals for this student tend to be language related, particularly written language. Typically the most common classroom adjustments for the student are preferential seating and the use of visual materials. Seldom do these students need materials rewritten or the use of notetakers or interpreters.

We must stress the importance of rapport with school personnel because that makes it easier to integrate the individual child into the school program (Swenson, 1995). The primary goal of the itinerant teacher is to achieve a good working relationship with the classroom teacher in which the classroom teacher recognizes the itinerant teacher's expertise (Affolter, 1985).

To be successful as an itinerant teacher or teacher consultant, you must collaborate with a variety of teachers and specialists. Collaborative consultation is an interactive approach to providing information to the general education teacher. You, as the consultant, have to recognize that you do have useful information. To begin with, you define yourself as a person who knows the potentials of deaf and hard of hearing children and not as a cataloguer of limitations. In collaborating you need to search for mutual problems, that is, issues that both you and the general education teachers see as problems. In response to a mutually defined problem, you will develop a creative solution. To be successfully implemented, this solution has to be practical with respect to time and effort to design and implement.

In the box titled "What Itinerant Teachers Can Ask General Education Teachers," there is a list of questions that itinerant teachers can use to begin a conversation with the general education teacher. These questions are critical to establishing a professional rapport between the two teachers that will help both of them address the many challenges that they will face with their deaf students.

The itinerant teacher serves as a consultant to the general education teacher and will not usually get involved in direct instruction. Consulting typically takes the form of advice on how to correct nonstandard language forms and to facilitate communication in the classroom. Some specific suggestions from the itinerant teacher to the general education teacher include the following (Luckner & Denzin, 1998):

1. *Seat student in best place to permit attending and participating.* Generally, this will mean getting the deaf or hard of hearing student to the front of the room. If the student is accompanied by an interpreter, it will mean arranging the seating so the student has a view of the teacher, the blackboard or overhead screen, and the interpreter without having to significantly move his or her head.

2. *Use a semicircular seating arrangement.* The issue of seating arrangement is one of visibility. The sight lines for a deaf or hard of hearing student are simpler in a semicircle than in a conventional system of rows of seating. The concept is easy to explain but will take some practice with the general education teacher in order for him or her to get used to it. Moreover, it might not be physically feasible in classrooms with a large number of students relative to the amount of space available.

What Itinerant Teachers Can Ask General Education Teachers

Itinerant teachers must work closely with their deaf students' general education teachers. Because of their large caseloads and the amount of time that they spend on the road, it is important that itinerant teachers make wise use of the time they do get to spend with the general education teacher. One way to do this is to always be prepared with a list of questions to ask the general education teacher. Following is a list of such questions.

Openers
- What topics are you planning to cover this week?
- What kind of help could I provide for those activities?
- How do you normally plan for the student?
- Can we brainstorm some options for working with this student?
- Would you be willing to try . . .?

Specifics
- How typical has the student's performance been this week?
- What is the objective of the lesson?
- How will the lesson be evaluated?
- How and when will progress be measured?

Operational Responsibilities
- What can I do to help?
- How much adaptation can your lesson plan tolerate for this student?
- How and by whom will the different parts of the lesson be presented?
- Who will have responsibility for evaluating which students?
- Who will communicate with parents?
- When should we meet again?
- Do we need to include anyone else in the future?

Although most discussions between the itinerant teacher and the general education teacher occur face-to-face, there are some itinerant teachers who maintain contact with general education teachers by using e-mail. We caution, however, against too heavily a reliance on e-mail because there may a degree of intimacy that arises when people talk directly to one another that may be lost via electronic dialogue on the Internet.

The above is an adaptation of a set of questions developed by Vargo (1998).

3. *Stand where the student can read lips.* This is the other side of the semicircular seating arrangement and especially important for students who depend upon speechreading to understand their teacher. However, many teachers are "pacers"; either for classroom management purposes or out of personal habit, they like to move about the room. If the teacher says she needs to keep moving to check on the class, mutual adjustments need to be made. For example, if the teacher will not stop moving, you need to encourage him or her to pause so that the deaf or hard of hearing student can be signaled and ready to attend before the teacher addresses the whole class.

4. *Face the student when talking*. This is a variation on the previous accommodation and speaks to the need for both awareness and commitment to practice. The teacher may be aware of the need to do it, but simply does not have enough practice, experience, or a reminder system for doing it. Remember that general education teachers often run on autopilot because of the number of students they have to deal with. Therefore, they need a way to work new behavior into their system.

5. *Use an overhead projector*. General education teachers are often trained to write on the board without looking at it because long sessions with their back to the students can result in unpleasant situations. The overhead solves this problem. In addition, if the general education teacher prepares overheads in advance it is much easier to make copies for notes. You can be especially effective if you encourage the general education teacher to use a word processor or presentation software to prepare overheads because it permits him or her the opportunity to prepare detailed notes or to prepare skeleton outlines so that students can practice taking notes. Either way, it gives you and the deaf or hard of hearing student an extra bit of help in the form of lecture notes.

In addition to the above accommodations, there are testing-related issues that general education teachers need to be aware of. When testing deaf students, the following should be considered:

- Provide extra time to complete tests and quizzes.
- Provide additional information to explain test questions and instructions.
- Provide graphic cues (e.g., arrows, stop signs) on answer forms.
- Teach test-taking skills.

Teaching in a Team Teaching Situation

This section deals with the notion of team teaching in the general education setting, although we do acknowledge that other team teaching situations exist (e.g., two teachers in a classroom at a school for the deaf).

In working in a team teaching or coteaching situation, curriculum pace is set by the overall progress of the class. Additional communication access to the material is provided by the teacher of the deaf signing during her presentations, by an aide or interpreter if needed, and frequently by the general education teacher, who often begins to learn signs when the deaf students use them as their main means for communicating with others. Signs are taught to the hearing students both formally and informally. In addition, a variety of unique solutions are derived locally (e.g., the use of a buddy system) to solve communication problems in the classroom.

A unique variation on this theme is the Tripod Program in Burbank, California. In this approach, co-enrollment, which is a more inclusive concept than team teaching or coteaching, is used (Kluwin, 1999). Co-enrollment does not involve modifying the curriculum nor changing methods of instruction but, rather, focuses on changing the classroom environment. From the beginning deaf and hearing children are placed on an equal footing.

The approach involves establishing specific co-enrollment classes with a carefully selected teaching team, reduction in overall class size, and the use of sign language by everyone.

The difference between co-enrollment and co-teaching is one of duration. Although many schools have attempted co-teaching deaf and hearing children together, few of them have lasted over an extended period of time. The Tripod Program, on the other hand, has conducted the co-enrollment approach over a long period of time with stable class situations.

Working as a Member of a Team: Some Key Concerns

Team teaching requires a lot of work for the people involved because more collaborative time for planning is required. A key ingredient in successful team teaching is for one person to take responsibility for getting certain things done. In addition, the teachers must agree upon commonly defined or accepted goals and spend adequate time together discussing their class arrangements.

One of the basic sources of friction in a team teaching situation is the problem of which teacher will make what decisions. Most difficulties can be resolved through mutual regard for each other's ideas and friendship. However, many difficulties can be resolved more readily with preplanning.

A pivotal issue is often the lack of commonly defined or accepted goals other than the desire to "make it work." Misunderstandings can be the result of individuals trying to achieve laudable but incompatible goals. Also, team teachers may fall into the trap of not being on the same page language-wise, such as when they are talking about similar issues while using different words. Developing a common vocabulary is an early part of team building.

Shared planning time can prevent problems; however, this can be awkward because the teacher of the deaf can have additional administrative duties that cut into her time for mutual planning. These extra duties relate to attendance at individualized educational plan meetings, meetings with parents of the deaf students, and meetings with other support personnel such as audiologists and interpreters.

A teacher's classroom is sacred ground and to allow another person to use part of that space is always a sensitive issue. Typically, one teacher is moved into the other teacher's classroom. While this may be done for good administrative reasons, the second person is put into a subordinate position. There can be constant tension from an unstated feeling of "this is mine but you can have this." When personality differences arise, there is no easy way to smooth the normal amount of human friction since the classroom is already one person's space.

An Example of Team Teaching

The following comes from the experiences of one of the authors, who has evaluated several team-taught or cotaught classrooms for deaf and hearing students (Kluwin, Gonsher, Silver, & Samuels, 1996). In this example, we describe the development of a team teaching situation at the kindergarten level.

One of the first decisions that was made in the development of a team taught kindergarten classroom involved the selection of the hearing students to participate in a team taught classroom. The staff discussed at length whether students should be selected based on ability, interest, and other factors; or whether the selection should be purely at random. After considerable discussion, random selection won out and students were assigned to the newly named E.T. class (Education Together) in the same way as they were assigned to all kindergarten classes (that is, somewhat randomly with a balance for race and gender).

Curriculum concerns emerged next, with the deaf teacher advocating for implementation of a whole language philosophy and the general education teacher believing that the E.T. class should mirror the curriculum and strategies (and work papers) that were used in the traditional kindergarten classes at the school. Compromises were made with both teachers integrating ideas as the curriculum evolved into a teacher-directed but child-centered approach. The hearing students and their parents felt comfortable that there was nothing they were missing by being in the E.T. class, while the teachers felt comfortable that they were able to focus class time on activities more meaningful to their mixed group.

The class followed a typical kindergarten schedule. Students were involved with center activities, reading and writing activities, science and social studies theme activities, and enrichment classes (e.g., art, music, physical education). The deaf students were not assigned to one group within the class, rather they were scattered throughout. As much as possible, all instruction was done using sign communication simultaneously with speech.

Resolving Communication Problems. A common first reaction to a person who has a profound hearing loss is "I can't talk to this person." One approach to this concern is to teach hearing individuals to use sign language. Use of the total communication philosophy, which espouses the use of any mode of communication that is appropriate to the skills of the child and the need to communicate, was adopted for the E.T. class. Everyone would try to learn to communicate with everyone else. Hearing students and the general education teacher would learn to sign while the teacher of the deaf and the speech teacher would reinforce speech skills with the deaf children.

The hearing children turned out to be communicative sponges. Within a year, many of them were as skilled at signing as the average deaf child was at the start of the year (Kluwin et al., 1996). The general education teacher expressed early and consistent dissatisfaction with her signing skills although she showed progress. The deaf children never became fluent speakers as a result of this experience, but no one expected that. What amazed the staff of the deaf program was the degree to which the deaf children's language grew and the way their vocabularies expanded. The deaf children's utterances increased in length, and they showed a willingness to use the colloquial expressions of their hearing peers.

Discipline: Whose Standard Do We Use? A primary activity of the first few weeks of kindergarten is the teaching of the rules about how to "do school." The writer who claimed he learned everything he needed to know in kindergarten was not too far off the mark since about half of the teacher's utterances during the first six weeks of kindergarten are devoted to either articulating or reinforcing the classroom rules.

The first symptom of discipline problems in the team taught kindergarten came with the noise level of the classroom. Individuals unfamiliar with the deaf assume that all is silence; however, deaf children make a variety of nonlinguistic noises, which are not moderated by a hearing person's social concerns. In addition, overt physical behavior such as tapping, which generates noise and is not necessarily suppressed in a self-contained deaf classroom. This behavior spilled over into the E.T. class.

The second instance of discipline problems came in the definition of what constitutes inappropriate behavior. Because general education kindergartens are large group experiences where noise can interfere with concentration, little additional movement or activity is tolerated. Sitting quietly means both not talking and not moving. In self-contained classes for the deaf students, physical movement is less restricted for a variety of reasons. First, given the smaller numbers, more individual activity can be tolerated. Further, the children often arrive in kindergarten with little or no previous group social experience. Oftentimes, a behavioral goal for a deaf child is simply to get the child to stay in one place and attend to the teacher. Given both the generally lower social skills of many deaf kindergartners and the greater flexibility of smaller classes associated with teaching deaf students, the teacher of the deaf in the E.T. class was prepared to tolerate more "misbehavior" from the children.

The best solution to the problem turned out to be a process of making each child responsible for his or her behavior and rewarding acceptable behavior rather than punishing inappropriate behavior. Since the peer group structure in the classroom developed early, peer pressure and peer support began slowly to reduce the range of unacceptable behavior from the deaf students.

By November, all but one of the deaf children had caught on to the general strictures and rules of the classroom.

Curriculum: What Do We Teach and At What Rate Do We Teach It?
For a period of time prior to the start of this team-teaching situation, the whole language approach to early literacy instruction was popular among educators of the deaf because it reduces the emphasis on children learning phonics or other speech-based approaches to reading and stresses expanding the child's range of experiences. The teacher of the deaf in the E.T. class subscribed to this approach. However, at the start of the E.T. class there existed a continuing emphasis in general education and, in fact, in some locales, a rededication to basal approaches to reading. Thus, there was a conflict in approaches to language development between the team teachers that persisted throughout the project.

For the deaf program staff, curriculum pace was a major concern since between one-third and one-half of the deaf children were operating with little language base compared to their hearing peers. Even the most linguistically facile of the deaf children were at a disadvantage relative to many of their hearing peers. The solution hit upon by the teacher of the deaf was to provide additional instruction in needed areas during the afternoon time slots when the students were segregated for specific activities, such as when some of the deaf children left the classroom for speech training.

Some General Suggestions for Deaf Students in the General Education Classroom

Throughout this book, we have talked about teachers being cognizant of a deaf student's overall educational needs and integrating the teaching of subject matter across the curriculum. We have also emphasized the need for teachers to help deaf students acquire competence in the language of each subject matter and providing opportunities for deaf students to express themselves verbally. Much of these discussions have focused on teachers of the deaf in whatever teaching situation they might be in.

But there are also teaching strategies that are directly applicable to the general education subject matter teacher who has a deaf student in the class. These teachers need to be told about these teaching strategies, and teachers of the deaf are the most likely candidates for doing this. Several of the teaching strategies that might be shared with a general education teacher are listed below.

1. If the deaf student is using an interpreter, discuss the location of the interpreter relative to the seating of the student. This should be discussed with both the deaf student and the interpreter. Where the interpreter is placed will depend upon the nature of the class. Is it a lecture or a demonstration? Does the teacher move from one part of the classroom to another? Are the students mobile during the lesson or do they remain seated at their desks? What is the lighting of the room like? These factors and others will affect where the interpreter is placed (see Seal, 1998 and Stewart et al., 1998 for a comprehensive discussion of the importance of interpreter placement during classes). Although teachers are not expected to know the best placement, they should take measures to ensure that placement is discussed and that the deaf student is satisfied with the placement of the interpreter.

Also discuss the nature of the lesson and experiments that will occur in the classroom. Interpreters who have advanced knowledge of the subject matter terminology that will be used in a class are better able to prepare for the actual task of interpreting. For example, if the demonstration of a science experiment involves the introduction of many new vocabulary terms, an interpreter might wish to share these terms with the student before the demonstration in order to insure that the signs and fingerspelling or the speech movements associated with these terms will be understood.

2. Discuss with the deaf student a format for including the student in classroom discussions. Whether there is or is not an interpreter, or whether a student has a profound deaf or moderate degree of hearing loss, participating in classroom discussions is a difficult endeavor. This is related in part to the delay in receiving messages from an interpreter or in understanding a message that is received directly through audition and speechreading. It is also related to the fact that deaf students may be too shy to participate; perhaps this is because they are not used to doing so or do not wish to be embarrass themselves in the event of providing a wrong answer. These are not reasons to maintain the status quo of the deaf student remaining silent. Rather, they are characteristics of a student a teacher should attempt to accommodate. Examples of some accommodations are making direct eye contact with the student and agreeing upon a visual cue that will signal a student's willingness to answer a question; writing key terms on the board or an overhead to help the student follow the flow of the discussions; writing questions on the board or an overhead; and rephrasing questions if the student indicates that he or she is confused.

3. If a class involves much student participation, pair a deaf student with a hearing classmate who is sensitive to the communication needs of deaf and hearing people interacting with one another in the presence or absence of an interpreter.

4. Create a chart that outlines the main steps of an experiment or science activity. The major benefit of such a chart is that it takes the guesswork out of a deaf student's attention to the class. Knowing the steps of an activity also clues the deaf student to what a teacher is likely to be talking about. (See Chapter 3 for an example of such a chart that was designed for a cooperative learning activity.)

5. When possible, make lessons a visual and hands-on learning experience. Deaf students are visual learners. This notion of visual learning should also be carried over to the area of evaluation; portfolio assessment is one way of accomplishing this.

6. Get to know the deaf student. Initiate an ongoing dialogue with the student so that information can be gained about the student's interest in a particular subject matter, knowledge of what is being taught, and thoughts about how the subject is being taught.

7. Work closely with the deaf student's teacher consultant, resource room teacher, or teacher of the deaf (if the student leaves a self-contained class to attend a mainstreamed class). This will help general education teachers learn more about the learning style of a particular deaf student as well as alert them to some general considerations for teaching deaf students. It is also a good opportunity for the general education teacher to provide information relating to the science class that can be taught or reinforced outside of the science classroom. Science vocabulary, textbook readings, and report writings are examples of tasks with which a teacher of the deaf can help.

Conclusion

We have met few prospective teachers of the deaf who have told us that their career goal is to work as a resource room teacher or as an itinerant or teacher consultant. Some have liked the idea of team teaching a mixed class of deaf and hearing students. Others have expressed a preference for team teaching deaf students only. But by far, prospective teachers of the deaf want their own class of deaf students. Yet when we meet up with these teachers a few years after they have graduated, many of them are either in a resource room or are working as an itinerant teacher.

The dynamics that effect the work of itinerant teachers, resource room teachers, and team teachers are markedly different from that of teachers of the deaf in a self-contained classroom. The differences occur mainly in the actual classroom configuration (individualized versus teaching to a group), instructional approach (tutoring and supportive instructions versus lesson and unit teaching), and roles (works with or in support of other teachers versus works alone).

KEY WORDS AND CONCEPTS

itinerant teacher/teacher consultant: A teacher of deaf students who are located in more than one school. These teachers typically teach each student on a one-to-one basis in a pull-out setting and travel from school to school on a daily basis. The instruction tends to be direct. The caseload for this type of teacher varies according to state requirements, and a teacher could be responsible for a specific grade level of students (e.g., elementary only) or all students within a particular geographic level.

resource room: Classroom instruction in which the student leaves the general education classroom for assistance in a particular subject area, a pull-out instructional setting; the teacher collaborates and consults with the regular classroom teacher.

team teaching: Also referred to as co-teaching; in this situation, two teachers in the same classroom provide instruction. Usually one of the teachers is a clear leader for certain activities. Both can instruct the same lesson or take turns teaching.

QUESTIONS

1. Create a list of similarities and differences between the itinerant/teacher consultant, resource room, and team teachers. How can these three professions assist one another?

2. Of the four types of teaching options (i.e., self-contained, resource room, itinerant/teacher consultant, team), which would you prefer as your career choice? Explain your answer.

3. Based on Kluwin, Stewart, and Sammons' (1994) research with resource room teachers, how can you help to improve the teaching situation for those who are not "Happy Campers"?

4. As an itinerant teacher (teacher consultant), how can you use the time spent on the road driving from one school to the next to your advantage? In other words, rather than seeing the traveling time as lost time, how can you use it to help you prepare for teaching or meeting your students' goals?

5. Develop a list of seven activities that can be used to build group skills that you can incorporate into your classroom to help create a sense of community.

6. Develop a list of five rules for a class of deaf students that you would like to use in your classroom.

7. What are some of the ways in which a general education teacher can be better prepared to teach a class that has a deaf student in it?

8. What are some of the things that a resource room teacher or an itinerant teacher can do to help deaf students in the area of science?

ACTIVITIES

1. Observe a classroom teacher for twenty to thirty minutes (in your practicum, internship, or as a visitor). Make a note of all the disruptions to the flow of instruction and describe how the teacher deals with them.

2. Contact the special education office in a rural and urban school district. Inquire about the number of deaf students that are served in the district and their placement according to the type of teacher by whom they are served. That is, how many deaf students are seen by an itinerant teacher or a resource room teacher and how many are taught in a team teaching situation with hearing students or in a self-contained classroom?

3. Make arrangements to spend one-half day accompanying an itinerant teacher. Record what the teacher does during this time and include information about the nature of meetings with the students and general education teachers, distance traveled between schools, length of time spent in a school, and any other pertinent information.

CHAPTER

12 Diversity in Deaf Education

CHAPTER OUTCOMES

After reading this chapter, you should be able to:

1. Show sensitivity to the challenges faced by teaching minority deaf students through thoughtful interactions with these students and their families.
2. Use your understanding of cultural diversity in the structuring of instructional activities.
3. Respond to variations in help-seeking behaviors across cultures that might impact your interaction with deaf children's parents and significant others.
4. Respond to variations in the learning styles characteristic of different cultural groups.

Let's go back in time to 1935, when Mary Herring Wright was just a youngster and in her first year at a school for the deaf. In her book, *Sounds Like Home*, her brief description of the school she went to captured how **diversity** in deaf education was dealt with at that time:

> The North Carolina School for the Blind and Deaf was for Black children. When I was there, it could handle about 300 children altogether. At that time, however, I think we had more deaf students than blind students. The school for White blind children was in town and the school for White deaf children was in western North Carolina. Although we had our own principal, our school and the school in town were under the same superintendent, George Lineberry, who was White. (Wright, 1999, p. 95)

Today, diversity is very much a part of the classroom. Students in the same classroom can differ by ethnicity, race, language preference, socioeconomic status, academic performance, and more. Their teachers, too, bring to the classroom diverse backgrounds. Society has recognized that such diversity will require the introduction of new approaches to teaching and consequently, new ways in how we prepare teachers. This all falls under the purview of multicultural education, an area that in the past thirty years has spawned an impressive collection of literature devoted to defining diversity and to identifying best practices in the education of all students.

After all of the attention, are minority students doing better in school today? Although we can say that some are and some are not, we simply do not, as yet, have a definitive answer of the overall progress (Banks, 1997). In fact, in recent years, reports of dissatisfaction about the education performance among minority groups has led to the establishment of charter schools that attempt to address diversity by giving certain groups of children the option of attending a less diverse school such as one with an Afrocentric focus. But even this solution has its detractors, who claim that this type of separation isolates students from the realities of a culturally diverse society (Wortham, 1992).

When we add deafness or the presence of a disability to the diversity soup, the pedagogical considerations become more complex. We are only now just learning what it means to be culturally sensitive to the educational needs of a deaf child whose parents come from Vietnam or Cuba or some other country. Moreover, responding to minority deaf children's educational needs also means learning how to talk to their parents. Always, there is the question of how to get parents involved in their deaf child's schooling when such involvement might run contrary to the cultural expectations of the parents—especially in light of the fact that parental involvement is an indicator of deaf children's success in school.

We still have a long way to go in addressing diversity in our schools. But we are making progress, and there are strategies for dealing with diversity in the classroom that can be helpful.

The Impact of Diversity on Teaching

Minority group deaf children constitute a larger proportion of the deaf school age population than you might expect. The present overall U.S. population is about 21 percent African American, Hispanic, or Asian, while 36 percent of the children in programs for the deaf are members of one of these ethnic, linguistic, or racial minorities (Cohen, Fischgrund, & Redding, 1990; Schildroth & Hotto, 1993).

Minority-group deaf children are less likely to be placed in an appropriate communication situation, less likely to be moved out of a restrictive educational environment, and less likely to achieve well in school when compared to white students (Allen, 1992; Kluwin & Stinson, 1993). According to Kluwin and Stinson (1993), African American students show the greatest amount of variability in program placement—that is, they are more likely to be moved among several different communication systems during their early education than are white deaf students.

Minority deaf youth are more likely to be kept in a special class. (Allen, 1992; Kluwin & Stinson, 1993). Kluwin and Stinson (1993) reported that a deaf child's placement in a less restrictive environment is related to the child's race, parental education, and family income. White children of more affluent and better educated parents were twice as likely as poor minority students to be mainstreamed.

In 1975 Jensema reported that African American and Hispanic deaf students scored significantly below white deaf students on the vocabulary, reading, and mathematics subtests of the Stanford Achievement Test Hearing Impaired Version. Allen (1986), a decade later and using a similarly drawn sample, reported the same results. As Allen (1986) pointed out, the poor school achievement of most minority-group deaf students is not a new phenomenon but one that has been fairly stable over the last twenty years.

Kluwin (1993) made the point that race is a major contributor to achievement differences both in ninth grade and in twelfth grade for deaf students. He reported greater academic slippage for Hispanic students than for African American students during high school (Kluwin, 1993); however, ethnic differences appear to be cumulative rather than short-term effects. In studies of achievement of one year's duration, race contributed to differences (Kluwin & Moores, 1985, 1989) but not significantly. But, over a four- to eight-year time frame, race becomes a significant contributor to achievement differences (Kluwin, 1993; Kluwin & Stinson, 1993). In other words, minority deaf students start school behind their white peers and continue to fall behind each year.

Minority-group deaf children are less likely to receive early and appropriate diagnosis of a hearing loss (Cohen et al., 1990; Strong, Clark, Berliner, Walden, & Williams, 1992) because they tend to come from families that are less affluent and less well-educated than the families of white deaf children (Kluwin & Stinson, 1993). Consequently, they have less access to social services and are less likely to be identified early or treated appropriately. Typically, white deaf children are diagnosed, on the average, at 17 months of age while African American or Hispanic deaf children are not diagnosed until 19 months of age (Strong et al., 1992). Further, on several measures of social or economic class membership, the families of Hispanic deaf children are more disadvantaged than the families of deaf African American children (Cohen et al., 1990; Kluwin & Stinson, 1993).

Deaf children from racial, linguistic, or ethnic minorities arrive in school programs with fewer language skills than their white counterparts, even when adjustments for other demographic differences are made (Strong et al., 1992). Typically, an African American or Hispanic deaf child will have a score that is only 75 percent of a white deaf child's score on a measure of expressive or receptive language at the start of a school program (Strong et al., 1992). Although some school programs have been shown to be equally effective for both minority and nonminority young deaf children (Strong et al., 1992), the delayed start carries on throughout the child's entire educational career (Kluwin & Stinson, 1993).

There are at least three issues in considering how to work with non-white or non-English deaf populations other than the simple facts that they form a large proportion of the student population and have serious educational problems. These three issues are:

1. Teachers need to be sensitive to cultural differences that interfere with interacting with minority children or their parents.
2. Teachers need to be aware of learning style differences that might interfere with learning.
3. Teachers need to be aware of help-seeking differences because parents have varying degrees of willingness to ask for assistance.

Implied Differences Between Cultures

In its broadest sense, **culture** is all of the things that people in a group do or believe in. It is comprised of the values, beliefs, behaviors, activities, and language of a group of people. As such it includes a group of people's art, music, religion, and literature. It also includes the group's medical practices, justice system, attitude toward charity, and attitude toward people who do not conform to group norms. Sports and leisure activities likewise fall under the rubric of culture.

Culture is an abstraction, just like language is an abstraction. Culture is also just as real as is language. Culture and language are abstractions because there is no one tangible thing called English or Ojibway or American Sign Language. There is simply the collection of the linguistic and physical behavior of numerous individuals who can understand each other. In the same way, culture is an abstraction because it is the behavior common to a group of individuals.

Four dimensions of culture that impact on what teachers do are historical, behavioral, functional, and symbolic. The key points of each of these dimensions are shown in Figure 12.1. When different groups of people exhibit differences in their culture, these differences are usually associated with one of the foregoing four dimensions.

Culture as history implies the transmission of traditional ideas, values, and beliefs. A large part of what we do as teachers is to communicate the cultural history of a group.

Historical		Behavioral
Transmission of ideas, values, and beliefs		Group norms Group-defined actions
	CULTURE	
Functional		**Symbolic**
Problem-solving approaches		Values and meanings of objects and language

FIGURE 12.1   An illustration of four dimensions of culture.

One of the fundamental problems we confront when trying to teach "American" culture is that the rather amorphous idea of American culture includes an assembly of different cultures. Deaf people too comprise an amorphous group of people. In Chapter 5, we talked about the importance of teaching about the lives of all deaf people, including those people who identify themselves as being Deaf as well as those who are hard of hearing and late-deafened.

Culture as behavior is the adherence to a group norm or mode of conduct. Deaf people who regularly attend social events in the Deaf community or use ASL as the primary language when speaking to their children, deaf or hearing, are exhibiting a behavior that is unique to the culture of the Deaf community. A recent teen style among boys, deaf and hearing, is a shaved head covered by a baseball cap. This is significant because it shows group identity or allegiance that has implications for the kinds of rules that a school might establish for the wearing of headgear in the classroom. Many schools, for example, do not permit students to wear any kind of head coverings because to many members of the adult population, it shows a lack of respect.

Culture as function is the person's approach to problem solving. The basic idea is that there is always more than one way to do anything, and some groups tend to prefer one solution over another. For example, virtually all cultures give children names. However, the age when a child is named, the number of names a child will have during his or her life, the sequence of names (e.g., clan, family, and personal), and the rationale for selecting a name vary greatly from one culture to another.

Culture as symbol is a potent part of U.S. education, particularly with younger children. In the general notion of culture, it is the assignment of meaning to objects and events. The Deaf President Now movement at Gallaudet University in 1988 was a revolutionary event that symbolized the "drive for self-determination that has long been characteristic of deaf people in the United States and elsewhere" (Christiansen & Barnartt, 1995, p. 227). There can, however, be multiple interpretations of the symbols. For example, are the "Stars and Bars" on the flag of the Confederacy a symbol of oppression or a monument to a glorious heritage? Can we celebrate George Washington as the father of our country or must we teach that he was a slave owner? In one culture an ax is just a tool; in another, it is a symbol of masculine power; in another, it is an emblem of an oppressive regime. Thus, a part of culture is assigning values and meanings to objects and events.

Culture embodies both content and process. As content, culture includes the ideas, behaviors, events, and products of a group of people. As a process, culture is something that is learned and shared.

How Culture Becomes a Barrier to Minority Parent Involvement

The education of deaf children is firmly anchored on two assumptions: First, the earlier educational intervention occurs in the life of the deaf child, the more successful the child will be in school. Second, parents are an integral part of the early education of deaf children. These assumptions are useful in planning for services for deaf children. Their value, however, is based on the willingness of parents to participate (Kluwin & Corbett, 1998).

Boone (1992) suggested several barriers to minority parent participation in the educational process of their deaf children, including a lack of parent information about the process, general communication problems between parents and schools, and parents harboring fear or resentment in response to previous encounters with the schools that included a fear of learning something negative about their child or a fear of being blamed. These barriers develop through the interaction of members of one group with the members of another group who hold different values and beliefs from the first group.

Cultural barriers between families and school programs can arise from different family traditions, different concepts of family pride, and cultural patterns of interaction with professionals or nonfamily members. Further complications to the response of a teacher to this situation arise because there are variations not only between ethnic groups but within ethnic groups as well.

Deafness must also be entered into the cultural equation. With deafness, responses to culture are not as straightforward. Stewart (1991) noted this in his discussion of the identity of elite athletes participating in international sport events. To explore the question of self-identity, he asked "Does the deaf Black sprinter see himself as a Black person first and a Deaf person second?" One response to this was given by Rohan Smith, a Deaf athlete:

> Where I grew up in Jamaica I always saw myself as a deaf person because there were so many Black people living there. Later, when I moved to Canada, I began to see that I am a Black person, which was how I identified myself. This is because there are a lot of white people living in Canada. Now that I am at Gallaudet University, I see myself as a Black Deaf person. (Stewart, 1991, p. 69)

In Rohan's case, the social milieu in which he was in influenced his self-identity. Translated to the school system, the issue of self-identity raises such questions as will a Hispanic mother who is deaf and living in Los Angeles exhibit different group affiliation and cultural beliefs than the Hispanic mother who is deaf and living in Lincoln, Nebraska? Although we do not have an answer to this question, it is reasonable to say that the strength of the identity and cultural affiliation of a deaf parent of various ethnic and racial backgrounds might not be readily apparent.

Several areas of differences can be identified that can potentially impact the responses of minority-group parents to current models of service delivery including the following key characteristics:

- Marital status or immediate family structure
- Kinship support versus general social support systems
- Decision making in the family
- Status of older people
- Importance of tradition for its own sake
- Response to convention and authority

Table 12.1 shows a comprehensive list of relevant characteristics pertaining to family structures and social values.

TABLE 12.1   Culture as Collections of Behavior

	Category	Definition
	Marital status	Married Divorce rate Unmarried head of household Female head of household
	Kinship system	Nuclear Extended
Family structure	Decision making	Single Negotiated Role-assigned
	Status of elderly	Ignored Respected Revered
Social values	Traditional views	Held Ignored
	Response to authority	Respect Fear Defiance

Marital Status or Immediate Family Structure

Family structure can be defined by several measures including divorce rates, the percentage of unmarried heads of households, or the percentage of female heads of households. African American families tend to have more single-parent households than the national average (Wilkinson, 1993). In a longitudinal study of a national population of deaf students in local public schools, Kluwin and Stinson (1993) reported that 43.2 percent of the children in their sample were from single-parent families. While about 33 percent of the white or the Hispanic children were from single-parent families, 72 percent of the African American children came from single parent families. In addition, across African American families, the rate of single-parent households is inversely related to family income (Wilkinson, 1993). The key issue is the degree to which a parent, usually the mother, must deal with a deaf child on her own. Being a single parent is a significant factor in a mother's ability to respond to the diagnosis of a severe disability regardless of ethnicity. If a particular group has a higher percentage of single parents, then this added challenge may be in delivering services to children from this group.

Kinship Support Versus General Social Support Systems

The issue of kinship support revolves around the degree to which family members other than the biological parents take on a specific role related to the child's upbringing. There is a national pattern of extended African American families that is characterized by a high degree of family cooperation, interaction among family members, loyalty, and residential propinquity in which blood relations may carry as much weight as conjugal relationships. Although variation is seen regionally and economically, the fundamental system as just described appears to be characteristic of African American families (Wilkinson, 1993).

The implications of this issue have been described by Dunst and Trivette (1990), who pointed out that a person's perceived need for social support impacts his or her interactions with early intervention services for a child with a disability. In other words, if a person has a large extended family system and no particular value for involving nonfamily members, that person might be less likely to seek the help of formal systems such as social services or the schools. Thus, when this person is reluctant to meet with a teacher, he or she is not necessarily rejecting the teacher's expertise. Rather, the teacher simply does not register within the person's system for organizing the world.

Decision Making in the Family

Decisions in a family can be made by a single individual. Or they may be negotiated between two equals. Or they may be divided on the basis of the domain of the decision (Blood & Wolfe, 1960). In dual-career, middle-class American families, economic issues are not the sole province of the father. Yet, these financial decisions tend to be the province of the father in Mexican American families (deValdez & Gallegos, 1982; Martinez, 1993). Martinez (1993) remarked that paternal decision making was more characteristic of Mexican American families than of African American or white families. However, Puerto Rican women, both on the island and on the U.S. mainland, have been more accustomed to working outside the home and taking responsibility for economic decisions than Mexican American women (Wilkinson, 1993). This variation in families as to who makes what decisions has implications for teachers. A teacher might try to interact with a parent who is not able to make a decision. If the teacher tries to suggest a service option, such as using sign language in the home, he or she might at the outset be less effective because the family member being talked to cannot make the decision.

Status of Older People

A difference between white middle-class American culture and many other cultural groups is that other groups hold the elderly in higher regard. This regard for older individuals ranges from simple respect, which is a common value among Chicano, traditional African, and native American groups, to reverence for the elderly, which is more characteristic of Asian cultures (Benton, 1996; Chiang, 1993; Rios, 1990). It is not uncommon for African American families to be built around a matriarch or grandmother figure who will raise more than one generation of children and who has a strong influence on the action of the family. For example, her opinion on the appropriateness of certain individuals as marriage partners is taken very seriously by the other family members.

In schools, conflict can arise when the school does not present the elderly in a positive light or does not show the older person the degree of respect they receive in the community when the older individual comes to the school (Kluwin & Corbett, 1998). We will see some of this conflict later in this chapter in the section on help seeking.

Importance of Tradition for Its Own Sake

Because of the relative newness and background of middle-class American culture, adherence to tradition has not been seen as a particular value. There has always been the lure of "the frontier" or "headin' West," a mentality that seeks change in the face of adversity. As a result, cultures such as Asian cultures, which have a higher regard for traditional practices, have often been stigmatized as being backward or stubborn.

Coggins (1996), in a study of a small number of Ojibway families, suggested that a mother's adherence to traditional values may help a minority child succeed in a mainstream school. What is particularly interesting about this study is that Coggins (1996) did not report any positive effects for a father's adherence to traditional values.

Medina, Jones, and Miller (1998), studying Navajo families, reported that varying beliefs about individuals with disabilities existed. Traditional views about the cause of disabilities often center around the breaking of taboos or not obeying traditional cultural ways. On the other hand, other traditional views supported the belief that individuals with disabilities had a special "gift" or were "blessed."

Response to Convention and Authority

There are at least three possible responses to authority: respect, fear, or defiance. There is a long tradition of enslaved Africans in America resisting authority in subtle ways similar in many ways to the resistance of Irish Catholics to English or Anglo-Irish landowners in colonial days. Many Central American immigrants exhibit open fear in the face of authority, either because they have suffered political persecution in their own countries or are in the United States illegally. As part of the governmental structure, teachers in schools should not be surprised if parental attitudes toward authority in general transfer to the parents' responses to educational programs.

While it is possible to speak of cultural barriers as arising from "a culture" or to define a cultural group as an organized system, culture in fact consists of a collection or assemblage of specific values, thought patterns, and forms of behavior. Consequently, automatically labeling parents or children as members of groups is not only potentially racist in that the individual's real needs could be subordinated to a response to a label, but it also ignores the underlying sources of the actual dynamics of the interaction between the parent and the service provider. In other words, not all Latino parents should be expected to hold the same views about the value of parental support in assisting with homework or attending parent-teacher conferences. Similarly, not all Deaf parents hold the same views about the educational role of ASL, English sign systems, speech, hearing aids, and cochlear implants. At another level, it may be that a mother is not ignoring a question that a teacher has asked but rather does not understand because of the way the question was phrased.

Thus, values or patterns of thought within a cultural group produce instances of behavior that do not correspond to the expectations of behavior held by a member of another group. In this conceptualization, a cultural barrier does not have to imply the implacable conflict between members of different groups but can account for misunderstandings between human beings on the basis of smaller-scale differences of perspective over a single issue. With greater understanding of cultural differences and their underlying reasons, teachers can learn to manage cultural barriers. This holds true for all types of cultural barriers including those that are derived from conflicts between Deaf and hearing perspectives.

Diversity in Help-Seeking

Help-seeking describes a person's willingness to obtain a service for a deaf child. As such it represents a potential source of conflict between parents and the teachers trying to serve deaf children and their families.

Help-seeking covers a range of human responses. It is a useful way to capture the explanation for why some people go to the emergency room every time they sneeze, and other people would rather stay home in great pain than go to the doctor. In the classroom, an analogy would be students who plead for help each time they stumble on a challenging problem and students who are reluctant to accept help from the teacher even when it is offered. Hence, it is crucial that a teacher understands that different groups have different tolerances for help seeking in general and for the individuals from whom they will seek help.

Often, the African American community underutilizes the services of professional helpers such as mental health and school counselors (Wilkinson, 1993). Part of the explanation for this phenomenon may lie in a differing approach toward seeking help among African Americans. The church, for example, is one of the primary places that African Americans seek help. In addition, it is often considered more appropriate within the African American community to seek help from family, extended family, or friends rather than to go to "strangers" for advice.

The issue of help-seeking becomes more complicated when an African American family member is deaf because African American parents tend to look first within their own community for information and resources. Also, experiences with racism and oppression may inhibit these African American parents from seeking help from professionals outside of their communities (Wilkinson, 1993).

Hispanic families can vary widely in their responses to help seeking depending on income, history of the group within the United States, marital status, and gender of the individual. For example, recent Spanish-speaking arrivals may be wary of government programs because they are fleeing poverty or political oppression at home or may be in the country illegally or both. In contrast, eighth- or tenth-generation Mexican Americans in

Texas may be more concerned with traditional value conflicts such as women working outside the home, which in, turn may impact the access of deaf girls to vocational training (Kluwin & Stinson, 1993).

Finally, three possible explanations for why some members of a minority group might find it difficult to work with the school systems in the education of their deaf children are institutional racism, ignorance of the system, and inadequate services (Kluwin & Corbett, 1998).

Institutional racism means that there is something intrinsically confrontational between white middle-class service providers and parents of a minority group. This implies that the system is designed or operated without consideration for the unique culture of these parents.

Ignorance of the system means that the parents of a minority group have insufficient knowledge of how the special education system works, so that they are unable to take full advantage of services.

Inadequate services means that the parents of a minority group need additional support in order to cooperate with the school system. For example, they may require transportation, or they may need day care or meeting times outside of normal working hours for school staff if they are to attend meetings.

Kluwin and Corbett (1998) interviewed 105 African American, Hispanic, and white parents who were generally categorized as "uncooperative" or "unresponsive" by school staffs in five cities around the United States. The parents had deaf children aged 2 to 14 years and had been identified for and scheduled for some form of service for at least one year. In three-quarters of the interviews, the interviewers spoke with the mother of the child while in one quarter of the interviews the interviewers talked to someone else, such as the father or grandparent.

On the basis of these interviews the authors identified five distinct groups of subjects: younger mothers who were high school dropouts, older mothers who were high school dropouts, older mothers who were high school graduates, mothers who had done some college work, and older respondents.

There were considerable differences between these groups, with parents differing not only on the basis of external measures such as age, income, and education, but also in the types of responses they can make to programs such as going to meetings, visiting the classroom, answering school-generated paperwork, and getting involved in the IEP process.

Parents, however, are not monolithic in their backgrounds and certainly not simplistic in their responses to educational programs. The Kluwin and Corbett (1998) study emphasized the importance of designing programs to serve deaf children that recognize the beliefs, values, educational background, experiences, and education of the families.

Reaching Out to Parents

No program or teacher can expect to successfully reach all types of parents of deaf children using a single approach. It is critical to have multiple approaches and to experiment until one approach succeeds. When it comes to communicating with parents or other caregivers about their deaf children, we suggest three parameters as a way to begin to organize multiple approaches:

- Form
- Content
- Audience

Form includes the format and the language of the communication. The format can be written, spoken, or signed. The language can be the language of the school or the language of the home. A message that is compatible in format and language with the home will be better received. For example, if parents do not read notes in English, a member of the community phoning the parents in the home language will be more effective. If messages are conveyed communally, posting flyers in the home language in the local church might go farther than sending them home with the children. If the bus driver knows every parent or caregiver on the route, then messages sent home that way might be one way of ensuring that information from the school reaches the parents. Use of interpreters for Deaf parents can help the communication process too.

Content in a school-generated message is system-centered, child-centered, or parent-centered. Schools are institutions and as such have institutional needs. There are bits of information that the institution needs to convey such as opening and closing dates, hours of business, and how to access various service providers. This information is important to parents but only in so far as it impacts the welfare of their child. It may be very important to you as a member of the organization, but for a parent it can be just one more bit of trivia of which to keep track. Involved parents are concerned about information that directly impacts their child, for example, the child's progress in learning, the child's emotional adjustment, or immediate safety. Another category of information that can be conveyed is information for the parents so that they can better help their child. This type of information essentially asks the parents to become more involved in some manner with their children. Parents might be asked, for example, to take their child to the doctor, focus on certain language structures in conversations with their child, or assist on a field trip. See Table 12.2 for examples of parental responses to school requests for information or participation and actions that teachers can take.

Providing information to parents is an important way that schools help families. Information itself can be hierarchical in that some types will be read with interest by the parents while other types will be disregarded. In general, information of immediate impact to the child will be attended to first. Information of general help to the parent comes in second. Institutional information like IEP meetings often comes in last. When you say, "But this is important for the kids," *you* are defining it as important. The parents may not. The parents might perceive the information that you are trying to convey as only being indirectly beneficial to their deaf children because it serves the school's purposes.

Audience is the likely recipient of the message. Audience can be illustrated with a little anecdote. One of the authors was interviewing a mainstream kindergarten teacher as part of a formative evaluation of a deaf education program. The teacher mentioned that some parents were not involved with their children. Every child had a backpack, and the teacher always put all communications into the children's backpacks herself. Every so often she would find a child's backpack filled with unopened messages. The teacher's assumption was that the purpose of the backpack was to convey things from school to home and back again. This assumption is supported by those parents who clearly saw the backpack as a way for the

TABLE 12.2   Parents' Responses to School Requests

Parent Response	What Is Being Said	Possible Action
I can't do that.	I am physically unable to do it.	Provide alternative forms of support, e.g., day care
	I am emotionally unable to do it.	Establish a support group
	I am unwilling to do it.	Explore reasons why
I don't know how to do that.	I don't have the knowledge you have.	Provide information
	I can't figure out how to include this in my life.	Explore possible resources
	I am unwilling to do it.	Explore reasons why
I'd like to.	I am willing but can't figure out how to do it.	Explore possible solutions
	I am unable to commit to solution.	Explore reasons why

child to take things to school. On the other hand, some parents may have seen the backpack as a necessary but nonfunctional school rule, which may have accounted for the unopened messages. Just because the teacher or school policies see a communication system as working in a particular way does not mean that the parents will see it in the same way.

When designing a communication system, you must recognize who the audience really is and how the audience perceives the message. You cannot assume that because you want the system to work a particular way that it will in fact work that way. Chapter 14 explores various ways of communicating with parents.

Learning Styles in a Cultural Context

Learning style is a flexible construct whose meaning can range from those people who are better at listening to information to those people who prefer to see information presented as a picture. It can also include the setting in which the learning takes place, such as public or large group instruction versus private or tutorial settings. Pacing, too, is important because learning can take place at a set rate or it can be controlled by the individual learner.

Learning style is heavily influenced by a child's first teachers: parents, grandparents, and people in the community. This is also how learning styles are linked to but not completely determined by cultural groups. Our first teachers are members of a cultural group. Because of the values and material content—stone axes or automobiles—of the culture, those individuals will tend to present information in a specific way. For example, if the culture and our first teacher organize locations in space on a written grid—a map—we will learn to navigate by street names in a two-dimensional space. If the culture and our first teacher navigates by landmarks—turn left at the big red rock—we will navigate by landmarks. If the culture and our first teacher remember journeys as stories, then we will learn verbal records for journeys. In this way a person can become a visual, a spatial, or a verbal learner.

Because personalities and abilities vary within any group, not every individual in every group is identical to ever other individual. Hence, a range of styles occurs in every cultural group. Since the cultural group has a preference for one style over another, the modal—most typical or frequently occurring—individual will tend to exhibit that particular style. Consequently, there is not one single learning style for each culture, but there may be a predominant form. Most important is that teachers are aware that problems or conflicts can arise because the learning style of one group of children is different from another or contrasts with the teacher's style of presentation.

Specific Learning Styles

Global Versus Analytic Learning.   Which does a student want first, the big picture or the details? A student who prefers a global approach does best when the overall concept is presented first. The analytic student wants learning cut into smaller pieces and gradually built up into a whole.

Verbal Versus Visual Learning.   Does a student want a dictionary definition or should the teacher draw a picture? The verbal learner will want verbal explanations, definitions of terms, and labels on objects because he or she stores the information as verbal content. The visual learner prefers diagrams, symbols, or charts. For these learners a picture is worth more than 1,000 words. In deaf education, we frequently use the term *visual learner* to describe deaf children's learning style.

Because ASL is a visual language, there might be a tendency among teachers to assume that ASL users are in fact visual learners. This is not necessarily the case because although ASL is visual and gestural, it nevertheless is still a verbal language. In fact, among deaf children, visual learning may not necessarily be more effective than verbal learning. Various kinds of mnemonics using phrases or sentences can be of assistance to students. For example, the phrase "fuzzy animals munch pretty plants" is a way to remember the biological kingdoms (i.e., fungi, animalia, mammalia, plantae, protozoans).

Concrete Versus Abstract.   Do students need to see something demonstrated before they can do it? Concrete learners need to have a frog in front of them before they can learn about frogs. Abstract learners can learn about frogs by reading about them and making generalizations about frogs based on their knowledge of other animals that are similar. This difference in style should not be confused with Piaget's concrete operations level, which is a developmental stage. Rather, the criterion here is the presence or absence of an actual object or event. For example, you may have taught a child the economic system of colonial

North America over and over, but until you take the field trip to Williamsburg, Virginia or to the Black Hawk Village outside Toronto, the concrete learner has difficulty grasping the significance of the idea of colonization.

Trial and Error Versus Reflective.   Would a student rather "just do it" or does the student have to be right? The trial and error learner prefers to "give it a try" and see what happens. This individual is a guesser who engages the new concept head on. This individual learns from mistakes and sees mistakes as a source of information. The quickest way to squelch this individual's enthusiasm for learning is to attach some kind of moral or social judgment to wrong answers. These learners are better served by more information about why their answer is wrong.

The reflective learner thinks about the answer and does not respond or offer to demonstrate competence until he or she feels confident that he or she is right. Thomas Aquinas was called "the dumb ox" by his classmates because he was so slow to respond, but he became perhaps the greatest philosopher of the Middle Ages in Europe.

Cooperative Versus Competitive.   Does a student need to be first? Some individuals are motivated by the intrinsic reward of knowing, the opportunity for human contact, or the sense of being part of a larger venture. Some individuals are motivated by knowing their place in a hierarchy or in receiving external rewards for success in learning.

Middle-class American culture, with an emphasis on the free market philosophy, lauds competition. This does not mean competition works for every white middle-class learner. Competition is certainly not always effective with Native American learners (Grossman, 1995).

Active Versus Passive.   "I can't sit still!" is not the battle cry of the hyperactive child but reflects a preferred learning style that is culturally transmitted. Kindergarten-age Amish children will sit more or less quietly for up to an hour playing with a matchbox and four or five beans, making up stories about the farm, the barn, the farmer, and the animals. Middle-class white boys of the same age raised on Nintendo and MTV appear to need a new visual stimulus every 60 seconds.

Like the concrete versus abstract style of learning, the active versus passive dichotomy reflects a need to engage the student with the content of the lesson directly or indirectly. The concrete passive learner will watch the frog, while the concrete active learner wants to hold it. But the concrete, active, trial and error learner will want to see how far the frog will jump. Active learners need to be involved in the learning; passive learners will permit the material to be presented to them.

Individual Versus Group.   The group learner prefers the protection and support of others when learning, while the individual learner prefers to learn or practice the information or skill with no one around. Traditional Native American cultures often stressed individual practice of skills before demonstration to the community. Mainstream American culture espouses a group mentality by organizing children into classes and teams with the admonition to "be a team player" or "a good citizen."

Learning Styles and Teaching Techniques

We can summarize all of the previous information in the chart in Table 12.3 that displays learning styles against some of the more common teaching techniques. It is clear is that no single teaching technique appeals to all types of learners. Each teaching method is slightly better with one learning style than another. This implies that teachers use a variety of methods when presenting material until they get a sense of the student's or the group's optimal or at least preferred learning style. Once the learning style is recognized, then the teachers are able to be more selective of the teaching methods to be used. The important point is for teachers to learn about each of their deaf student's learning style rather than make assumptions based on what they perceive to be the learning styles associated with deaf children in general.

Conclusion

The best response to diversity is variety. No teacher can develop a single approach that will meet all of the conflicting demands of different groups of individuals. But every teacher can develop an instructional program that uses multiple approaches including multiple forms of measurement. This is what diversity in the classroom and at home demands.

Diversity will never go away. There will always be children who are different from the majority. The best solution to the complex problem of diversity is good teaching. The good teacher has a large repertoire of skills and techniques that are thoughtfully and appropriately applied to specific situations. Becoming a skillful teacher means to know more than one solution to a problem. If you can attain this level of knowledge, then you will be able to meet the challenges of diversity that teachers of the deaf encounter in their classrooms.

KEY WORDS AND CONCEPTS

cultural barrier: A barrier that exists between families and school programs. Cultural barriers can develop through interaction of members of one group with the members of another group who hold different values and beliefs from the first group.

culture: All things that people in a group do or believe in, including their values, behaviors, activities, and language.

diversity: The many characteristics that shape the makeup and nature of a person. Diversity in a classroom of deaf students, for example, might be reflected in the ethnicity, language preference, socioeconomic status, academic performance, and degree of hearing of the students.

help-seeking: A person's willingness to obtain a service. In the context of a deaf child, help-seeking is evidenced, for example, when parents make contact with the teacher for advice about an IEP or a referral to an audiologist.

learning style: The conditions under which a person learns best. Terminology related to learning style includes global versus analytic learning, verbal versus visual learning, concert versus abstract learning, trial and error versus reflective learning, cooperative versus competitive learning, active versus passive learning, and individual versus group learning.

TABLE 12.3   Matching Teaching Techniques with Student Learning Styles

| | LEARNING STYLE | | | | | | |
TEACHING TECHNIQUE	Global/ Analytic	Verbal/ Visual	Concrete/ Abstract	Trial and Error/ Reflective	Cooperative/ Competitive	Active/ Passive	Individual/ Group
Advance organizers	Global	Verbal	Abstract	Reflective			
Analyze documents		Verbal					
Visuals		Visual	Concrete				
Physical rehearsing		Visual	Concrete	Trial and Error		Active	
Programmed instruction	Analytic			Trial and Error		Active	Individual
Large group							Group
Small group/competitive					Competitive		
Cooperative learning					Cooperative		Group

Except for the four techniques described below, the teaching techniques listed in this table are self-explanatory.

Advance organizers are abstract, often visual, representations of material prior to presenting the details.

Document analysis means looking in detail at words within a text as in literary analysis or history.

Physical rehearsal involves "walking through" a situation or using one's body to act out a concept.

Programmed instruction is the reduction of information to small bits that are learned piecemeal.

QUESTIONS

1. What can you do to provide parents with the information they need about services and access to information or programs in a manner that will be accessible to them as well as understood?

2. Delayed start in language acquisition negatively impacts a deaf child's language skills and academic career. Based on what you have read about minority students' additional delays in language, develop a list of ways to combat or compensate for this.

3. Minority groups may prefer to decline your help because your background or culture is different from theirs or you are perceived as a threat. Describe a plan to deal with this.

4. What are some strategies that you can use to acquire information about a deaf child's family that will help you in your communications with this family?

5. Is it possible to meet all learning styles in *every* lesson? Defend your answer.

6. Different cultures have different values and behaviors. What can you do to prevent barriers between yourself and the minority parents and families that you might work with?

7. How will your personal background and family structure affect your work with minority families and children? How will you explain yourself to them?

ACTIVITIES

1. Make a list of the various learning styles you can encounter in a classroom of deaf students. Develop a framework for a practical lesson plan that will appeal to or match all students in the classroom (assume a variety of learning styles are present).

2. Interview an administrator of a school with a culturally diverse student population. In your interview try to cover the following areas:

   ■ Percentage of students representing various ethnic and racial groups.
   ■ School plans for addressing diversity in the classroom through instruction, awareness programs, and other approaches.
   ■ Professional development activities for teachers to better prepare them for teaching a diverse mix of students.
   ■ Proportion of students who are identified as being in special education. Break this number down by ethnic and racial categories to determine representation in special education.
   ■ Qualifications that the administrator looks for in a candidate applying for a teaching position at this school.

3. Create a personal set of guiding principles and suggestions that will help you address diversity issues in a classroom of deaf students. Compare this with other students in your class or show it to a teacher of the deaf and ask for feedback.

13 Classroom Management and Learning Disabilities

CHAPTER OUTCOMES

After reading this chapter, you should be able to:

1. Describe some common classroom management techniques.
2. Make classroom management a critical component of teaching, such as planning instruction that aims to keep students engaged on tasks.
3. Differentiate between deafness and a learning disability.
4. Plan changes in instruction to respond to students with learning disabilities.

Classroom management has been identified as one of the most important factors related to effective teaching (Wang, Haertel, & Walberg, 1993). It is a broad term that includes establishing class rules, positioning of student desks, scanning of the classroom to ensure that students are working, using nonverbal signals, establishing meaningful reward systems, and communicating in a clear and effective manner.

Given the importance of classroom management, it might seem odd that each year more and more teachers of the deaf are encountering difficulty managing their classrooms, especially in the area of handling **discipline**. Some of these teachers reminisce in the staff room about the old days when deaf children had respect for teachers, parents, and other adults. When a "no" from the teacher was obeyed. When students feared being sent to the principal's office and feared even more that their incidences of misbehavior would be reported to their parents. These same teachers now have concerns about having to deal with more behavior management issues, and they wish that parents would institute stricter discipline at home. Their school principals, in turn, note that they are increasingly being called upon to step in and handle students who are out of control, and they wish that teachers would be more effective in their control of the classroom.

There may be some truth to all of the complaining. Take the mother of an 11-year-old deaf boy. The boy's teacher, who was a twenty-year experienced teacher of the deaf, reported him to the office for using exceedingly obscene signs in the classroom. The boy said that it was not fair that he was caught because he thought that the teacher was out of the classroom. He argued that he didn't hear or see her come back in. The mother came to a meeting with the principal and teacher where she openly agreed with her son's defense. She said that because the boy was deaf he should have been alerted that the teacher had returned. When the teacher said that other children in the class have a right to come to school and learn in a safe environment and not be subjected to such crude language in the classroom, the mother responded that "boys will be boys."

Perhaps there is some truth to what teachers are complaining about, but are the incidences of misbehavior more prevalent today than just thirty years ago? This question was posed to a deaf teacher of the deaf who was a product of the same school for the deaf in which he was currently teaching. He offered an astute observation of how teachers today viewed discipline. He said that the number of deaf students with additional disabilities such as **learning disabilities** and behavior disorders is essentially the same today as it was in the past. However, today's schools are more prone to label those students who constantly disrupt the class or who steadily fall behind their peers academically as having an additional disability. He felt that teachers use these labels as a reason for why they have trouble controlling their students because they do not have the training to help students with additional disabilities. He went on to explain that in the past, teachers did not have the "additional disability" label around to use as an excuse. Therefore, they were more inclined to treat their deaf students as people who required special management techniques and instructional strategies rather than people with "problems."

This is a fascinating hypothesis, but it won't alleviate the discipline issue at hand unless teachers of the deaf make a conscious effort to become effective at recognizing and acting upon misbehaviors before they escalate into serious disruptions of the learning process. They must also recognize that there are teaching strategies and behavior management techniques that can help students with additional disabilities learn.

In this chapter, the term classroom management is used in its global sense to refer to the organizing of the classroom, planning instruction, managing class time, and controlling the behavior of all students in the classroom so that an optimum environment for learning can be created. We examine strategies for controlling the behavior of students and the necessity of recognizing and designing lessons for deaf students whose additional disability is a learning disability.

Classroom Management

Teachers who practice effective management do so for the benefit of all children in the classroom. Their classes are characterized as having well-organized schedules, established rules, a fair and consistent reward system, and clear communication between the teacher and students. Effective classroom management also requires that teachers have a firm knowledge of the type of students who are in the classroom. An example of the importance of knowing about the characteristics of the students in the classroom is shown in the box entitled "What You Don't Know Can Hurt." This story illustrates the importance of teachers' taking the time to read their student files for information about student behavior that might not be readily discerned or accounted for in the classroom.

What You Don't Know Can Hurt

A male middle school teacher at a school for the deaf had a class of eight students. Three of the students had behaviors that required special attention on the part of the teacher and were low academic performers. The other five students were all in a college-bound program and posed little to no behavioral challenges for the teacher. This is all the teacher knew about the students at the beginning of the school year. Knowing that he had to take charge of the class from the beginning, he imposed strict classroom rules and spent considerable time during the first two weeks of school enforcing them. He planned group lessons for the entire class in social studies and separated the class for mathematics and language arts. The class ran smoothly for the first two months of the school year.

Then the teacher got mononucleosis and missed three weeks of school. The information he left for the substitute teachers was mainly about where the students were in various textbooks. Toward the end of his absence, a female substitute teacher was having difficulty getting the cooperation of one of the boys who had been identified as having behavior problems at the beginning of the school year. She did not, however, know this from the way he had been behaving in the class up to this point. Nor had anyone mentioned to her his past history of behavior problems in the classroom. The day he did misbehave she just thought he was having an off day because he did not want to do something on the blackboard. She decided to be firm in her demand that he complete his work. She approached him with a stern look and got very close to him physically, at which point the boy yelled out angrily and pushed her away. The boy was consequently expelled from the school for physically assaulting the teacher. When the regular teacher returned a few days later, he learned from the school's part-time psychologist that there was a note in the boy's school file about his fear of women. The fear was thought to be related to his having a single mother who was domineering and aggressive in her approach to raising him. The female substitute teacher, who was an experienced teacher of the deaf, admitted that she had cornered the boy in such a manner that she gave him few options for responding.

The moral of this story is the more you know about the students in your classroom, the better able you will be to prepare a suitable learning environment for them.

Another type of student that calls for special consideration when planning for classroom management is that student whose behavior is disruptive to his or her own learning and possibly to the ability of other students in the classroom to learn. Students who exhibit this adverse behavior are variously identified as being students with emotional impairment, emotional disorders, or behavioral disorders. Some of the characteristics attributed to this group of students and defined by the federal government (Hardman, Drew, & Egan, 1996) are the following:

- The inability to learn in the normal manner that cannot be explained by intellectual, sensory, or health factors
- The inability to acquire and maintain satisfactory relationships with peers and teachers
- A general mood of unhappiness or depression

■ An inclination to develop physical symptoms or fear associated with personal or school problems

Although each student in the classroom should be accounted for in a classroom management plan, the student who has a behavioral disorder may require extra time and effort on the part of teachers. But what to do with these students, and when to do it, is not a universal concept. Where some teachers might see a problem—a concern for discipline—others do not. In fact, research shows that teachers, parents, and students within the same school view different types of behavior as being a problem (Kluwin, 1985). Therefore, it is not unreasonable to say that using a problem-based approach to thinking about discipline is unproductive and results in little usable information.

Discipline

Kluwin (1985) illustrated the complexity of just one aspect of classroom management, discipline, in a perusal of the discipline records at five residential schools for the deaf. Three types of information were collected from each of the schools, including copies of actual disciplinary referrals; specific information about the students such as their age, sex, race, and degree of hearing loss; and academic achievement. He also examined background information on the teachers at the schools.

Analyses of this information revealed that the five schools did not share the same approach to discipline. Four of the schools used the traditional approach to discipline referrals. In these schools, for example, it was the teacher who decided that a student's behavior was such that the student would no longer participate in the class and was sent to the office. The fifth school used a different approach. Students were allowed to take themselves out of class if they felt that their behavior was disruptive to the learning process of the classroom. Thus, if students had difficulty paying attention or if they were too upset to participate in class, they could go to a counselor.

In the four traditional discipline schools, the typical student in need of disciplinary action was a 15-year-old male who had a severe hearing loss and was a poor reader. The racial makeup of these schools varied too much, so race did not enter into the analysis; however, anecdotally, it was noted that minority students tended to be disciplined more often than white students. It was also found that students who were doing poorly in school were also frequently in some kind of trouble, either within the school or outside of the school.

The surprise in the study was in the fifth school. When students referred themselves to the counselor rather than being sent out by the teacher, the typical deaf student who sensed that she or he had a problem, as opposed to the deaf student who was perceived as being a problem, looked considerably different: a 14-year-old girl who could be performing satisfactorily academically.

This particular study illustrates the difficulty in talking about discipline and classroom management. Different school constituencies define undesirable action by students in different ways. Student characteristics such as age, gender, race, and school achievement are tied into the mix in very complicated ways. Nevertheless, there are certain behaviors and characteristics that appear to be associated with students who constantly challenge teachers to react in some manner. Examples are sloppy appearance, poor study habits, lack of preparation for learning, talking, nonparticipation, inattentiveness, noncooperation, negative or hostile attitude, harassment of peers, harassment of teachers, and overt acts of violence. There are also factors external to the student, such as large group versus small group situations, that can impact on how students will behave.

Other considerations in the area of classroom management also arise from the dynamics of interpersonal encounters. "Personality clash" is an administrator's polite phrase for the issue of failed human interaction. Sometimes, a teacher and a student simply do not get along. Or perhaps a teacher might knowingly or unknowingly react to a student in a provoking manner, such as we saw in the box "What You Don't Know Can Hurt."

One approach to thinking about discipline in the classroom is consistency between expectations for student behavior and in the application of disciplinary action when student behavior calls for such a response. Additionally, teachers can benefit from adhering to such classic classroom management practices as preventing undesirable behavior, creating a sense of community and responsibility, following up on chronic but correctable problems, and revising instruction for student needs.

Preventing Undesirable Behavior

There are many ways in which teachers can prevent undesirable behavior. For example, in small- and large- group teaching situations teachers can present material to the class in a way that keeps them engaged. Or, in group activities, they can reinforce group membership so that each student has a stake in the success of the group. In this way, peer pressure is used to maintain appropriate behavior. Another strategy is for the teacher to have alternative teaching strategies on hand to respond to students who will not or cannot be directed through engagement in a task or inclusion in a group.

Keeping Students on Task. Kluwin (1984) looked at the presentation styles of high school teachers working in schools for the deaf. He delineated several elements relating to presentation style that were effective in keeping deaf students on task. These elements are shown in the box entitled "Keeping High School Deaf Students on Task."

Creating and Enforcing Routines. Routines are a valued part of almost every aspect of our lives. Books about how to be successful in business talk about the value of routines. Successful athletes adhere to strict routines in their training and preparation for major events. Successful teachers follow routines in their planning, instruction, and management of the class.

Effective routines are reasonable and the transition times between them are short. They should be created for instructional as well as noninstructional activities. Examples of routines that are associated with both of these activities follow.

Routines for Instructional Activities
- Routines that will help students prepare for a lesson in the few minutes before a lesson begins (e.g., students getting books, paper, and pen ready for a lesson).
- Routines for students with assistive listening devices (e.g., FM systems) that will help them ensure the availability of equipment and their working conditions. For students

Keeping Deaf High School Students on Task

A study of the discipline practices of teachers of the deaf working in schools for the deaf revealed the following effective management techniques:

1. Regularly praise students.
2. Use praise only for specific accomplishments.
3. Regularly offer public recognition of significant accomplishments.
4. Emphasize subject matter over emotional support.
5. Maintain regular contact with parents.
6. Give individual rewards and special privileges only for successful performance.
7. Make the structure of the lesson explicit at the start.
8. Persist with a student until real understanding is achieved.
9. Monitor student's actual understanding of the task.
10. Stop misbehavior.
    From Kluwin (1984).

in a mainstreamed program this might include carrying a microphone from one class to the next and giving it to the teacher.

■ Routines are needed for students who use an interpreter or a real-time captioner that relate to seating arrangements to ensure that the teacher and the interpreter or captioner can be clearly seen. The exact positioning of the interpreter relative to the student and teacher will, of course, be contingent upon the nature of the class. A shop class, a science lab, and a mathematics class would each require different accommodations.

■ Routines that a teacher regularly follows when introducing a lesson. These might include telling the students what the outcomes of the lesson are (e.g., "Yesterday at the museum each of you kept a journal of the activities you did, including some of the things you said or that you heard other people say. Today, we are going to translate this journal into a story.") and reminding them of their expected behavior during the lesson. Students can also be reminded about how they are expected to behave during the time when the teacher is instructing, when they might be working independently or in a group, and when they have completed their work. If rules for behavior are presented, then the teacher should also remind the students about the consequences for those who do not follow the rules.

■ Given the diverse range of communication skills that are often found in a classroom of deaf students, routines can be established that focus solely on communication related matters such as:

■ What students can do when they do not understand what a teacher or classmate had said

■ How they are to speak so that others can best understand their speech and/or signs

■ What activities can they engage in when they are learning new vocabulary in any of their subject areas (e.g., write the word down in a separate notebook, look up the dictionary definition, make a point in using the word in a sentence to the teacher).

Routines for Noninstructional Activities

- Routines for leaving the classroom that are specific for each place that the student can go to including the restroom, office, library, lunchroom, and other classes.
- Routines for showing their respect to others in the classroom and visitors. Deaf students may be delayed in their development of appropriate social skills, including how to acknowledge the presence of people and how to talk to them in an appropriate manner. Therefore, when teachers create routines that relate to showing respect, they might consider demonstrating when and how students can greet people who come to their classes. This demonstration might include the teacher's going over a list of things that are appropriate to talk about (e.g., what they like about school; their favorite place to visit) and inappropriate things to touch upon (e.g., personal information related to the family, derogatory information about other people).
- Routines for engaging in movement and activities during noninstructional period or free time that have been assigned in the class.

Great routines are only as good as the degree to which students understand them and to which they are able and willing to follow. High demands may result in a student getting frustrated and eventually rebelling against a routine. On the other hand, routines that are derived from input from the students might have a high chance of being followed. Help students understand the purpose of routines, why classrooms and, more generally, society, have rules. Write the routines out and post them in the classroom. Make a small notebook of routines that students can carry around with them or keep at their desks. Ensure that the students understand the language used in writing up a routine.

Managing Free Time. In a sense, the management of free time is a routine. Students are given specific instructions about what they can and cannot do between the time that they have finished their work and the time of their next instructional activity. But managing free time is not a simple matter. This statement stems from our observations of teachers of the deaf who tend to give their students too much free time during the day.

The average deaf student lags far enough behind his or her hearing peers in academic subjects that time should be one of the most valued components of the educational program. Yet, we have witnessed teachers of the deaf assigning fewer math problems, shorter compositions in a writing assignment, and fewer sentences to write when answering a social studies question, only to have these same deaf students complete their work with ten to fifteen minutes remaining before the end of the period. During this time, the students are allowed to do a range of activities including play activities for young children, games, and surfing the Internet. We have also watched teachers at all levels of school stop their classes ten minutes before the end of the period so that students can get ready for recess, lunch, or catching the bus at the end of the day.

But how does free time replace the time not spent on absorbing new knowledge or practicing academic skills? Although there might be some peripheral or incidental learning that takes place during free time, teachers should consider the educational risk to deaf students by comparing the benefits of students being engaged in free time at the expense of being engaged in a well-thought-out learning activity.

Thus, free time should be viewed within the context of a whole educational program. Before assigning free time, teachers might consider asking themselves, for example, if ten minutes of undirected exploration on the Internet is equal or more value than ten minutes of performing an explicit, goal-oriented Internet task. For those students who have a computer at home, free exploration of the Internet in the classroom is likely a poor use of school time. However, this might not be the case for students who do not have access to a computer outside of the classroom.

Preventing Misbehaviors.   Deaf students need to learn self-discipline during their early elementary years. They need to learn how to recognize the connection between certain behaviors and school learning and how to monitor and control their emotions. Such a program for doing this was developed by Greenberg and Kushché (1993). Called the PATHS (Promoting Alternative Thinking Strategies) Curriculum, the program was designed specifically for deaf students and aims to "(1) increase emotional awareness and social problem-solving skills, (2) improve behavioral adjustment, and (3) integrate affect, cognition, language, and behavior for better cognitive and academic performance" (Greenberg & Kushché, 1998, p. 50).

Briefly, the PATHS curriculum is based on taking deaf children through four steps that will lead to their acquiring more effective interpersonal problem-solving skills (Greenberg & Kushché, 1998). Space does not allow us to detail this program, but this information is readily available in the PATHS curriculum manual (Greenberg & Kushché, 1993). However, we will spell out the primary steps of the program, which are:

Step 1:   Teach deaf children to "Stop and Think." Implicit in this step is that the children are taught to use verbal thought for self-regulation.

Step 2:   Provide children with linguistic and communicative experiences and opportunities for talking to others. This will allow them to develop an understanding of self and others.

Step 3:   Provide children with experiences to analyze and solve problems. The key here is that the experiences encourage the children to integrate their emotional understanding with cognitive and linguistic skills.

Step 4:   Facilitate a carryover of skills learned in the program to meaningful social contexts such as in the lunchroom, on the playground, and anywhere else where the children will be interacting with others.

The PATHS Curriculum's emphasis on talking about things such as emotions, problems, and possible responses to them, and so forth, ties in with one of our themes that deaf children need opportunities for self-expression. In addition, the PATHS reliance on experiences matches with our theme of creating authentic experiences for deaf children as a means for helping them make connections between thoughts, language, and real-world concepts—connections that are mediated by the people around them. In light of social-cognition theories, these similarities in approaches to helping deaf children learn and teaching them about self-discipline are not unexpected. Both approaches take into account the effects of social and cultural factors on the processing of information.

Creating a Sense of Community and Responsibility

The Marines create a sense of group membership through constant mutual suffering during boot camp. Since the Marines are a military organization and school classes are not, you will need a different approach to building a sense of community in the classroom. The following eight techniques are examples of how this can occur:

1. *Provide consistent expectations and consequences with regard to classroom routines and rules.* Rules must apply every day in every situation to every student. Inconsistency breeds a sense of frustration because students will see one group or individual as favored and others as not favored. Ensure that students understand the rules by spending sufficient time teaching them at the beginning of the school year.

2. *Place general rules and behavior expectations on charts displayed in the room or on a sheet of paper placed on the student's desk.* What made Hammurabi and Moses famous was not that they invented the concept of law, but that they wrote it down so everyone knew what it was. When the rules are displayed, students cannot argue whether something is right or wrong, they can only dispute whether they did it.

3. *Use assignment books and/or folders to increase organizational and memory skills.* This combines the benefits of both of the previous two ideas. The material is public, and it is consistent. It has the additional benefits of teaching the students how to organize and keep their materials tidy and safe from getting lost or damaged.

4. *Provide regular feedback and check progress often.* The general rule is that the older and brighter the student, the longer time frame you can use for providing feedback. With early elementary children, materials checks, stars, and other reward systems come with each change of subject matter. For middle grade children, once a day for at least one subject is not too often. As students get older, weekly checks are sufficient, but checking depends on the subject matter and the student's ability. For example, mathematics can tolerate daily checks while weekly checks for English and social studies might be sufficient.

5. *Use corrective feedback.* Corrective or constructive feedback has the teacher saying to a student, "I would like you to take out a book and read when you finish your work" instead of saying "Stop bothering the person sitting next to you." The key is to emphasize the positive and offer something that will distract the student from whatever it is that is influencing his or her undesirable behavior. If a student sees himself or herself as being given an alternative to the present situation, then there is the possibility that the student will be intrinsically motivated to engage in this alternative option. This is especially effective when the alternative to misbehavior can be rewarding in itself, like free reading or the chance to do something creative but not disruptive.

6. *Increase frequency of descriptive praise.* An example of a descriptive praise is, "You really paid attention and stayed in your seat for the past fifteen minutes." But the praise must be meaningful because repeated teacher utterances that lack an authentic rationale become background noise. If you always say, "Great job," then no job is great. Praise appropriately and praise accurately. Simply repeating "Good" or "Fine" is insufficient for garnering cooperation. If the work is truly better than before, then say so. If some part of it is better, then inform the student about this part. Another benefit of descriptive praise is linguistic in nature because it is an opportunity for a teacher to model language to deaf students. It is more valuable for a teacher to say "You have completed the assignment and you used good sentences and vocabulary in your answers. Now please move on to the next assignment where you must answer questions relating to the impact of the steam engine on the industrial revolution" than to say, "You're done. Great. Now, move on to your next assignment."

7. *Use response procedures that emphasize the delay of rewards.* Examples of such responses are taking away privileges, points, or rewards. Punishment does not work well in most human situations. The philosopher Nietzsche observed, "That which does not destroy me only makes me stronger." In the classroom this translates to replacing punishment with delays in the rewards. Fishermen will spend hours waiting for a single strike and years stalking a special fish. If students truly desire a specific reward, they will wait for it.

8. *Use time-out.* Before placing a student outside of the classroom activity, question whether the student's behavior can best be handled by punishment, delay of rewards, or cooling-off time. Punishment often backfires, but delaying a reward because a student is in time-out can be a suitable alternative. A student in time-out cannot enjoy a reward. Taking a misbehaving student out of a learning activity only rewards bad behavior. The student thinks: "If I misbehave, I'll be put in time-out and won't have to do this work." Time-out is more effective if it means a delay in something positive.

The other side to time-out is that it presents the student with a period of cooling off. Anger has a chance to subside and reflection may set in. At the end of time-out, discuss with the student what had happened, why it happened, and what his or her future behavior should be. This follow-up discussion is critical because otherwise the time-out just becomes a rest period, which is an inappropriate reward for misbehavior.

Follow up on Chronic but Correctable Misbehavior

Every teacher encounters students who need extra attention and support in order to remain focused on schoolwork and to avoid acting up. Some of the more common indications of such students are listed below:

Type of Student	Associated Behavior
Unmotivated	Doesn't want to work
Slow worker	Can't finish on time
Unorganized	Can't find anything
Off task	Not working at the moment
Socially immature	Does not act his or her age
Disruptive	Personal actions interfere with others' work
Belligerent	Attacks or annoys others

Each of these types of student will require different approaches. Success cannot be expected if the same solution is applied to different student behaviors. Figure 13.1 provides a set of responses that might help each type of student. An elaboration of each of the response type now follows.

Parent Contact. For example, a teacher might write in a report a deaf child's need to learn new vocabulary words relating to foods. One suggestion might be to ask parents to spend more time talking about the names of different foods and then provide a list of critical vocabulary relating to foods. Another and more specific suggestion would be to provide specific instructions about what the parents can do to help build up their child's vocabulary. Some suggestions are:

- Provide a weekly list of the names of different foods that parents might focus on.
- Encourage parents to go shopping with their child to select different types of food (e.g., artichokes, broccoli, corn meal). They can then have their child help them prepare the food for a meal. At dinner, they can then talk about the shopping and cooking adventure during which time the name of the food has been used on many occasions.
- For deaf children who use sign language, teachers can provide a video or pictures of the signs that are associated with the foods.

Type of Student	R E S P O N S E S											
	A			B			C				D	
	1	2	3	1	2	3	1	2	3	4	1	2
Unmotivated		X					X				X	
Slow worker												
Unorganized		X			X	X	X					
Off task			X					X			X	
Socially immature									X	X		
Disruptive	X			X			X	X	X	X		
Belligerent							X		X			X

Legend:

A. Parent contact
  1. Daily home reports
  2. Signing homework
  3. Conferences
B. Self-monitoring
  1. Self-explanation of behavior
  2. Assignment pads/notebooks
  3. Folders for papers

C. External measures
  1. Positive reinforcement
  2. Nonverbal signals
  3. Teacher consistency
  4. Firm expectations
D. Instructional revisions
  1. Targeted material
  2. Opportunity for leadership

FIGURE 13.1 Responses to different types of student behaviors.

Signing Homework.   This is less paperwork than writing up a report to the parent. But, prior to sending a request to sign homework make some form of parent contact to see if the parents will cooperate. Also, it does no good for the parent to sign the homework sheet if a teacher does not check to see if the student has the work signed and has brought it back. This brief interaction gives the teacher an opportunity to explain the purpose of having parents sign homework. Some parents may not wish to sign homework, and teachers should respect this reluctance.

Conferences.   Teachers should meet with parents with a plan in mind. For example, they might structure the conference around a specific goal such as a home-school contract whereby when specific behaviors are demonstrated in school, the student receives a specified token of reinforcement at home. Flexibility is of the essence when teachers meet with parents. If a parent is not open to a teacher's plan, then an alternative should be suggested. Note that parental lack of cooperation may be a result of their misunderstanding of a teacher's goals or a lack of time or confidence on their part. All plans must be manageable for the parents to give a better chance of implementation.

Self-Monitoring.   Ultimately, we want deaf students to develop skills at self-monitoring, and students may need to be taught how to engage in this act. Some examples of self-monitoring behavior are as follows:

Self-Explanation of Behavior.   There is a difference between the rhetorical, "Why did you do that?" and self-explanation. In self-explanation, the individual is asked to give an account of what occurred. Asking a student to explain what has happened has the appearance of being less confrontive to a student than the threatening overtones of the request "Why did you do that?" Self-explanation is also an opportunity for deaf students to use language to develop their skills in self-expression.

Assignment Pads/Notebooks.   The use of assignment pads and notebooks is an excellent technique for developing self-discipline and can also give the students a sense of ownership in their schoolwork. The teacher can develop a checklist, a set of instructions, or a list of key words that can be glued or stapled to the inside cover to remind or help the child. A part of the process of education is learning "how to do school." If the child sees the material in the real world or if the parent knows that he or she can get the material while running other errands, it makes the process more real to the child. Therefore, having the parent take the child to purchase an assignment pad or notebook could lead to the child's being more motivated to use it. Doing this activity presents the parents with an opportunity to engage in meaningful communication with their deaf children.

Folders for Papers.   Some schools provide students with folders. If they do not, then it may be necessary for the parent and the child to go out to the store and make a selection. If one of the parents, a relative, or friend works somewhere that uses a corporate folder, then the teacher should try to obtain some for the child. Carrying around a folder with a corporate logo (or big brother's or big sister's college logo) can be a source of pride for the child.

A good management technique is to provide a list of things to be in the folder. A single sheet that starts, "I will keep . . ." put in one of the pockets is better than frequent reminders because instead of asking the child, "Did you remember your math homework?", you are asking him or her to run down the checklist for today and see if everything is there. This involvement of the child in monitoring his or her work is a strong step toward being an effective learner. Teachers do not help deaf children when they do things for them. It is far better if they create the means for deaf children to do things for themselves.

External Measures. External measures frame a number of teacher behaviors that are the basis of sound classroom management techniques.

Positive Reinforcement. Positive reinforcement involves a reward from the perspective of the subject, a set of conditions to be met, and a schedule to be followed. It is also only a temporary solution because the reward loses its potency over time. The goal is always to move the child from the reward system to intrinsic motivation and self-regulated action.

A reward is whatever appeals to an individual. To a first grader, it could be a cookie or a sticker. To a middle school student, it could be a point that can be accumulated toward a larger or a delayed reward, or one that the student can pick. We have seen middle grade teachers who have had special Friday afternoon sessions where children can bring in pillows, favorite reading materials, and snacks if they accumulate enough points during the week.

A set of conditions for receiving the reward that are clear, simple to follow, and above argument need to be established. Clarity means keeping the conditions to the level of finishing work on time, not talking, or not touching a neighbor. Examples of poor conditions—open to interpretation—are telling the students to behave themselves, be good, or work hard.

Reinforcement expectations must be consistent and clear to the students. In classrooms, random or erratic reinforcement is counterproductive, since it leaves room for argument and accusations of injustice. If the child performs the action, then the child is rewarded. If the condition-reward pair is too easy or becomes too easy, then you need to "up the ante" and rewrite the rules.

Nonverbal Signals. A nonverbal signal is a signal to the student that the current behavior is inappropriate. This process saves the teacher from giving constant verbal reminders to the student and from singling the student out in the classroom. Depending on the child, the classroom, and the behavior to be modified, the teacher of the deaf can use the usual attention getting signals such as desk tapping, hand waving, and foot stomping to alert the student. Instead of these signals, some other gesture can be substituted. For example, a flag or a button or a similar kind of object placed in the room or worn by the teacher could become the signal: The teacher wears a button with the logo of a baseball team. Every time the student is behaving inappropriately, the teacher gets the attention of the student and taps the button twice. This action reminds the student of the appropriate behavior. The signal can also be one that only the student and the teacher know about.

For this system to work, the teacher establishes with the student what kind of behavior is unacceptable and what the signal will be. At the start of using nonverbal signals, daily and frequent reminders may be necessary to establish the connection. If other students establish the connection before the target student, then another strategy needs to be considered.

Teacher Consistency.   This is one of those wonderfully vague admonitions that cooperating teachers, university supervisors, and building administrators love to throw out. Although it is difficult to define in practice, it has the ring of legitimacy. Consistency will occur when students will trust and obey teachers because they are certain that if they do their part, the teachers will do theirs. It is a contract between adults and children. Children need rocks to cling to as they climb toward maturity. Teachers need to be handholds made of granite. In addition, rules must hold for all students, at all times. When deviations to a rule occur, teachers should explain the reasons for them to the students. One key to consistency in teaching is simplicity. The fewer the number of rules, the easier it is for children to follow them. Actually, the fewer the rules, the easier it is for teachers to remember them and apply them consistently.

Firm Expectations.   Like consistency, firm expectations grow out of simplicity. Adults can devise very complicated schemes, but children need simpler schemes that are very clear. Suppose a teacher has assigned a specific task for the students to complete that is due by the end of the week. The teacher announces a deadline that is reasonable given the skills of the students.

The second task is to subdivide the project into smaller units with their own specific deadlines and responsibilities. For example, one day the students might conduct a brainstorming session around three or four topics. The next day, the teacher picks one topic and has the students brainstorm three or four supporting or clarifying ideas. A day later the students might write expansions of the supporting ideas. This is followed by a day to edit the paper. Finally, on the last day, the students hand in a clean copy. Built into each step is Plan B. Plan B is the alternative activity if the students have not been able to do the assigned work for that day. The alternative activity should focus on providing the time and the resources necessary so children can finish.

In sum, firm expectations work when the teacher expects the student to complete tasks appropriately. Students can expect that if they do what is asked, the task will be manageable.

Revising Instructions for Student Needs

Targeted Material.   In deaf education, teachers tend to focus on appropriateness and apply criteria such as:

- Does the reading level of the material match that of the student?
- Is the material sequenced in small enough steps?
- Are there opportunities for self-monitoring?

This process is known as *targeting materials* for the student. Another way of targeting material is to ask about interest levels. If a student is interested in cars or horses or sports, then materials are needed that incorporate this interest and yet teach the requisite concepts and present new concepts in a meaningful way. For example, teachers might try to teach "survival" skills, such as emphasizing simple arithmetic for the purpose of balancing a checkbook. However, balancing a checkbook has little or no meaning to many students in high school, which is a significant barrier to students' learning the targeted skills. Furthermore, the task of balancing a checkbook is quite complex when one considers the real-life issues that adults face such as what it is necessary to buy today, what should be saved before buying a costly but necessary item, and how can money be saved. To ensure that students have a solid idea about all of the processes involved in balancing a checkbook, the instructional task will have to be sequenced in small enough steps. It should also be tied to an authentic experience. For example, a reward system might consist of points that are given in the form of classroom money. Five points equals one dollar that is saved in a classroom bank account. Ten dollars earned can be used to buy fifteen minutes of reading time during the last period on Friday afternoon. Students write a check and balance their accounts when buying reading time. This type of reward system doubles as a transition activity.

Now, let's generalize the lessons learned in this activity by posing the question, "If you write a check, what are other things that you can get in return in the real world?" Student should answer this question in situations that simulate reality. The students might create a scrapbook with pages for "rooms" of furnishings, with tables for weekly or monthly budgets, pages for cars "I want to buy," and pages for cars "I can afford." The students can be given a weekly salary or allowance for household expenditures. Newspaper flyers and advertisements can be used for pricing and cost comparisons of things the students might purchase. Discussions can revolve around the need to purchase something and the merits of buying something affordable versus something that is a bit more expensive but is aesthetically more pleasing. A deaf person or some other person could visit the class posing as a furniture salesperson. Periodically, students can give "tours" of their "apartments." This entire activity ties in strongly with our themes for effective teaching. It is especially good because it creates many opportunities for the expressive use of language and for learning new vocabulary as well as some real-life concepts.

Opportunity for Leadership. All students need opportunities to learn how to self-monitor their work. Self-monitoring is actually a form of leadership in that the student assumes responsibility for his or her own success. For students who have experienced little success in school because of their penchant for misbehaving, their inability to focus on their schoolwork, or for other reasons, then self-monitoring may be their first step toward greater accomplishment in school. But it may take time to learn this skill, and it may be necessary to give the student opportunities to assume leadership roles with other students in a learning activity. By leading others, the student gains a sense of what it is like to lead in a positive way and also experiences the satisfaction that is often associated with leadership. One way to do this is to assign the student to be a group leader in a small-group activity or make that person responsible for contributing a design or an idea for a bulletin board for the class.

Learning Disabilities and the Deaf Student

Learning disabilities are by far the most prevalent disabilities among school-age children. According to the Individuals with Disabilities Education Act, a child's learning disability is determined by the discrepancy between what the child should be achieving educationally, given his or her age and intellectual ability, and what he or she is in fact achieving. The discrepancy is measured in one or more of the following areas (Hardman, Drew, & Egan, 1996):

1. Oral expression
2. Listening comprehension
3. Written expression
4. Basic reading skill
5. Reading comprehension
6. Mathematical calculation
7. Mathematical abilities

Applying this measurement to deaf students is not as straightforward as it is with hearing students. With deaf students there is the uncertainty of the contribution of deafness and its associated communication implications to any discrepancy noted. Indeed, one researcher has flatly stated that learning disabilities in deaf students are "neither clearly understood nor even recognized by many educators working with deaf students" (Marlowe, 1991, p. 283).

For the purpose of our discussions we are defining a deaf child as having a learning disability if it can be shown that the child's intellectual capacity limits his or her ability to function at the same level as same-age deaf peers. In other words, the norm for deaf students becomes the benchmark from which to measure the discrepancies listed above.

Even with this definition, we have limited information on the degree or nature of learning disabilities among deaf students. Van Vuuren (1995) studied sixty-eight deaf students aged 6 to 12 years with a normal nonverbal IQ and a severe hearing loss. She reported the following characteristics of an atypical group of students:

1. Very poor communication skills
2. Higher percentage of male students
3. Higher incidence of medical problems
4. Weak mother-child relationships
5. Low motivation
6. Weak visual perception
7. Weak integration processes
8. Passive activity level
9. Low concentration

Her description of this group suggested more complex problems than just learning disabilities. What is tantalizing about this single study is the possibility of a relationship between visual processing problems and other communication problems for these deaf students. It is possible that visual processing problems can have much more serious communication consequences for deaf children than for their hearing peers.

Other researchers have also sought to delineate the symptoms of learning disabilities in deaf students (see Mauk & Mauk, 1998, for a review of this literature), but not enough progress has been made to allow us to identify deaf students with learning disabilities early on and institute appropriate intervention measures. Nevertheless, there is widespread agreement that deaf children are adversely affected by the presence of a learning disability. Moreover, educators and researchers alike agree that something urgently needs to be done for this population of students to help them emotionally and in their schooling (Powers & Elliott, 1990).

The following points frame our discussion about deaf students with a learning disability:

- Deafness per se is not a learning disability.
- Deafness can result in experiential deficits that mimic the behavior and learning characteristics of hearing students with learning disabilities.
- Some deaf students will have learning disabilities.

The Challenges Posed by a Learning Disability

It is difficult to identify the reasons for a deaf student's lack of expected achievement. A deaf student's education is influenced by many factors including early intervention, effective communication strategies, involved parents, good study habits, real-life experiences, good teachers, and much more. Still, the need to determine whether a deaf child is not achieving because of some underlying intellectual incapacity is critical.

An important step in this direction is to distinguish between a perception problem and a processing problem. A *perception problem* is the result of the failure of all or part of a major sensory function. Color blindness or astigmatism or being hard of hearing are perception problems because a major sense organ is not operating properly. There can be degrees of perception problems and, in some instances, there are specific medical solutions to these problems.

A *processing problem* is the result of a failure of the brain to organize sensory input in a standard fashion. Learning disabilities are a class of processing problems. The child who sees or perceives the letter "d" but who processes it as the letter "b" is experiencing a processing problem. This particular processing problem is called *dyslexia*. Another similar type of processing problem is the transposition of numbers as in the child who sees "13" but says or computes "31." The senses function but the brain misinterprets the input or is unable to properly attend to the input.

A learning disability is a processing problem or, more specifically, a dysfunction of a basic psychological process involved in using language, which shows up as a specific problem in the ability to understand language, including reading, writing, or spelling as well as doing mathematical calculations. This assumes, however, that the child has at least average intelligence with a significant difference between the potential to learn and actual achievement, no evidence of mental retardation, no separate emotional disturbance, no cultural difference or lack of opportunity to learn such as extreme poverty. Finally, the underlying cause of the dysfunction is assumed to be a central nervous system dysfunction that excludes sensory limitations such as blindness or deafness. Figure 13.2 illustrates various types of learning disabilities that are the results of an intellectual dysfunction.

With deaf students a word of warning is necessary prior to the identification of a learning disability. Some deaf children may have been diagnosed and started in an educational

Nature of Learning Disabilities	Characteristics
Developmental arithmetic disorder (dyscalculia)	Significant lag in mathematics learning vis-à-vis other subjects. Severe problems with multiplication.
Developmental expressive writing disorder	Difficulty in composing written material and may make grammatical, spelling, and punctuation errors.
Developmental reading disorder	Significant lag in reading skills. Mixes up words. Makes substitutions or omits words.
Developmental expressive language disorder	Difficulty learning new words. Small vocabularies. Tendency to generalize, substitute, and omit words.
Attention-deficit disorder	Cannot pay attention. Constantly daydreaming or being distracted. Impulsive.
Attention-deficit hyperactivity disorder	Attention problems and cannot sit still. Fidgets, impulsive, won't wait for turn, disrupts others trying to work.
Sequencing disorder	Tendency to reverse the order of words and numbers.
Tracking disorder	Difficulty in visually following an object. Skips whole parts of sentence when reading.
Fine motor skills disorder (dysgraphia)	Good with large motor skills but problems with fine motor skills. Can shoot baskets but can't sew. Poor penmanship.
Visual foreground disorder	Fails to see a word on a page because he or she is distracted by pictures or numbers. Loses one object in a group of related objects.
Visual closure disorder	Trouble visually finishing an incomplete image.
Visual aphasia (alexia) Dysgraphia	Transposition of letters when reading or when writing.
Dyslexia	Collection of disorders that result in an inability to read.

FIGURE 13.2   Types of learning disabilities and their characteristics.

program after the critical language learning period has taken place. Or they may have had inadequate learning experiences due to poor communication at home or parents who did not engage them in many learning experiences outside the home. Or they may have gone through a number of programming changes and never acquired proficiency in any one modality or language (i.e., in English or American Sign Language). For these reasons and others, a deaf child may exhibit some characteristics of a learning disability without actually having one.

One way to understand how this can occur is to compare a child learning English as a second language (Fradd & Wiesmantel, 1989) and a deaf child. We can apply learning

Learning Disorder	Problems of Second Language Learner	Problems of Deaf Child
Discrepancy between verbal and performance IQ	Verbal skill is tested in L2 while nonverbal is not impacted by L1/L2 difference.	Inadequate language background in English or poor reading ability.
Academic learning difficulty	New abstract terms in L2 cannot map onto less sophisticated concepts in L1.	
Language disorders	Interference of L1 in acquisition of L2.	Inadequate language experience or ASL/English interference.
Perceptual disorders	Naming can be impacted by L2 language learning.	Inadequate language experience or ASL/English interference.
Social or emotional problems	Inadequate expressive vocabulary; different social rules; cultural conflicts.	Inadequate social experience or reduced communication ability.
Attention or memory problems	Cannot tie new information to previous experiences or schema.	Incomplete or inappropriately applied schema.
Hyperactivity/impulsivity	Difficulty in understanding situation leads to restlessness or inattention.	Difficulty in understanding situation leads to restlessness or inattention.

FIGURE 13.3   **Learning disorder or lack of proficiency in a language: The complexity of diagnosing deaf children and children who are second language learners.**

disability categories to either child's behavior and be wrong in the diagnosis because of the problems posed by either child's trying to learn or not knowing enough of the school language. The complexity of diagnosing these children is illustrated in Figure 13.3.

Thus, a child learning a second language or a deaf child may exhibit the characteristics of several different learning disorders but not necessarily have a learning disorder. Before applying the term *learning disability* to a deaf child, we must be sure that all other explanations have been eliminated.

Diagnosis and Referral

Given that many deaf children can appear to have a learning disability, teachers are faced with two challenges. Potentially, they can overdiagnose children and clog the system, which can lead to those who truly need intervention and support not being served. Or they can disregard symptoms because they do not wish to clog the system and, again, those who are in need will not be served. To avoid either eventuality, a preliminary screening procedure is needed. Figure 13.4 is a sample of such a form.

Powers and Hibbet (1998) recommended that no attempt be made to do formal diagnosis and referral but rather to use forms to coordinate instruction. In other words, instead of attempting to label the child, the child stays within the regular system but has instruction tailored to his or her needs. They also stressed authentic or functional assessment, that is, assessment that uses realistic tasks as a way to measure performance. They recommended a list of categories—such as attention, visual motor or perceptual behaviors, and memory processes—that are measured both through standardized tests and teacher observations. Eldredge and Coyners (1998) also recommended using a battery of different tests coupled with teacher observations. They included in their referral process a clinical interview as a first step in the process. Their approach is much more in the tradition of formal evaluation whereby a problem is identified in a step-by-step procedure and specific interventions are recommended.

Both procedures (Powers & Hibbet, 1998, and Eldredge & Coyners, 1998) use a strong teacher observation or recommendation component in making the diagnosis, therefore beginning teachers need to be careful in offering an opinion before they have had sufficient experience with a variety of deaf children.

At present, the search for a specific diagnosis of learning disability for a deaf child may be more art than science, although formal assessments in intellectual skills, cognitive processing, linguistic and cultural knowledge, emotional state, diversity of experience, and academic achievement need to be considered.

Principles of Instruction

Once the deaf student has been diagnosed as having a learning disability, a departure from the general principles of teaching that we have espoused in this book will likely need to be considered, given that the child needs to learn to overcome a specific processing problem by overlearning specific skills that will compensate for the processing problem. In this spirit we can consider McNamara's (1998) recommendations for some general principles when teaching students with a learning disability:

- There is no single right way.
- All other factors being equal, the newest method should be used.
- Some type of positive reconditioning should be used.
- Complete and accurate information about learning strengths is essential.

The individual needs of the student should be the starting point for instruction. What works with that particular student should be how learning will proceed. For a deaf student who is also learning disabled, failure has been a part of the educational landscape. To eradicate negative feelings toward school and learning, each successful step needs to be rewarded. Intrinsic rewards will take over later when deaf students are actually successful, but until they experience real success an active reward system is needed.

Child's Name: _____ Date: _____

Grade: _____ Teacher's name: _____

Personal and Social Behavior

	Disruptive in class		Fidgety, can't stay seated
	Talks out of turn		Disruptive while others are organized
	Constantly seeks attention		Overly aggressive to peers
	Fights		Impulsive
	Shy, timid		Quiet
	Does not make friends		Limited expression of feelings
	Worried, seems anxious		Cries easily, pouts, sulks, seems sad
	Fearful		Does not take risks
	Depends too much on others		Disorganized
	Difficulty following directions		Poor concentration, limited attention span

Academic Behavior

	Significant lag in math and/or reading		Good with large motor skills but problems with fine motor skills
	Difficulty in composing written material		Difficulty in visually following an object
	Transposes letters or numbers when reading or writing		Average or above average ability but below average achievement

Background data:

A. Standardized tests

Percentile rank on nonverbal intelligence measure: _____

Percentile rank on standardized reading test: _____

Percentile rank on standardized mathematics test: _____

B. Communication Information

Age of onset of hearing loss: _____

Age of identification: _____

Preschool / early intervention communication mode: _____

Home language: _____

Child's preferred mode of communication: _____

Mother's mode of communication with child: _____

FIGURE 13.4 **Sample of a preliminary diagnostic evaluation by a teacher.**

The other side of the picture is the behavior of the teacher who must learn to adopt new ways of teaching. To get a sense of how to function as a teacher of a learning disabled deaf child, we can turn to Lochner and McNamara (1989), who described several traits of effective teachers who work with learning disabled students:

- Plan for small increments of change.
- Use modeling, prompting, and shaping.
- Provide for practice, review, and generalization.
- Provide feedback and reinforcement.

As mentioned earlier, the decision to categorize a deaf child as learning disabled is an important one because effective instruction for these deaf children will be significantly different from the general principles we have described elsewhere in the book. The emphasis shifts from a cognitive psychological approach to a behaviorist approach. Broad outlines and general structures are replaced with small, specific steps that are rewarded immediately if achieved. For example:

- If, with the other deaf students, weekly reviews are needed, then it may be necessary to shift to daily reviews with the student with a learning disability.
- If the standard reward system is smiley faces or stars on finished papers, then this reward system may have to be provided at each step until the finished paper.
- If the deaf students go through four steps to complete the assignment, the assignment now must be broken down into four separate assignments for the student with a learning disability. Each step must have its own monitoring procedure and reward plus a fifth integrating activity so that the child sees everything go together.
- If the teacher normally requires the deaf students to complete twenty math problems before she or he will check them, then a smaller number of problems to be completed before checking will be required for the deaf student with a learning disability. This student needs at least as many repetitions as the deaf student without a learning disability, but needs the repetitions in smaller increments with checking in between.

Finally, it is helpful for all teachers to remember that there are experts in the field of special education who are knowledgeable about students with learning disabilities as well as other disabilities. If a teacher of the deaf suspects that a deaf student might have a learning disability, then he or she might consider contacting the teacher consultant who has an endorsement in the area of learning disabilities. The consultant can be brought in to diagnose the student and provide suggestion for how the teacher of the deaf can adapt instructions for this student.

Bringing a consultant into a situation where a student is already being served by a teacher of the deaf might not be an easy task in some school districts and especially in those districts where consultant loads are stretched thin. To counter this situation, a teacher of the deaf can request on a student's IEP that the student must be seen by a teacher consultant with expertise in learning disabilities. If this route is taken, the IEP should clearly spell out the responsibilities of the teacher consultant. Examples of some of the responsibilities that might be included are:

- The learning disabilities teacher consultant will conduct an evaluation of the student within thirty days of the start of the school year.
- If a learning disability is diagnosed, then the learning disabilities teacher consultant will meet with the student's teacher within two weeks of this diagnosis and provide directions on how this teacher can address the instructional implications posed by the learning disability.
- The teacher consultant will contact the student's teacher once a month to review the student's progress.

This approach to using expert consultants can be applied to the presence of disabilities in a deaf student other than a learning disability. Autism, mental retardation, and severe multiple disabilities in deaf students present special challenges to a teacher of the deaf because of the educational implication posed by each of these disabilities and the further complications of communication and language educational issues associated with deafness. Therefore, seeking help with these types of students can be considered part of a well-balanced classroom management plan.

Conclusion

We are going to end this chapter by raising to the surface that most fundamental teaching skill of all—communication. If classroom management is to succeed, then teachers must be able to communicate effectively with their students in order to convey their expectations and deliver their instruction. They must also be able to understand what their students are saying, because feedback from the students is essential to helping teachers improve in all areas of teaching.

These statements about communication are seemingly obvious, yet a stroll through various classrooms of deaf students will reveal instances in which the potential exists for disruptions to the flow of communication. Students may lack the communication skills to adequately convey their thoughts in signs and/or speech to their teachers. Some teachers may have communication skills that are below those of their students, a situation that can arise when a teacher's proficiency in ASL is less than that of his or her students. It can also arise during crises in classroom management if the emotions of a student or a teacher short circuit the communication process because one of them begins to speak in a manner that is unclear to the other. Therefore, it bears repeating that attending to the effectiveness of communication is a critical element of classroom management.

A second important point about communication is that it is not limited to the discourse that flows between the teacher and student. When working with students with other disabilities such as a learning disability, teachers of the deaf will benefit from contact with people who have expertise in this disability area. This is not an area that many teachers of the deaf have engaged in nor do many of them feel comfortable doing so. However, at the present time, our knowledge base about the diagnosis of learning disabilities in deaf students is scant. The same can be said about how we can best address the learning disabled deaf student with learning disabilities in the classroom. Therefore, communication with outside professionals is an important part of being a successful teacher.

KEY WORDS AND CONCEPTS

classroom management: All activities that a teacher engages in to teach a class. It includes activities prior to teaching such as the designing of lesson plans and the establishing of classroom rules and activities during teaching such as scanning the classroom to ensure that students are on-task and using effective communication.

discipline: The act of gaining control through the imposition of rules and schedules that enforce obedience. In the classroom, good discipline usually refers to well-mannered students. Poor discipline, on the other hand, is associated with a teacher who has little control of the classroom.

learning disability: The discrepancy between what the child should be achieving educationally given his or her age and intellectual ability, and what he or she is in fact achieving. The discrepancy is measured in one or more of the following areas: oral expression, listening comprehension, written expression, basic reading skill, reading comprehension, mathematical calculation, and/or mathematical abilities.

QUESTIONS

1. Describe a traditional and a nontraditional approach to discipline referrals.

2. Why is it important to keep students on task and what can teachers do to accomplish this?

3. Reread the box "What You Don't Know Can Hurt." The box talks about a substitute teacher not having information that a certain boy in the classroom has had a history of behavior problems. Draw a list of the pros and cons of providing this information to substitute teachers.

4. Compare the relative merits and disadvantages of punishment and delay of rewards as ways to disciplining a student.

5. Describe why free time can be disruptive to the learning process. What can a teacher do to ensure the time allotted for free time has educational merit?

6. Describe four different types of routines a teacher can incorporate into the classroom management plan that relate to instructional activities.

7. Why is it important to have routines for noninstructional activities?

8. Define the term *learning disability*.

9. What are some of the obstacles in determining whether a deaf student has a learning disability?

10. Describe some key principles when structuring instructions for a deaf student with a learning disability.

ACTIVITIES

1. Create a list of five classroom rules that can help students stay on task and avoid behavior that is disruptive to their learning and that of other students.

2. Survey five teachers of the deaf to find out what classroom management techniques they have found to be most helpful for their work with deaf students. Compile all of this information then rank the three most popular techniques.

3. Interview a teacher of the deaf who has a deaf student who has been identified as having a learning disability. Include the following questions in your interview:

   - What student behavior led to a diagnosis for learning disability?
   - What instructional adaptations does the teacher make for this student?
   - How has the student responded to these instructional adaptations?
   - Does the teacher harbor any doubts as to whether the student's discrepancy in learning is linked to a specific intellectual incapacity as opposed to communication and language abilities?
   - How did the teacher prepare for teaching the student?

CHAPTER

14 Involving the Families

CHAPTER OUTCOMES

After reading this chapter, you should be able to:

1. Respond to parents' needs and requests in a manner that is sensitive to the tasks they face raising and educating a deaf child.
2. Set up an open line of communication with parents while maintaining a professional relationship with them.
3. Devise a plan for involving the family in activities that occur in your classroom or school.
4. Provide parents with tips about watching captioned programs with their deaf child.
5. Provide parents with tips about how to help their deaf children learn to read.
6. Convince parents about the value of spending time helping their deaf children gain valuable experiences and enriching these experiences by talking about them.

L̲et's take a look at the long-term effect of having a deaf child on two family members.

Gwen: You can catch Gwen every Sunday morning at the 10:30 Mass in the local Catholic Church. Her deaf son, who is now almost 30 years old, has long since graduated from the National Technical Institute for the Deaf and has a job and leads a good life. But Gwen has not relinquished her connections to deaf children. She still interprets at Mass and teaches religion to deaf children every Sunday like she has since her son was making his First Communion. This weekly event typifies the commitment she made to her deaf child years ago. Her little congregation waxes and wanes over the years but includes deaf people from toddlers to septuagenarians who often come long distances because she so obviously cares about them as she cared enough years ago to be involved in her child's education.

Rebecca's Grandmother: Rebecca's grandmother is another regular fixture in the community. She has volunteered at Rebecca's school, sat through every one of Rebecca's basketball games, and has delivered the Girl Scout cookies Rebecca has sold around town. When people first see the two of them together they are impressed that Rebecca's grandmother can communicate well with her deaf granddaughter. The grandmother has committed herself to helping Rebecca experience life as fully as possible. This was the same sort of commitment that she gave to her own deaf daughter, Rebecca's mother, years ago.

In the first part of this book we talked about the importance of experiential knowledge in learning subject matter. Although a teacher can design activities and field trips to give children a chance to gain knowledge, the bulk of time available for children to get experiences is outside of school hours. Mervin Garretson (1995) made the following observation:

> After teaching some twenty years, I became interested in knowing how much of and what part of the 365 days in the year were spent in a classroom. In taking account of all the time spent out of the classroom: walking down the halls; during recess; in the bathroom; during the lunch break; during after school hours; counting the time spent out of school for Thanksgiving, Easter, Christmas, and other holidays, and the long summer vacation; the actual time spent in the classroom for the average child, whether deaf or hearing, came to just eight percent of the total year. This means that 92 percent of their learning is taking place through communication outside of the classroom. (p. 72)

Parents and other family members are in a position to have a tremendous impact on deaf children's learning because of their influence on how these children will spend their time outside of school:

- Will this time be spent with video games and the TV or will it be spent going places and interacting with people?
- Will the child be given the option of joining sports and other recreational activities in the community?
- Will the parent monitor and assist a child doing homework?

These questions and more lead to decisions that can directly impact a child's education.

Some people think that questions like these are for parents to ask and answer; that teachers need not be involved in monitoring or guiding the relationship between deaf children and their families. There are many parents who take the steps necessary to enrich their child's life and, hence, add to the growth of their child's experiences. However, there are also many parents who can benefit from the guidance and suggestions of professionals.

Moreover, not all parents acquire a realistic perspective of their child's deafness. Some never come to accept that their child is deaf or that this will be a lifelong condition. McCay Vernon and Jean Andrews (1990) illustrated how this denial process typically reveals itself in a family:

> With deafness, the less intimate the relationship to the deaf child, the greater the tendency to deny. Thus, close relatives deny more than parents. The mother who tends to be with the child all day is generally less denying than the father. In fact, fathers often escape from the environment of deafness and its implications by spending more time away from the home. Such behavior makes denial easier and contributes directly to the father's failure to face the implications of deafness in his child, and thus he avoids fulfilling a basic paternal responsibility. (p. 127)

Denial from any quarters has the potential to adversely affect the relationship between members of a family and the deaf child. Furthermore, if denial leads to escape, as noted by Vernon and Andrews, then these parents will likely spend far less time with their deaf children.

Some parents lack confidence in their ability to raise a deaf child. Others are overwhelmed by the information that they are given about the effect of deafness on a person's education, career possibilities, and lifestyles. All parents face decisions about the type of communication that they are going to use (e.g., signs or speech or both), language (e.g., English, American Sign Language, and/or the native spoken language of a non-English speaking home), school placement (e.g., general education class in a public school, school for the deaf), and community involvement (e.g., local community, Deaf community, ethnic community, or some combination of these). None of these decisions are easy for parents to make.

Whatever decisions parents make, there is one decision that will stand out above all others. This is the decision of whether they will be actively involved in their deaf child's education. In Chapter 12 on diversity in deaf education, we talked about the barriers to parental involvement. In this chapter, we will talk about the ways in which a teacher can facilitate parental involvement.

Building a Good Relationship with Parents

It is imperative that teachers seek ways to forge strong, positive relationships with parents. The thrust of this section is in establishing a professional relationship that will (1) allow the parents to talk to teachers without fear of intimidation and (2) enable teachers to retain their professional role and act responsibly toward parents.

Recognizing the Challenges Faced by Parents

If you are planning to help parents get involved in the education of their deaf children, then you need to be sensitive to the struggles that they experience being parents. A first step toward developing sensitivity is to become aware of the challenges that parents face when raising a deaf child.

The first challenge is how parents respond when they find out that their child is deaf. Vernon and Andrews (1990) offered the following list of coping reactions of parents who have come to a full realization that their child is deaf:

- Denial
- Guilt
- Seeking many opinions or cures
- Feelings of impotence
- Questioning the reason for the deafness
- Isolation of affect (e.g., deafness is accepted at an intellectual level, which may lead to an absence of a period of grieving)
- Turning to religion

- Blaming the doctor
- Blaming the other parent
- Increased motor activity (e.g., attempts to reduce stress by engaging in physical activities such as excessive smoking, walking, insomnia, overeating)
- Fears for the future
- Complete overt rejection
- Pregnancy
- Reading medical literature
- Reaction formation (i.e., where parents equate deafness as being a gift)
- Grief and depression

Many of these reactions usually occur before the parents meet their deaf child's first teacher. And the last one, grief and depression, is actually seen as part of an overall healthy response to deafness—a stage that, once passed, helps parents face the reality of raising a deaf child (Vernon & Andrews, 1990). In whichever manner parents react, the most productive outcome is for them to accept that their child is deaf.

Another challenge for parents stems from the many decisions that they have to make relative to the communication and education that they want for their deaf child. Although all parents must make educational decisions for their children, parents of children with disabilities are faced with the additional stress of preparing for and attending meetings to develop their child's Individualized Education Plan.

Given these challenges and others that parents face, teachers need to be understanding and supportive. This does not mean that they have to agree with everything that the parents say or do. It does mean that they have to be good listeners to what the parents have to say, that they have to be prepared to direct parents to sources for further information and help when necessary, and foremost, that they respect what the parents believe or desire and that they share their opinions with parents without intimidation. Doing this will help teachers earn the respect of parents and will enable them to be trusted as teachers.

First Steps in Building a Good Parent-Teacher Relationship

Following are some principles that can help you gain the respect of your students' parents and will pave the way for a long and fitting parent-teacher relationship:

1. *Be a good listener.* There are not many people to whom parents can comfortably talk about their deaf child's education. Parent support groups are one outlet for expressing concerns about education. But not all parents have access to such a group. Still, parents need someone to whom they can talk about their children because the very act of talking serves as an important emotional safety valve for them. Oftentimes, all parents need is for someone to listen to them; someone who will listen without offering criticism.

2. *Ask parents for advice about the best way for you to communicate school matters with them.* In our discussion about diversity in Chapter 12, we talked about the danger of making assumptions about how parents will respond to your efforts to share information with them about their deaf children. Unless they ask first, teachers have no assurance that a daily note in a backpack or an e-mailed message will be read by parents. At the beginning of the year, teachers should ask parents how they can best communicate with them about school matters. Suggest to the parents a number of options and be prepared to accept a reasonable alternative request by them.

3. *Present your opinions without intimidation.* If you must express your beliefs to parents then let these beliefs stand on their own merits. There is no need to discredit other people's beliefs because they may contradict yours. See the box titled "Intimidation Has No Place in Our Schools" for examples of how teachers might inadvertently say something that is intimidating to a parent.

Intimidation Has No Place in Our Schools

Although having beliefs about raising and teaching deaf children is acceptable, it is inappropriate to disparage others who do not adhere to the same beliefs. Following are some examples of beliefs that carry a strong flavor of intimidation when presented to parents. These are actual quotes that we have heard from educators along with the context in which they were expressed:

- "Your child does not have to grow up being deaf."
  - A deaf education administrator explaining why a cochlear implant is a good choice.

- "If you want your child to make it in a hearing world, then he has to know English."
  - A teacher of the deaf explaining why English signing is a better choice than ASL.

- "English in signs is not a language."
  - A teacher of the deaf explaining why ASL should be used instead of English signing systems.

- "She doesn't have to grow up in a Deaf ghetto. She can have hearing friends."
  - A special education supervisor describing why a deaf child should be placed in a mainstreamed program rather than in a school for the deaf.

- "Mainstreamed deaf children grow up feeling isolated, and they don't have many friends."
  - A teacher of the deaf explaining why going to a school for the deaf is the best option for a deaf child.

The problem with each of these statements is twofold (at least). First, as blanket statements they are wrong in either what they mean or in what they are implying. Second, they insinuate that there is something wrong if a parent does not agree with them. This is unwarranted intimidation. It is damaging to a parent-teacher relationship.

4. *Respond promptly and courteously to a parent's question or request for information.* Parents of deaf children may be under a lot of stress, and your prompt responses to their questions or requests for information will mean a lot to them. If you are unable to provide the information quickly, then let them know that you will be responding as soon as you are able.

5. *Show your positive side.* Let parents know that you enjoy teaching their deaf children. Find something positive to say about your deaf students each time you meet their parents. Doing this will make it easier to speak to the parents about some specific concerns that you might have about their child's learning.

6. *Be a good resource person.* Being a resource person means knowing the answers to questions that parents might have about the education of their deaf child or knowing where to go to look up information to bring back to the parents. But having all of the answers will not always be in the cards for you. Therefore, a good resource person also knows where to send parents so that they can get the answers to their questions or seek more information about a particular topic.

All parents face challenges when they are raising children. As a teacher, use these foregoing principles to show them that you understand what they are going through and that you are there for support when needed.

Steps to Maintain Positive Relationships with Parents

When you meet parents for the first time, it is important that you portray yourself as an effective and knowledgeable teacher, well-prepared to teach their deaf children. As you get to know the parents, you must make an effort to establish and maintain a positive relationship with them. It helps if you have a healthy perspective about your relationship to the parents. Following are some principles that might be helpful in shaping and maintaining this perspective:

1. *Maintain a professional relationship with the parents of your students.* Your primary responsibility to the parents is to teach their deaf child. Parental demands and student performance will cause some amount of stress on your ability to teach. This amount of stress will be heightened if your relationship with the parents borders on friendship.

2. *Respect the manner in which parents have chosen to raise their deaf child.* What parents do in their home and community is their business. As long as there is no indication of abuse, it is within their right to raise their children as they see fit. Your expectations of how a deaf child can best be raised can cloud your judgment of parents if these expectations clash with what you think the parents are doing. Included in this concept of raising a deaf child are the choices made with respect to use of communication and school placement. Remember, no matter what you might think is the "right way," there are people somewhere who have successfully raised a deaf child doing it in a "different way."

3. *Let your instructional behavior be guided by objective and sound pedagogical principles.* You teach in a certain way because you believe it is best for your deaf students. In some instances, your school might subscribe to a particular instructional approach such as thematic teaching, cooperative learning, or an interactive approach to language acquisition. Consistency in teachers' use of a particular approach is important to its success; therefore, you and other teachers in a program agree to use this approach in your classrooms. Parents must be informed about your teaching principles and instructional approaches. However, some of the most disastrous teacher-parent relationships that we have witnessed stemmed from parents trying to impose their philosophy of teaching on teachers—parents who have essentially said, "This is the way I want you to teach my deaf child." One set of parents told their two deaf children to look away from the teacher when she was teaching language using a particular approach. They were adamant in their demands that the teacher change her way of teaching. Yet, all of the other deaf students in this same classroom benefited from the approach the teacher used. Your classroom is your home. Keep it that way.

4. *Keep an open line of communication with parents.* Let parents know that they can talk to you about their child's progress. Provide them with options for communicating with you such as meeting in person, corresponding by mail, fax, or e-mail, or conversations via telephone. Be clear, however, about the limits of your accessibility. Discourage the practice of parents calling you at your home. Observe protocol when it comes to the time and length of meetings. If you have to reschedule for parent's convenience, it may be necessary to make arrangements for compensation with your supervisor. Finally, be clear about the length of time that you are available to meet. Long, emotionally charged meetings are counterproductive to the establishment of an effective parent-teacher relationship.

5. *Send home a regular classroom newsletter.* Keep parents informed about what their children are learning, what they can be doing to help at home, and upcoming school events. You can create a template for a newsletter using computer programs like those described in Chapter 8. Some teachers send weekly newsletters home while others prefer sending them once a month. At the lower grade levels you may wish to attach homework assignments and activities that parents can do with their children. For all grade levels, include tips for involving parents with their children such as helping children do their homework, increasing their self-esteem, and participating in community activities. There are many books and web sites that contain information for parents. Use them for ideas about what to put in your newsletter. See box titled "Developing Respect and Responsibility in Your Children" for examples of tips that can be included in a newsletter. You may also wish to include works of your deaf students in the newsletter. If you do this, then ensure that the display of work is balanced out for all of the students over the course of the year.

6. *Be sensitive to the parents' backgrounds and at-home responsibilities.* Your image of the "perfect parent" might just be that—an image, with no connection in real life. The good work that one parent is doing will not necessarily be a good thing for another parent to do. Just as we treat children as individuals with special educational needs, we should approach their parents in a similar fashion.

Developing Respect and Responsibility in Your Children

Many schools regularly include brief inserts in their newsletters to parents about raising children. They range from science activities and tips for helping children learn mathematics to the development of social skills and confidence-building activities. Below is an example of a possible insert relating to the development of responsibility and respect. These principles were taken from the book *Raising Self-Reliant Children in a Self-Indulgent World* by Glenn and Nelsen (1989):

1. Avoid strictness (excessive control).
2. Avoid permissiveness (excessive autonomy, too little structure and follow-through).
3. Convey unqualified love, care, and respect (distinguish action from people and avoid using love, praise, and approval as rewards).
4. Give clear feedback ("I feel . . . about . . . because . . .").
5. Structure consequences (teach children the relationship between cause and effect—for example, responsibility and privileges).
6. Be firm (say what you mean and mean what you say).
7. Maintain dignity (avoid projecting anger or other feelings onto the child. Be an actor rather than a reactor; choose to deal with things when you are at your best rather than at your worst).
8. Teach with respect (clarify what the child has caused to happen rather than what you have done to punish the child). (p. 189)

This message is simple, quickly typed up, and informative. Will it help the parents of your deaf children? It may. But if it helps just one set of parents, then you have performed an invaluable service. Will it help a teacher? Each of these principles by itself or with slight modification can be found in a list of good classroom management strategies.

A Plan for Family Involvement

There are many ways in which parents and other family members can be involved in the education of a deaf child. We highly recommend that deaf education programs have a plan to facilitate this involvement. This Family Involvement Plan would be appropriate for any program that has at least one class of deaf students and is an absolute must for large deaf education day programs and schools for the deaf. The Family Involvement Plan should begin with a set of beliefs that will serve as guidelines for plans that actually involve the parents. Following are examples of possible belief statements:

- All parents are a welcomed asset to the school.
- All children have achievements that can be celebrated.
- When possible, effort will be made to accommodate all reasonable parental requests to become involved in the school.

■ Guidance for involvement will be given so that parents have positive avenues for contributing to their children's education.

■ Parents will be kept informed on a timely basis of all activities occurring at the school.

Once a selection of belief statements has been made, your classroom or program may want to develop procedures to ensure that these beliefs are acted upon. Here are some examples of procedures for involving the family:

1. Every preschool and elementary school classroom will have at least one designated room parent. The primary responsibility of the room parent is to help the teacher with traditional classroom parties (e.g., Halloween, Christmas, Valentine's Day) and to provide assistance on field trips. The nature of the assistance will be negotiated between the classroom teacher and the parent. The room parent will also serve as a hospitality parent to parents of new students who might be coming to that classroom or school program.

2. Arrangements will be made for those parents who desire to make a specific contribution to a classroom. This contribution is broadly defined to include activities that foster the educational process in a positive manner. For example, some parents may wish to talk about their jobs, demonstrate an appreciation for artwork, or make a short presentation designed to instill a sense of self-awareness in the students. This type of contribution must be negotiated with the teacher. Not all activities can be accommodated, and the merit of each activity needs to be considered in light of the overall program for a classroom or program.

3. Parents and other family members will be encouraged to participate in one-on-one situations with other deaf children in the program. The one-on-one situation might be during school hours or after school. Activities will be decided by the teacher and can include tutoring, reading books, working on an art project, and playing educational games.

4. A monthly parent package will be sent home with all deaf students. The package will contain reports of what has happened at the school, a list of upcoming events, instructions about what students will be learning in class, and how this work can be supported or supplemented at home. This package should be used to encourage parents to participate in sport events, participate on field trips, help with fund-raising events, and other school activities.

This set of procedures can be used in any school program with any number of deaf students. In schools for deaf children and large deaf education programs in public schools, it might be desirable to set up a small committee consisting of teachers, parents, and administrators. This committee would be responsible for reviewing the family involvement plan and making suggestions for changes and coordinating parental involvement activities.

An elaborate family involvement plan might not be necessary in those instances in which only one or two deaf students are in an entire school. Nevertheless, a plan of some sort is needed if parental involvement is to be a valued part of a deaf child's education. For those students in a general education class, the itinerant teacher or the resource room teacher, with input from the general education teachers, could take responsibility for involving the parents.

Getting Parents Involved in the Education of Their Deaf Children

Once teachers have established a strong, positive relationship with parents, they will be in a better position for helping parents influence their deaf children's education. There are numerous ways in which this can occur. We have selected three areas in which teachers can help parents get involved with their deaf children and in so doing contribute to their children's education. These areas are closed-captioning, reading, and gaining experiences in the home and community.

Closed-Captioning and the Parent

Many parents will confirm the benefits that reading captions has on the reading skills of their deaf children. Deaf adults too, speak highly about the value of captioning in helping them improve their English skills. And the value is not all related to reading and English skills. Television is a cultural icon and as such is a significant provider of information about one's own society and that of others. Because of the complex nature of captioning, it is important for teachers to take responsibility for making parents aware of the potential advantages that closed captions (and open captions) have for deaf children.

Getting to Know Captions.   There are two exercises that can help parents understand both the upside of reading captions and the challenges that captions present to deaf children. The first one involves turning the sound off and watching a TV program without captions. Encourage parents to do this for a long period of time by creating a chart that will guide them in this experience. The purpose of this chart is to highlight the importance of visual information to a deaf person's comprehension and enjoyment of a TV program. Exercise 14.1 shows an example of such a chart.

In this exercise, parents choose programs that their deaf child typically watches as well as those that they themselves are accustomed to watching. Speechreading a person on TV is a difficult task. Parents should attempt to speechread the characters on TV and note how much information they are able to get in this modality. Likely, very little information will be received this way, but when some words or sentences are understood, the parent should note why they were able to understand them; was it, for example, their understanding of the context of the program that allowed them to anticipate what was going to be said? The faces of actors provide visual cues about their emotions and can indicate changes in the atmosphere of a program or events that might be occurring away from the screen. For instance, depending upon the context of the program, a surprised look might reveal that an actor has heard something, has come to a sudden realization, or is anticipating that something is about to occur.

There are other visual cues that can help a viewer understand a program. Slow motion often accompanies an exploding bomb, an approaching tragic accident, and the appearance of a rapid sequence of events. A fuzzy or wavy outline around the screen is typically associated with someone dreaming or thinking about something. Visual graphics are excellent for helping people understand what is being said. The names and descriptions of people speaking on the screen is another example of valuable information.

EXERCISE **14.1**

Experience Chart for Watching TV Without Captions and Sound

Name of TV Program	Ease of Speech-reaching	Use of Facial Cues	Nature of Other Visual Cues	Overall Comprehension	Overall Enjoyment

While filling out the chart in Exercise 14.1, parents should be encouraged to stay with a program for its entire length. At the end, they should indicate on their chart their overall comprehension of the program (e.g., very low, low, half, most) and their enjoyment of the program itself. Following completion of this activity for several programs, parents should compare the programs to determine which type offers the most enjoyment in the absence of sound and captions. Sports programs, for example, can usually be enjoyed without accompanying dialogue. Indeed, there are some deaf adults who choose to watch sports without captions because they find that the captions interfere with the action taking place in a game.

But a game in progress is not all that captions might interfere with. A few years ago, one of the authors was watching an afterschool cartoon with four deaf children ages 7, 12, 13, and 14. All of the children were performing average to above-average academically in school and all of them had Deaf parents. After a few minutes, the author realized that the captioning was turned off. He asked the children about this and the response was "The captioning interferes with the action in the cartoons." This brings up the second activity, illustrated in Exercise 14.2, that parents should be encouraged to do.

In this exercise, the parents watch TV programs with the captioning turned on but no sound. Again, selection of programs should be a mixture of those that the parent's deaf child watches and those that the parents usually watch. The main purpose of this activity is to demonstrate that reading captions involves factors that are related to the viewer, such as command of language and reading ability. It also involves factors connected to the nature and display of captions. The chart in Exercise 14.2 shows some of the more critical factors. A few minutes watching national news or live coverage of a debate will show how much can be missed when the captions appear on the screen for just a brief period of time. There are certain programs that tend to have rapid-fire conversations and therefore quick captions.

EXERCISE 14.2
Experience Chart for Watching TV with Captions but Without Sound

Name of TV Program	Speed of Captions	Accuracy of Captions (spelling, etc.)	Visual Cues Presented by Captions	Complexity of Language and Vocabulary	Overall Enjoyment

Moreover, not all captions and especially real-time captions (i.e., captions that are being created during a live broadcast as opposed to captions that are created from a script) contain correct spelling. Words might be missing, and there might be characters that have been inadvertently inserted that confuse the reader. As technology improves, however, we should see an increase in the accuracy of captions.

Over the years, captioning companies have created a number of visual cues to alert the viewer to sounds being made in a program such as a phone ringing, knocking on a door, a gunshot, music, barking, or a baby crying. Another important factor is the complexity of the language spoken on a program and the difficulty of the vocabulary. This category is often the key to determining whether a deaf child likes a program.

Parents (and teachers!) who complete both of the above exercises should be more aware of the advantages and limitations of captioning. At the very least, they should be better prepared to help their deaf child benefit from captioning. The box titled "Tips for Parents About Captioned Programs" describes a number of things that parents can do.

What Parents Can Do to Help Their Deaf Child Learn to Read

In recent years much attention has been given to the role of literacy in the development of deaf students' language skills. This attention cuts across all methods of communication as researchers are exploring literacy strategies with deaf students in English signing programs, ASL-oriented programs, Cued Speech programs, and oral programs. Notions about the value of literacy instruction, however, are not new. Reading and writing have always had a prominent role in the education of deaf children, although it is just one of the pieces critical in the development of a whole child.

Tips for Parents About Captioned Programs

Even the best of readers can experience difficulty understanding all of the captions on TV or video. Moreover, if a child does not have strong reading skills then he or she might be inclined to watch a TV or video program without the captions so that there is no interference with the picture. Indeed, reading captions, like reading books, is a skill that must be nurtured. Following are some tips to guide parents to help their deaf child meet the challenges of reading captions:

1. Leave the captions turned on at all times. Show that captioning is a part of the family's TV culture and not just something that is turned on in the presence of deaf children. Leaving the captioning on whenever the TV is turned on demonstrates to deaf children that their communication needs are a valued part of how the family functions.
2. Watch TV and videos with your deaf child. Find out which programs are your child's favorites and take the time to watch some of them. If the timing of the program does not allow you to watch the program, then you might wish to tape the program and watch it later. Taping a program gives you the opportunity to watch a program more than once, to stop the program at any time to talk about what is happening, and to review words and sentences.
3. Explain to your deaf child what is happening in a show. This will make it easier for the child to understand the captioning, and it will certainly make it easier for him or her to follow the show.
4. Explain the meaning of visual cues that appear as a part of the captioning. These cues come in a variety of forms such as musical notes to indicate music or text in parentheses to describe action that can be heard occurring elsewhere, such as a dog barking or a siren blaring.
5. If the captions help you understand what is being said on TV, then tell this to your deaf child. Provide real examples, such as the captions helped you learn the spelling of a name or word or it helped you understand what was being said because you could not understand what the speaker was saying.
6. Use captioned programs as a way of directly communicating with your deaf child. Captioned TV by itself is not an adequate substitute for direct communication. However, the time you spend with your child discussing a program is an excellent language-learning opportunity.

What can parents do to help their deaf children learn to read? Much has been written about how parents can help their children read. In general, parents are encouraged to:

- Value reading as an intellectual and leisure activity.
- Model reading habits by reading on a regular basis at home.
- Read regularly to children.
- For younger children, read the same books over and over again.
- Talk about the stories they have read.
- Explain words and concepts that children might not understand.
- Have plenty of books, magazines, and other reading materials at home.

- Set aside a time for quiet reading.
- At all times, make reading an enjoyable activity.

These suggestions for reading at home apply to all children, deaf and hearing, young and old. They are also applicable to the classroom, and teachers should incorporate them into their reading approach.

The process of reading to deaf children might not be as straightforward as it is when reading to hearing children. The process is further complicated when signing is involved. Parents see reading to deaf children as a complex process that raises many questions. Following is just a short list of the many questions that we have been asked by both deaf and hearing parents of deaf children:

- How much of what I read aloud will be heard and understood?
- Should my child watch my lips, look at the pages in a picture book, or do both?
- When do I ask my child if he or she is understanding what I am reading?
- When do I explain the meaning of words? If there are too many words to explain, should I just keep reading?
- Do I make my child practice reading along with me?
- My child wants me to read the same book over and over again and is always interrupting me when I am reading. What do I do?
- How can my child follow the words in a book while I am reading?
- Should each word be signed or just the gist of each sentence?
- Should I use my voice only when reading?
- Should I read the book to myself first, then just tell the story to my child?
- Should my child be told the story first and then read the book?
- Should words that have to be fingerspelled be omitted or substituted?
- What do I do about long words that need to be fingerspelled?
- I can't sign well, so why should I read books to my child?
- Should some words that have signs be fingerspelled so that my child is introduced to the concept of English spelling in preparation for reading?
- My child just got a cochlear implant. Should I stop signing when I am reading a book to her?
- What do I do when my child keeps looking away from me?

These questions plus many more might seem trivial to experienced teachers but they are serious questions for parents. They also indicate that not only is the process of reading a book to a deaf child complicated, but that there are many options for doing so.

There are several strategies for reading that teachers can share with parents. Some of these strategies are good for all parents irrespective of the communication mode they will use for reading. Barbara Luetke-Stahlman is a professional in the field of deaf education and a parent of two deaf children. She has compiled a list of activities that parents can do at home to help deaf children read. These activities are shown in Figure 14.1. Note how Luetke-Stahlman has included suggestions for parents to help teachers in their reading program. These suggestions included collecting pictures and materials such as story props that a teacher can use when reading a particular story. This idea is an excellent one also for helping teachers create a reading center.

1. Read the story and be mindful of the content. Talk about related content when opportunities arise at school, home, or out in the community.
2. Upon request by a teacher, gather the materials that might be needed to tell the story at school. Parents' willingness to hunt up items allows the teacher time to concentrate on other aspects of reading the story and gives the parents the satisfaction of assisting.
3. Upon request by a teacher, collect pictures needed to augment a story.
4. Adults can rent videos or secure them from The National Captioning Institute. Research suggests that multiple exposure to the same stories benefits students.
5. Adults can buy single copies of the stories that are bound in the basal text or can check them out from the public library. This allows the students the opportunity to reread the story at home and share it with others.
6. Provide a quiet time and a comfortable spot for reading on a daily basis. Sit near the child and read independently too.
7. Provide experiences mentioned in stories.

FIGURE 14.1   Involving families in the reading process.*

*This is a condensed version of a list of suggestions from Luetke-Stahlman, B. (1999a). *Language across the curriculum: When students are deaf or hard of hearing* (pp. 485–486). Hillsboro, OR: Butte Publications. In the original version, the author's suggestions were aimed at both teachers and parents, and readers should read this version for a more detailed explanation of some of the suggestions shown in this figure.

One concern that faces parents with deaf children who rely on signing is what to do about the signing component when reading aloud. The first step is obviously to improve signing skills to a level of fluency where signing is not a hindrance to the flow of the book. But even deaf teachers who are native signers may struggle when it comes to reading in signs because books are written with the vocabulary and syntax of English and the cadence of this language may be critical to the flow of the story when reading aloud or even silently.

Reading in signs is an art in itself that takes much practice over and above having a proficient command of the signs that one uses. David Schleper is a literacy coordinator at the Laurent Clerc Deaf Education Center at Gallaudet University. He synthesized from the literature a list of strategies used by deaf adults when reading to deaf children. This list is shown in Figure 14.2. Note that this list is a compilation of principles based on strategies used by different deaf readers and is not meant to imply that all deaf adults readily embrace these principles.

What Parents Can Do to Help Their Deaf Child Gain Experiences

Throughout our earlier discussions about teaching academic subjects, we emphasized the role that prior experiences have in helping children learn the content of their academic subjects. We also pointed out the challenges that deaf children have in getting these experiences. The primary source of experiences for all children is and should be the family. In this respect, there are two things that parents must do with their deaf children. First, they must make the effort to expose their children to experiences that include experiences that they

---

Deaf adults read to deaf children using the following principles:

1. Translate stories using American Sign Language.
2. Keep both languages (ASL and English) visible.
3. Elaborate on the text.
4. Reread stories on a "storytelling" to "story reading" continuum.
5. Follow the child's lead.
6. Make what is implied explicit.
7. Adjust sign placement to fit the story.
8. Adjust signing style to fit the character.
9. Connect concepts in the story to the real world.
10. Use attention maintenance strategies.
11. Use eye gaze to elicit participation
12. Engage in role play to extend concepts.
13. Use ASL variations to sign repetitive English phrases.
14. Provide a positive and reinforcing environment.
15. Expect the child to become literate.

FIGURE 14.2   How deaf adults read to deaf children.*

* Taken from Schleper, D. R. (1997). *Reading to deaf children: Learning from deaf adults* (pp. 3–4). Washington, DC: Pre-College National Mission Programs.

share with their children alone and those in which their children are with other people (e.g., camps, community sports programs). Second, deaf children must have opportunities to talk about these experiences.

Building up Experiences.   Experiences of all sorts are valuable for all children. When parents are encouraged to expose their deaf children to lots of experiences, they should know that the bulk of these experiences are simple and require little or no planning. Following is a number of suggestions that can be shared with parents:

1. *Take your deaf child with you when you do activities related to everyday necessities and living in general.* Deaf children should accompany you when you go shopping for groceries, to get a haircut, to get an oil change, to buy a new faucet for the kitchen sink, to see a lawyer, to renew your driver's license, for a walk, to talk to your neighbor, to the dentist or doctor, to the corner store to buy milk, to buy a present, for the newspaper, to mail some letters, to the bank, to a produce market, to an insurance agent, for a coffee and donut, to the library, to take the garbage out, to look for a new couch, and hundreds of other places. If you think all of this sounds obvious, then the next time you are doing one of them look around to see how many children are with their parents.

2. *Involve your deaf child in small jobs that you might normally do yourself.* The key here is to increase the amount of time that you spend with your child. Your deaf child can help mow the lawn, clean up the garage, put tools away, pull weeds in the garden, clean out the fish tank (*News Flash!* Recent research has found that college students who grew up with pets, and especially with fish, performed higher on standard college entry examinations such as the Scholastic Aptitude Test than those students who never had pets), clean the dishes, take clothes to a Goodwill or charity organization, ride a bike, count and package loose change, rearrange the kitchen pantry, and so many other small jobs. Make sure there is something for your child to do everyday.

3. *Go special places with your deaf child.* These are places you go to because you enjoy visiting them or because you think it might be a nice adventure. The zoo, art gallery, library, park, mall, theater, and museum are places that many people think about when planning to "do something." They are great places for talking about things in a relaxing atmosphere. But how about going to view open houses that are for sale because they provide a good opportunity to talk about likes and dislikes? Or houses still under construction that will allow you to talk about ceiling joists, studs, vents, electrical wiring, plumbing, floor plans, particle board, plywood, floor coverings, prices, and mortgages? Take a trip through the industrial part of town to show where things are manufactured, food packaged, computers assembled, and items are stored in large warehouses. If you live near the ocean then see what longshoremen do for a living and visit the docks where fishing boats unload their catches or a cannery where the fish are cleaned and packed. Wherever you live, there are many fascinating places to see. Do not make the assumption that just because you are familiar with something that perhaps your child might be bored with it. Better to give them the opportunity to show you that they are bored.

4. *Play games.* Playing games is an experience, too. Think about books in which the main character is playing a particular game. Understanding what a particular game is about may help your child understand a passage in a book where the game is mentioned. So, have a crack at one of your child's computer or video games. Show him or her that you are interested in his or her entertainment and ask him or her to explain the games to you. But do not forget other games that are slowly being eased out of the family recreation room. A lot of these games are good because they can be better paced than the high excitement and highly visual games on computers, are inexpensive, require the participants to say something, and teach valuable academic skills. Cribbage is a good game for learning how to quickly add up numbers and to see patterns in cards. Rumoli teaches about patterns, numbers, and strategies as well as the benefits and perils of borrowing money (or chips) to continue playing a game. Mankata requires less strategy than many other games, but it is one that is easily learned and can be played by people of all ages. The board game Clue has movies and books that can reinforce the excitement of playing it. There are the board games such as chess and checkers and many card games such as hearts and gin rummy. You might be surprised at how much children will enjoy playing them. All of these games have the potential to elicit lots of communication between parent and child.

5. *Check with your child's teacher or with your child to see what is being studied in school and plan an activity that can reinforce this learning at home.* Do you have a child taking tenth-grade biology who is studying plant diversity or a child who is learning about plants in the fourth grade? Either age can benefit from a trip to a horticulture garden, to a tree nursery, or a walk through the woods. If you live in a dry area, consider a trip to an acid pond that is drying up. There are plant species that appear as the pond shrinks, with different plants growing at specific distances from the water's edge. From the road, it might look

like there are only a few plants growing, but up close you might find up to thirty different plants within fifty feet of the pond. Is your child studying life in the early eighteenth century? Visit an antique shop to search for furniture from this period. Learn how to make soap at home from ashes (lye is a good substitute), suet (animal fat), and spices. Whatever you do will benefit your child back in the classroom.

6. *Talk.* Talk about anything and everything. If you watch sports on TV, there is much that you can talk about. You can talk about the players and some of the things that you might have read about them in the newspaper. Determine how much time is left in a period of hockey or a quarter of football. Predict the time that a game will end and the final score. Calculate how many yards a football team has to move to score a touchdown (e.g., if they are on their own 38 yard line then they have to move the ball 62 yards in American football; and 72 yards if they are playing on a Canadian football field, which is 10 yards longer.) Talk about news on TV and find out if your child knows the location of different states and countries. Does he or she understand which cities are the largest in the United States and Canada; that Mexico City and São Paulo are two of the largest and fastest growing cities in the world? What do the terms *economy* and *marketplace* mean to your deaf child? Do not use language as an excuse not to talk but rather as the reason why you are talking. Maintain reasonable language expectations in your conversations with your child.

Tackling Communication Concerns. There are at least two main concerns about communication that parents have: what kind of communication to use and when to use it. We are not going to discuss the pros and cons of various types of communication because each type has experienced a certain degree of success with some deaf children. In addition, we feel that it is the role of teachers to simply inform parents in an impartial manner about the different types of communication that are available and describe what they use in their classroom. They should also refer parents to readings and other resources that examine issues relating to communication.

For example, one handy book for parents who have concerns about signing is *The Signing Family: What Every Parent Should Know About Sign Communication.* This book describes the popular types of sign communication used in the classroom: ASL, Signed English, Signing Exact English, and contact sign. It shows how parents can use this knowledge of signing to create goals that revolve around the educational and social needs of their deaf children. There are also sections in the book that describe how parents can build partnerships with schools and the following advice is one that parents should well heed (Stewart & Luetke-Stahlman, 1998):

> Schools and parents must strive to work together. Ask your child's teachers what you can do at home to supplement the work being done at school. If you have the time, offer to help out in the classroom now and then. Whatever you do, stay involved in your deaf child's education. Think of your involvement as part of the total educational package.
>
> Your deaf child's education is your education too! (p. 155).

This is the type of quote that might be put in a newsletter to parents. It helps keep parents informed of their role in the education of their children.

The other big concern relating to communication is the actual act of communicating. No matter what type of communication parents might use with their deaf children, they should use it at every opportunity. Indeed, it is the talking-to-your-child part of the communication equation that many parents of deaf children find most challenging. Simple things like getting a child's attention, cutting back on distractions, and becoming more animated in their use of facial expressions and body language can be a very disheartening endeavor for some parents. Parents need to know that communication is a challenge for all parents, deaf and hearing, and that there are strategies to help.

In the book *My Turn to Learn* by Lane, Bell, and Parson-Tylka (1997) answers are given to many questions that parents have about communication. There are also strategies described that can help parents become effective communicators. For example, there is a section in the book about how parents can modify the complexity of their messages to reflect the command of language that their deaf child has. This section and others like it help parents build up their confidence in communicating—irrespective of the mode and language of communication they chose. In another section, they demonstrate how parents and other family members can model language. This demonstration is shown in Figure 14.3. When parents make a habit of expanding upon a deaf child's language they turn mere exposure to events into linguistically rich learning experiences.

In sum, parents must make the effort to expose their deaf children to lots of experiences and provide opportunities to talk about them. Doing this will translate into greater success in the classroom. This will be evident in the deaf child's learning of new vocabulary terms because they will more likely have had prior experiences with the concepts asso-

Child	Grandfather
"Fish"	"Fish swimming. Fish swimming *fast*."
"Swimming"	"Yes, fish swimming. Two fish swimming."
"Uh, oh. All gone."	"The fish are all gone. They swam away. Bye bye fish."

Child	Mother
"Look, Mommy, boat."	"That's a tugboat. See, it's pulling the ship."

Child	Sister
"Birds! Birds eating."	"The birds are eating bread. Look, two birds are fighting. They want the bread."
"Birds eating bread."	"Yes, lots of birds eating bread. Those birds are called seagulls."

FIGURE 14.3   Making family outings a linguistically rich experience—in any mode or language of communication.*

*Adapted from Lane, S., Bell, L., & Parson-Tylka, T. (1997). *My turn to learn: A communication guide for parents of deaf or hard of hearing children* (pp. 277–279). Surrey, BC: Elks Family Hearing Resource Centre.

ciated with new words. These experiences should also lead to a better chance of absorbing new concepts and to be able to generalize these new concepts to things that they do or observe in their life outside of the classroom.

Conclusion

Schools do not have the full responsibility for educating deaf children. This is true whether deaf children are in a general education classroom full-time, in a self-contained classroom with a teacher of the deaf, or in a school for the deaf. There are not enough hours in school for teachers to be deaf children's only source of learning. If we are going to shape the educational environment such that it optimizes the opportunities for deaf children to learn, then parents, or more generally, families, must be involved in their children's education. Being informed is one way of being involved. Open communication between parents and teachers keeps parents informed and gives them an ongoing means for providing input into the educational process.

Another angle in the area of communication is the need for parents to actively pursue talking to their children, in whatever modality (signs, speech, print, or audition) and language (English and ASL) fit the family's needs. A child's hearing loss must not be viewed as a hindrance to the initiation and sustaining of an act of communication. Furthermore, only with communication can parents enrich deaf children's exposure to language—which better prepares these children for learning in school.

In addition to communication, parents must become active in building up their child's experiential background by stimulating his or her intellectual growth. Going places and doing things with their child is a good way to gain experiences. But some parents might not have the confidence to do this. These parents and others need guidance from their child's teachers, and a family involvement plan is an excellent way of doing so.

Finally, in thinking about their relationship with parents, teachers may benefit from heeding the following words of advice given to parents of deaf children on how they should relate to their children's teachers (Stewart & Luetke-Stahlman, 1998):

> Some parents tell us that they hate to make demands of their child's teachers because they want everyone to be friends. Some fear that teachers will "take it out on the child." We have never found any justification for this fear, but we do know that friendliness doesn't do the trick. You may be friendly with your car dealer, but when things go wrong with the car, you need to bring it in and explain the problem. When things go wrong at school you should take the same approach, with confidence that you are simply being a good consumer. (p. 155)

Parents see teachers as professionals. Be one.

QUESTIONS

1. Name eight responses from parents who come to realize that they have a deaf child.

2. Why do teachers need to be sensitive to the tasks that parents face when raising a deaf child?

3. What are two challenges that parents face when sending a deaf child to school?

4. What five principles can teachers follow that will help them establish a good relationship with their students' parents?

5. What is meant by the principle "Respect the manner in which parents have chosen to raise their deaf child"?

6. Why is it important to keep an open line of communication with parents? How does a newsletter help keep an open line of communication and what are some other benefits of having a newsletter about your classroom?

7. Give an example of two belief statements and describe why such statements are important in the development of a Family Involvement Plan.

8. Why is it important to inform parents about the importance of captioning to deaf children?

9. Why is it important for parents to talk to their deaf children about what they are doing, things they have seen and done, the meaning of certain events, and other things?

10. What can parents do to help their deaf children gain experiences that will help them in school?

ACTIVITIES

1. Design a newsletter for parents for each of the following classroom situations:

   a. fourth-grade class in a school for the deaf
   b. self-contained seventh-grade class in public school
   c. tenth-grade mainstreamed deaf student who is seen by an itinerant teacher twice a week

2. Complete the charts indicated in Exercises 14.1 and 14.2.

3. Plan an outing for a parent and a deaf child and include the following:

   a. type of place that will be visited (e.g., farm, train station, art gallery, etc.)
   b. things that will be observed at this place
   c. concepts that could be learned from a visitation
   d. questions related to the concept that parents can ask a deaf child
   e. questions that are related to the visitation in general

4. In small groups, discuss possible responses to the questions asked by parents related to reading books to deaf children. These questions are shown on page 327.

REFERENCES AND BIBLIOGRAPHY

Affolter, M. (1985). *Working with hearing impaired students in rural areas*. Technical Report. Bellingham, WA: Western Washington University. National Rural Development Institute.

Airasian, P. (1987). *Classroom assessment* (3rd ed.). New York: McGraw-Hill.

Allen, T. (1986). Patterns of academic achievement among hearing impaired students: 1974 and 1983. In A. Schildroth & M. Karchmer (Eds.), *Deaf children in America*. Boston: Little, Brown & Co.

Allen, T. (1992). Subgroup differences in educational placement for deaf and hard of hearing students. *American Annals of the Deaf*, *135*(7), 381-388.

Allen, T.E. (1996). *Stanford Achievement Test, 9th Edition, and WISC-III and their use with deaf and hard of hearing students: Progress Report* [World Wide Web document]. URL: http://www.gallaudet.edu/~cadsweb/satprogr.html.

Anderson, R., & Pearson, P. (1984) A schema theoretic view of the reading process in reading comprehension. *Handbook of reading research* (pp. 255–291). New York: Longman.

Applebee, A. (1984) . Writing and reasoning. *Review of Educational Research*, *54*(4), 577–596.

Bailes, C., Searles, S., Slobodzian, J., & Staton, J. (1986). *It's your turn now!* Washington, DC: Gallaudet University.

Banks, J.A. (1997). *Teaching strategies for ethnic studies* (6th ed.). Boston: Allyn & Bacon.

Barba, R.H. (1995). *Science in the multicultural classroom: A guide to teaching and learning*. Boston: Allyn & Bacon.

Batson, T. (1993). ENFI research. *Computers & Composition, 10*(3).

Biddle, S., & Armstrong, N. (1992). Children's physical activity: An exploratory study of psychological correlates. *Social Science in Medicine*, *34*(3), 325–331.

Bennett, A. (1988). *Schooling the different: Incorporating deaf Hispanic children into special education*. London: Taylor & Francis.

Benton, S. (1996). Grand entry: A new ceremony derived from the Old West. *Tribal College*, *8*(3), 10–14.

Bitter, G., & Person, M. (1999). *Using technology in the classroom* (4th ed.). Boston: Allyn & Bacon.

Blood, R.O., & Wolfe, D.M. (1960). *Husbands and wives: The dynamics of married living*. New York: The Free Press.

Bodner-Johnson, B. (1986). The family environment and achievement of deaf students: A discriminant analysis. *Exceptional Children*, *52*(5), 443–449.

Bolte, A. (1989). Cloze techniques: Opening doors to understanding. *Perspectives in Education and Deafness*, *8*(2), 6–8.

Boone, R. (1992). Involving culturally diverse parents in transition planning. *Career Development for Exceptional Individuals, 15*(2), 205–221.

Borg, W.R., & Gall, M.D. (1989). *Educational research* (5th ed.). New York: Longman.

Brunt, D., & Broadhead, G.D. (1982). Motor proficiency traits of deaf children. *Research Quarterly for Exercise and Sport*, *53*(3), 236–238.

Burton, A.W., & Davis, W.E. (1992). Assessing balance in adapted physical education: Fundamental concepts and application. *Adapted Physical Activity Quarterly*, *9*(1), 14–46.

Burton, V., & Campbell, M. (1997). The seven "E" teaching model. *Science Scope, 20*, 32–34.

Butterfield, S.A. (1986). Motor proficiency traits of deaf children. *Perceptual and Motor Skills*, *62*, 68–70.

Caccamise, F., & Lang, H. (1995). *Signs for science and mathematics: A resource book for teachers and students*. Rochester, NY: National Technical Institute for the Deaf, Rochester Institute of Technology.

Calfee, R.C., & Pointkowski, D. (1981). The reading diary: Acquisition of decoding. *Reading Research Quarterly*, *16*(3), 346–373.

Carney, A.E. (1986). Understanding speech intelligibility in the hearing impaired. *Topics in Language Disorders*, *6*(3), 47–59.

Chiang, L.H. (1993). *Beyond the language: Native Americans' nonverbal communication*. Paper presented at the Annual Meeting of the Midwest Association of Teachers of Educational Psychology, Anderson, IN, October 1–2.

Christensen, K.M., & Delgado, G.L. (1993). *Multicultural issues in deafness*. White Plains, NY: Longman.

Christiansen, J.B., & Barnartt, S.N. (1987). The silent minority: The socioeconomic status of deaf people. In P. Higgins & J. Nash (Eds.), *Understanding deafness socially* (pp. 171–196). Springfield, IL: Charles C. Thomas.

Christiansen, J.B., & Barnartt, S.N. (1995). *Deaf President Now! The 1988 revolution at Gallaudet University.* Washington, DC: Gallaudet University.

Clark, C., & Peterson, P. (1985). Teachers' thought processes. In M.C. Wittrock (Ed.), *Handbook of research on teaching* (pp. 255–296). New York: Macmillan Publishing.

Clark, G.M., & Kolstoe, O.P. (1995). *Career development and transition education for adolescents with disabilities* (3rd ed.). Boston: Allyn & Bacon.

Clarke, B.R. (1983). Competence in communication for hearing impaired children: A conversation, activity, experience approach. *British Columbia Journal of Special Education, 7,* 15–27.

Clarke, B.R., & Stewart, D.A. (1986). Reflections on language programs for the hearing impaired. *Journal of Special Education, 20*(2), 153–165.

Coggins, K. (1996). *The traditional tribal values of Ojibwa parents and the school performance of their children: An exploratory study.* Technical Report. Ann Arbor, MI: University of Michigan.

Cohen, E.P., & Gainer, R.S. (1995). *Art: Another language for learning* (3rd ed.). Portsmouth, NH: Heinemann.

Cohen, O., Fischgrund, J., & Redding, R. (1990). Deaf children from ethnic, linguistic, and racial minority backgrounds: An overview. *American Annals of the Deaf. 135(2).*

Collet-Klingenberg, L.L. (1998). The reality of best practices in transition: A case study. *Exceptional Children, 65*(1), 67–78.

Dance away stress. (1998). *Prevention, 50*(3), 144.

Daniele, V. (1993). Quantitative literacy. *American Annals of the Deaf, 138*(2), 76–81.

Delpit, L. (1995). *Other people's children: Cultural conflict in the classroom.* New York: The New Press.

deValdez, T.A., & Gallegos, J. (1982). The Chicano families in social work. In J.W. Green (Ed.), *Cultural awareness in the human services.* Englewood Cliffs, NJ: Prentice-Hall.

Dietz, C.H. (1995). *Moving toward the standards: A national action plan for mathematics education reform for the deaf.* Washington, DC: Pre-College Outreach Programs.

Dockterman, D. (1998). *Great teaching in the one-computer classroom* (5th ed.). Watertown, MA: Tom Snyder Productions.

Dummer, G., Haubenstricker, J., & Stewart, D.A. (1996). Motor skill performances of children who are deaf. *Adapted Physical Activity Quarterly, 13,* 400–414.

Dunst, C.J., & Trivette, C.M. (1990). Assessment of social support in early intervention programs. In S.J. Meisels & J.P. Shonkoff (Eds.), *Handbook of early childhood intervention.* New York: Cambridge University Press.

Edwards, B. (1979). *Drawing on the right side of the brain.* Los Angeles, CA: J.P. Tarcher.

Eldredge, N., & Coyners, L. (1998). Differential diagnosis and assessment of learning disabilities with deaf students. In H. Markowicz & C. Berdichevsky (Eds.), *Bridging the gap between research and practice in the fields of learning disabilities and deafness.* Gallaudet University: College for Continuing Education, Washington, DC.

Elliott, S.N., Kratochwill, T.R., & Schulte, A.G. (1998). The assessment accommodation checklist: Who, what, where, when, why, and how? *Teaching Exceptional Children, 31*(2), 10–14.

Ellis, M.K., & Darby, L.A. (1993). The effect of balance on the determination of peak oxygen consumption for hearing and nonhearing female athletes. *Adapted Physical Activity Quarterly, 10,* 216–225.

Emig, J. (1971). *The composing processes of twelfth graders.* Urbana, IL: National Council of Teachers of English.

Eraut, M. (1988). Management knowledge: Its nature and its development. In J. Calderhead (Ed.), *Teachers: Professional learning* (pp. 196–204). London: Falmer Press.

Erickson, H.L. (1998). *Concept-based curriculum and instruction: Teaching beyond the facts.* Thousand Oaks, CA: Corwin.

Erting, C. (1994). *Deafness, communication, social identity: Ethnography in a preschool for deaf children.* Burtonsville, MD: Linstok.

Evans, J.M., & Brueckner, M.M. (1990). *Elementary social studies: Teaching for today and tomorrow.* Boston: Allyn & Bacon.

Ewoldt, C. (1981) A psycholinguistic description of selected deaf children reading in sign language. *Reading Research Quarterly, 17*(1), 58–89.

Ewoldt, C., & Saulnier, K. (1995). When teachers and children share good books. *Perspectives in Education and Deafness, 13*(3), 4–8.

Ferguson, A. (1999). Inside the crazy culture of kids' sports. *Time Magazine, 154*(2), 52–60.

Foster, S. (1992). *Working with deaf people: Accessibility and accommodation in the workplace.* Springfield, IL: Charles C. Thomas.

Fradd, S., & Wiesmantel, M. (1989). *Meeting the needs of culturally and linguistically different students: A handbook for educators*. Austin, TX: Pro-Ed.

French, M. (1999). *Starting with assessment: A developmental approach to deaf children's literacy*. Washington, DC: Pre-College National Mission Programs.

Fridriksson, T., & Stewart, D. (1988). From the concrete to the abstract: Mathematics for deaf children. *American Annals of the Deaf, 133*, 51–55.

Furney, K.S., Hasazi, S.B., & Destefano, L. (1997). Transition policies, practices, and promises: Lessons from three states. *Exceptional Children, 63*(3), 343–355.

Gajar, A., Goodman, L., & McAfee, J. (1993). *Secondary schools and beyond: Transition of individuals with mild disabilities*. New York: Merrill.

Gallaudet Research Institute. (1996, November). *Stanford Achievement Test 9th Edition, Form S: Norms booklet for deaf and hard-of-hearing students*. Washington, DC: Gallaudet University.

Gannon, J.R. (1981). *Deaf heritage: A narrative history of Deaf America*. Silver Spring, MD: National Association of the Deaf.

Gardner, H. (1983). *Frames of mind: The theory of multiple intelligences*. New York: Basic Books.

Garretson, M.D. (1995). Developing communication in the family. In D. Medwid & D.C. Weston (Eds.), *Kid-friendly parenting with deaf and hard of hearing children* (pp. 70–72). Washington, DC: Clerc Books.

Gaustad, M.G. (1997). *Inclusive education for deaf and hard of hearing students: Intervention with mainstream students and teachers*. Annual meeting of the Council for Exceptional Children, Salt Lake City, UT.

Gaustad, M.G. (1999). Including the kids across the hall: Collaborative instruction of hearing, deaf and hard of hearing students. *Journal of Deaf Studies and Deaf Education, 4*(3), 176–190.

Glenn, H.S., & Nelsen, J. (1989). *Raising self-reliant children in a self-indulgent world*. Rocklin, CA: Prima.

Glomb, N., & Morgan, D. (1991). Resource room teachers' use of strategies that promote the success of handicapped students in regular classrooms. *Journal of Special Education, 25*(2), 221–235.

Greenberg, M.T., & Kushché, C.A. (1993). *Promoting social and emotional development of deaf children: The PATHS Project*. Seattle: University of Washington Press.

Greenberg, M.T., & Kushché, C.A. (1998). Preventive intervention for school-age deaf children: The PATHS curriculum. *Journal of Deaf Studies and Deaf Education, 3*(1), 49–63.

Griffin, S. (1988). Students activities in the middle school: What do they contribute? *NASSP Bulletin, 72*, 87–92.

Grigal, M., Test, D.W., Beattie, J., & Wood, W.M. (1997). An evaluation of transition components of Individualized Education Programs. *Exceptional Children, 63*, 357–372.

Grossman, H. (1995). *Special education in a diverse society*. Boston: Allyn & Bacon.

Gutowski, T.W. (1988). Student initiative and the origins of the high school extracurriculum: Chicago, 1880–1915. *History of Education Quarterly, 28*, 49–72.

Halpern, A. (1988). Transition: A look at the foundations. *Exceptional Children, 57*, 479–486.

Hamm, M., & Adams, D. (1991). Portfolio assessment: It's not just for artists anymore. *The Science Teacher, 58*(5), 18–21.

Hanson, M.J., Lynch, E.W., & Wayman, K.I. (1990). Honoring the cultural diversity of families when gathering data. *Topics in Early Childhood Special Education, 10*(1), 112–131.

Hardman, M.L., Drew, C.J., & Egan, M.W. (1996). *Human exceptionality: Society, school, and family*. Boston: Allyn & Bacon.

Harry, B. (1993) Making sense of disability: Low income Puerto Rican parents' theories of the problem. *Exceptional Children, 59*(1), 27–40.

Hastad, D.N., & Lacy, A.C. (1998). *Measurement and evaluation in physical education and exercise science* (3rd ed.). Boston: Allyn & Bacon.

Jansma, P., & French, R. (1992). *Special physical education*. Englewood Cliffs: Prentice Hall.

Jensema, C. (1975). *The relationship between academic achievement and the demographic characteristics of hearing impaired children and youth*. Gallaudet College: Office of Demographic Studies. Series R. #2. Washington, DC.

Johnson, D.W., & Johnson, R.T. (1994). Learning together in the social studies classroom. In R.J. Stahl (ed.), *Cooperative learning in social studies: A handbook for teacher* (pp. 51–77). Menlo Park, CA: Addison-Wesley.

Just, M., & Carpenter, P. (1987). *The psychology of reading and language comprehension*. Boston: Allyn & Bacon.

Kelly, L. (1995). Processing of bottom-up and top-down information by skilled and average deaf readers and implications for whole language instruction. *Exceptional Children, 61*, 318–334.

Kelly, L., & Ewoldt, C. (1984). Interpreting nonverbatim cloze responses to evaluate program success and diagnose student needs for reading instruction. *American Annals of the Deaf, 129*(1), 45–51.

Kluwin, T. (1984). Keeping secondary school hearing impaired students on task. *Journal of Educational Research, 78*(1), 45–50.

Kluwin, T. (1985). Profiling the deaf high school student who is a problem in the classroom. *Adolescence, 20*, 863–875.

Kluwin, T. (1993). The cumulative effects of mainstreaming on the achievement of hearing impaired adolescents. *Exceptional Children, 60*(1), 73–81.

Kluwin, T. (1996). Getting hearing and deaf students to write to each other through dialogue journals. *Teaching Exceptional Children, 28*(2), 50–53.

Kluwin, T. (1999). Co-teaching deaf and hearing students. *American Annals of the Deaf, 144*(4), 339–344.

Kluwin, T., & Corbett, C. (1998). Parent characteristics and educational program involvement. *American Annals of the Deaf, 143*(5), 425–432.

Kluwin, T., & Gaustad, M.G. (1991). Predicting family communication choices. *American Annals of the Deaf, 136*(1), 28–34.

Kluwin, T., & Gaustad, M. (1992). How family factors influence school achievement. In T.N. Kluwin, D.F. Moores, & M.M. Gaustad (Eds.), *Defining the effective public school program for deaf students*. New York: Teachers College Press.

Kluwin, T., & Gonsher, W. (1994). Social integration of deaf and hearing children in a team taught kindergarten. *The ACEHI Journal / La Revue ACEDA, 20*(4), 16–30.

Kluwin, T., Gonsher, W., Silver, K., & Samuels, J. (1996). The E.T. Class: Education together! Team teaching hearing impaired and hearing students together. *Teaching Exceptional Children, 29*(1), 11–15.

Kluwin, T., & Kelly, A. (1991). The effectiveness of dialogue journal writing in improving the writing skills of young deaf writers. *American Annals of the Deaf, 136*(3), 284–291.

Kluwin, T., & Kelly, A. (1992). Implementing a successful writing program in public schools for students who are deaf. *Exceptional Children, 59*(1), 41–53.

Kluwin, T., & Moores, D.F. (1985). The effect of integration on the achievement of hearing impaired adolescents. *Exceptional Children, 52*(2), 153–160.

Kluwin, T., & Moores, D.F. (1989). Mathematics achievement of hearing impaired adolescents in different placements. *Exceptional Children, 55*(4), 327–335.

Kluwin, T., Moores, D.F., & Gaustad, M. (Eds.). (1992). *Toward effective public school programs for deaf students*. New York: Teachers College.

Kluwin, T., Stewart, D.A., & Sammons, A. (1994). The isolation of teachers of the deaf and hard of hearing in local public school programs. *The Association of Canadian Educators of the Hearing Impaired Journal, 20*, 16–30.

Kluwin, T.N., & Stinson, M.S. (1993). *Deaf students in local public high schools: Backgrounds, experiences, and outcomes*. Springfield, IL: Charles C. Thomas.

Kohler, P.D. (1993). Best practices in transition: Substantiated or implied? *Career Development for Exceptional Individuals, 16*, 107–121.

Kounin, J.S. (1970). Observing and delineating technique of managing behavior in classrooms. *Journal of Research & Development in Education, 4*(1), 62–72.

Ladson-Billings, G. (1997). Crafting a culturally relevant social studies approach. In E.W. Ross (Ed.), *The social studies curriculum: Purposes, problems, and possibilities* (pp. 123–135). Albany, NY: State University of New York.

Landers, D.M. (1994). Performance, stress, and health: Overall reaction. *Quest, 46*(1), 123–135.

Lane, H., Hoffmeister, R., & Bahan, B. (1996). *A journey into the Deaf-World*. San Diego, CA: DawnSignPress.

Lane, S., Bell, L., & Parson-Tylka, T. (1997). *My turn to learn: A communication guide for parents of deaf or hard of hearing children*. Surrey, BC: Elks Family Hearing.

Lang, H.G. (1994). *Silence of the spheres: The deaf experience in the history of science*. Westport, CT: Bergin & Garvey.

Lang, H.G. (2000). *A phone of our own: The Deaf insurrection against Ma Bell*. Washington, DC: Gallaudet University Press.

Lang, H.G., & Albertini, J.A. (2000). *The role of writing in the construction of meaning: A study with deaf students in science*. Section of Final Report to the National Science Foundation on Grant No. HRD-9550468.

Lang, H.G., & Meath-Lang, B. (1985). *The attitudes of hearing-impaired students toward science: Implications for teachers*. Paper presented at the Convention of American Instructors of the Deaf, St. Augustine, FL, June.

Lang, H.G., & Meath-Lang, B. (1995). *Deaf persons in the arts and sciences*. Westport, CT: Greenwood.

Lang, H.G., & Propp, G. (1982). Science education for hearing impaired students: State of the art. *American Annals of the Deaf, 127*(7), 860–869.

LaSasso, C., & Metzger, M. (1998). An alternate route for preparing deaf children for BiBi programs: The home language as L1 and Cued Speech for conveying traditionally spoken languages. *Journal of Deaf Studies and Deaf Education*, *3*(4), 265–289.

LaSasso, C., & Mobley, R. (1998). National survey of reading instruction for deaf or hard-of-hearing students in the United States. *Volta Review*, *99*(1), 31–58.

Leu, D., & Leu, D. (1999). *Teaching with the Internet: Lessons from the classroom*. Norwood, MA: Christopher-Gordon.

Lindsey, D., & O'Neal, J. (1976). Static and dynamic balance skills of eight-year-old deaf and hard of hearing children. *American Annals of the Deaf, 121*, 49–55.

Lochner, P., & McNamara, B. (1989, April). *Meeting the needs of the atypical learner*. Paper presented at the annual convention of the C.E.C., Toronto, Ontario, Canada.

Luckner, J. (1991). Competencies critical to teachers of students with hearing impairments. *Teacher Education and Special Education, 13*(2), 135–139.

Luckner, J., & Denzin, P. (1998). In the mainstream: Adaptations for students who are deaf or hard of hearing. *Perspectives in Education & Deafness, 17*(1), 8–11.

Luckner, J., & Miller, K. (1994). Itinerant teachers: Responsibilities, perceptions, preparation, and students served. *American Annals of the Deaf, 139* (2),111–118.

Luetke-Stahlman, B. (1999a). *Language across the curriculum: When students are deaf or hard of hearing* (pp. 485–486).

Luetke-Stahlman, B. (1999b). *Language issues in deaf education*. Hillsboro, OR: Butte.

Hillsboro, OR: Butte Publications.

Luetke-Stahlman, B., & Luckner, J. (1991). *Effectively educating students with hearing impairments*. White Plains, NY: Longman.

Lynch, E., & Stein, R. (1987). Parent participation by ethnicity: A comparison of Hispanic, Black, and Anglo families. *Exceptional Children, 54*(2), 105–111.

Madaus, G.F. (1993). A national testing system: Manna from above. *Educational Assessment, 1*(1), 9–26.

Mahshie, S. (1995). *Educating deaf children bilingually*. Washington, DC: Gallaudet University Pre-College Programs.

Markowicz, H., & Berdichevsky, C. (1998) *Bridging the gap between research and practice in the fields of learning disabilities and deafness*. Gallaudet University: College for Continuing Education, Washington D.C. Resource Centre.

Marlowe, B. (1991). Learning disabilities and deafness: Do short-term sequential memory deficits provide the key? In D.S. Martin (Ed.), *Advances in cognition, education, deafness* (pp. 279–288). Washington, DC: Gallaudet University Press.

Marschark, M. (1997). *Raising and educating a deaf child*. New York: Oxford University Press.

Martinez, E. (1993). Parenting young children in Mexican American/Chicano families. In H.P. McAdoo (Ed.), *Family ethnicity*. London: Sage.

Mathison, S. (1994). Assessment in social studies: Moving toward authenticity. In E.W. Ross (Ed.), *The social studies curriculum: Purposes, problems, and possibilities* (pp. 213–224). Albany, NY: State University of New York Press.

Mauk, G.W., & Mauk, P.P. (1998). Considerations, conceptualizations, and challenges in the study of concomitant learning disabilities among children and adolescents who are deaf or hard of hearing. *Journal of Deaf Studies and Deaf Education, 3*(1), 15–34.

McNamara, B. (1998) *Learning disabilities*. Albany, NY: State University of New York Press.

Meadow-Orlans, K.P. (1987). Understanding deafness: Socialization of children and youth. In P. Higgins & J. Nash (Eds.), *Understanding deafness socially* (pp. 29–58). Springfield, IL: Charles C. Thomas.

Medina, C., Jones, D., & Miller, S. (1998). *Traditional versus contemporary Navajo views of special education*. Paper presented at American Council on Rural Special Education (Charleston, SC, March 25–28).

Medwid, D., & Weston, D.C. (1995). *Kid-friendly parenting with deaf and hard of hearing children*. Washington, DC: Clerc Books.

Michigan Department of Education. (1996). *Michigan curriculum framework*. Lansing, MI: Author.

Miller-Lachmann, L. (1995). *Global voices, global visions: A core collection of multicultural books*. New Providence, NJ: R. R. Bowker.

Miller-Nomeland, M., & Gillespie, S. (1993). *Deaf studies curriculum guide*. Washington, DC: Gallaudet University Pre-College Programs.

Moores, D. F. (1992). An historical perspective on school placement. In T.N. Kluwin, D.F. Moores, & M.M. Gaustad, (Eds.), *Defining the effective public school program for deaf students*. New York: Teachers College Press.

Moores, D.F. (1996). *Educating the deaf: Psychology, principles, and practices* (4th ed.). Boston: Houghton Mifflin.

Moores, D., Kluwin, T., & Mertens, D. (1985). *High school program for deaf students in metropolitan areas*. Gallaudet Research Institute Monograph No.3, Washington, DC: Gallaudet University.

Morningstar, M. (1997). Critical issues in career development and employment preparation for adolescents with disabilities. *Remedial and Special Education, 18*(3), 307–320.

Morrison, G., Lowther, D., & DeMeulle, L. (1999). *Integrating computer technology into the classroom*. Upper Saddle River, NJ: Merrill.

National Academy of Science-National Research Council. (1996). *National Science Education Standards*. Washington, DC: National Academy Press.

National Science Resource Center. (1997). *Science for all children*. National Academy Press.

Neiss, M. (1992, March). Winds of change. *The Computing Teacher*, 32–35.

Padden, C., & Humphries, T. (1988). *Deaf in America: Voices from a culture*. Cambridge, MA: Harvard University.

Padden, C., & Ramsey, C. (1993). Deaf culture and literacy. *American Annals of the Deaf, 138*(2), 96–99.

Pagliaro, C.M. (1998). Mathematics preparation and professional development of deaf education teachers. *American Annals of the Deaf, 143*(5), 373–379.

Parker, R. (1994). *Desktop publishing and design for dummies*. Foster City, CA: IDG Books Worldwide.

Patton, J.R., Cronin, M.E., & Jairrels, V. (1997). Curricular implications of transition: Life skills instruction as an integral part of transition education. *Remedial and Special Education, 18*(3), 294–306.

Paul, P. (1998). *Literacy and deafness: The development of reading, writing, and literate thought*. Boston: Allyn & Bacon.

Perkins, D. (1992). *Smart schools: Better thinking and learning for every child*. New York: The Free Press.

Porter, K.F., & Bradley, S. (1985). A comparison of three speech intelligibility measures for deaf students. *American Annals of the Deaf, 130*(6), 514–525.

Powers, A.R., & Elliott, R. Jr. (1990). Preparation of teachers who serve hearing impaired students with additional mild handicaps. *Teacher Education and Special Education, 13*(3), 200–202.

Powers, A.R., & Hibbet, C. (1998). A framework for selecting instructional strategies for learners who are deaf or hard of hearing and mildly learning disabled, mentally retarded, and/or behaviorally disordered. In H. Markowicz & C. Berdichevsky (Eds.), *Bridging the gap between research and practice in the fields of learning disabilities and deafness*. Washington, DC: Gallaudet University, College for Continuing Education.

Ravitch, R. (1995). *National standards in American education*. Washington, DC: Brookings Institute.

Reed, C.M. (1990). An I-Search quest. *Perspectives in Education and Deafness, 9*(2), 10–12.

Reed, R. (1987). Process approach to developing language with hearing impaired children: An overview. *Teaching English to Deaf and Second-Language Students, 5*(3) 1–9.

Rios, A. (1990). *The Hispanic family: The decade of change*. Paper presented at the Annual Wisconsin Conference on the Hispanic Family (Milwaukee, WI, November 2).

Roerden, L. (1997). *Net lesson: Web-based projects for your classroom*. Sebastopol, CA: O'Reilly & Associates.

Ross, E.W. (Ed.). (1997). *The social studies curriculum: Purposes, problems, and possibilities*. Albany, NY: State University of New York.

Rumelhart, D. (1977). Toward an interactive model of reading. In S. Dornic (Ed.), *Attention and performance VI*. Hillsdale, NJ: Erlbaum.

Sammann, P. (1998). *Active youth: Ideas for implementing CDC physical activity promotion guidelines*. Champaign, IL: Human Kinetics.

Schein, J.D. (1989). *At home among strangers*. Washington, DC: Gallaudet University.

Schein, J.D., & Stewart, D.A. (1995). *Language in motion: Exploring the nature of signs*. Washington, DC: Gallaudet University.

Schildroth, A., & Hotto, S. (1993). Annual survey of hearing-impaired children and youth: 1991–92 school year. *American Annals of the Deaf, 138*(2), 163–168.

Schildroth, A.N., & Karchmer, M.A. (1986). *Deaf children in America*. San Diego, CA: College-Hill.

Schirmer, B.R. (1994). *Language and literacy development in children who are deaf*. New York : Merrill.

Schleper, D. (1996). Talking about books. *Perspectives in Education and Deafness, 14*(3), 7–10.

Schleper, D.R. (1997). *Reading to deaf children: Learning from deaf adults* (pp. 3–4). Washington, DC: Pre-College National Mission Programs.

Schmidt, W.H., McKnight, C.C., Cogan, L.S., Jakwerth, P.M., & Houang, R.T. (1999). *Facing the consequences: Using TIMSS for a closer look at U.S. mathematics and science education*. Boston: Kluwer Academics.

Schmidt, W.H., McKnight, C.C., & Raizen, S.A. (1997). *A splintered vision: An investigation of U.S. science and mathematics education*. Boston: Kluwer Academics.

Scott, J. (1992). *Science language and links*. Portsmouth, NH: Heinemann.

Seal, B.C. (1998). *Best practices in educational interpreting*. Boston: Allyn & Bacon.

Shelly, G., Chasman, T., Forsythe, S. (1998). *Corel Word Perfect 7: Complete concepts and techniques*. Cambridge, MA: Course Technology.

Shelly, G., Chasman, T., Green, S., Boetcher, M., & Sebok, S. (1998). *Microsoft Power Point 97: Complete concepts and techniques*. Cambridge, MA: Course Technology.

Sherrill, C. (1993). *Adapted physical activity, recreation and sport: Cross disciplinary and lifespan* (4th ed.). Madison, WI: Brown & Benchmark.

Shulman, L. (1987). Knowledge and teaching: Foundations of the new reform. *Harvard Educational Review, 57*, 1–22.

Siedentop, D. (1998). *Introduction to physical education, fitness and sport* (3rd ed.). Mountain View, CA: Mayfield.

Sperry, R.W. (1973). Lateral specialization of cerebral function in the surgically separated hemispheres. In F.J. McGuigan & R.A. Schoonover (Eds.), *The psychophysiology of thinking* (pp. 209–229). New York: Academic.

Stahl, R.J. (Ed.). (1994a). *Cooperative learning in social studies: A handbook for the teacher*. Menlo Park, CA: Addison-Wesley.

Stahl, R.J. (1994b). Cooperative learning: A social studies context and an overview. In R.J. Stahl (Ed.), *Cooperative learning in social studies: A handbook for teacher* (pp. 1–17). Menlo Park, CA: Addison-Wesley.

Stanley, W.B., & Nelson, J.L. (1994). The foundations of social education in historical context. In W.B. Stanley (Ed.), *Review of research in social studies education: 1976–1983* (pp. 309–399). New York: St. Martin's.

Stanovich, K. (1980). Toward an interactive-compensatory model of individual differences in the development of reading fluency. *Reading Research Quarterly, 16*, 32–71.

Statewide Transition Project. (1995). *Fundamentals of transition*. Lansing, MI: Michigan Department of Education, Office of Special Education.

Staton, J. (1984). *Student attitudes toward dialogue journals* (Dialogue Journal Project, report #3). Washington, DC: Linguistics Research Laboratory, Gallaudet College.

Stewart, D. (1995). Bi-Bi to MCE? *American Annals of the Deaf, 138*, 331–337.

Stewart, D. (1998). *American Sign Language the easy way*. Hauppauge, NY: Barron's Educational Series.

Stewart, D., Bennett, D., & Bonkowski, N. (1992, January/February). Books to read, books to sign. *Perspectives in Education and Deafness, 10*(3), 4–7.

Stewart, D.A. (1991). *Deaf sport: The impact of sports within the Deaf community*. Washington, DC: Gallaudet University Press.

Stewart, D.A. (1992). Toward effective use of ASL in the classroom. In M. Walworth, D.F. Moores, & T.J. O'Rourke (Eds.), *A free hand* (pp. 89–118). Silver Springs, MD: TJ Publishers.

Stewart, D.A., & Ellis, M.K. (1999). Physical education for deaf students. *American Annals of the Deaf, 144*(4), 315–319.

Stewart, D.A., & Hollifield, A. (1988). A model for team teaching: Using American Sign Language and English. *Perspectives for Teachers of the Hearing Impaired, 6*, 15–18.

Stewart, D.A., & Luetke-Stahlman, B. (1998). *The signing family: What every parent should know about sign communication*. Washington, DC: Clerc Books.

Stewart, D.A., McCarthy, D., & Robinson, J. (1988). Participation in Deaf sport: Characteristics of Deaf sport directors. *Adapted Physical Activity Quarterly, 5*, 233–244.

Stewart, D.A., Robinson, J., & McCarthy, D. (1991). Participation in Deaf sport: Characteristics of elite deaf athletes. *Adapted Physical Activity Quarterly, 8*, 233–244.

Stewart, D.A., Schein, J.D., & Cartwright, B. (1998). *Sign language interpreting: Exploring its art and science*. Boston: Allyn & Bacon.

Stewart, D.A., & Stinson, M.S. (1992). The role of sport and extracurricular activities in shaping socialization patterns. In T.N. Kluwin, D.F. Moores, & M.G. Gaustad (Eds.), *Toward effective public school programs for deaf students* (pp. 129–148). New York: Teachers College Press.

Stinson, M. (1994). Affective and social development. In R.C. Nowell & L.E. Marshak (Eds.), *Understanding deafness and the rehabilitation process*. Boston: Allyn & Bacon.

Stinson, M.S., & Whitmire, K. (1992). Students' views of their social relationship. In T.N. Kluwin, D.F. Moores, & M.G. Gaustad (Eds.), *Toward effective public school programs for deaf students* (pp. 149–174). New York: Teachers College Press.

Stokoe, W. (1960) Sign language structure: An outline of the visual communication systems of the American Deaf. *Studies in Linguistics: Occasional Papers 8*, Revised 1978, Silver Spring, MD: Linstok Press.

Strong, C., & Clark, T., Berliner, D., Walden, B., & Williams, S. (1992). *SKI*HI home-based programming for children who are deaf or hard of hearing: Project report.* Logan, UT: Dept. of Communicative Disorders, Utah State University.

Strong, C.J. (1992). *SKI*HI home-based programming for children with hearing impairments.* Project Report. Dept. of Communicative Disorders, Utah State University, Logan, UT.

Suggs, T. (1999, July). NC administrator calls ASL "Child Abuse." *DeafNation, 4*(10), 1, 8.

Swenson, A. (1995). Itinerant teaching: An insider's view. *RE:view, 27*(3), 113–116.

Toliver, P., & Kellog, C. (1997). *PC's for teachers* (2nd. ed.). Foster City, CA: IDG Books Worldwide.

Townsend, J. (1996). Big books: Links to literacy for everyone. *Perspectives in Education and Deafness, 14*(3), 23–24.

Traxler, C.B. (1996). Frequently asked questions about the Stanford Achievement Test. [World Wide Web document: URL:http://www.gallaudet.edu/~catraxle/sat-faq.html.].

Treanor, L., & Housner, L. (1999). Shaping up physical evaluation. *The Education Digest, 64*(9), 58–61.

U.S. Equal Opportunity Commission. (1991). *Americans with Disabilities Act handbook.* Washington, DC: United States Government Printing Office.

U.S. Public Health Service. (1991). *Healthy People 2000: National health promotion and disease prevention objectives* (DDHS Publication No. PHS 91-50212). Washington, DC: U.S. Government Printing Office.

Van Vuuren, E. (1995). *The deaf pupil with learning disabilities.* ERIC Document Service. ED392177.

Vargo, S. (1998). Consulting: Teacher-to-teacher. *Teaching Exceptional Children, 30*(3), 54–55.

Vernon, M., & Andrews, J.F. (1990). *The psychology of deafness.* New York, Longman.

Voltz, D., & Elliot, R. (1990). Resource room teacher roles in promoting interaction with regular educators. *Teacher Education and Special Education, 13*(3–4), 160–166.

Wang, M.C., Haertel, G.D., & Walberg, H.J. (December, 1993). What helps students learn? *Educational Leadership, 51*(4), 74–79.

Wehman, R., Moon, M.S., Everson, J.M., Wood, W., & Barcus, J.M. (1988). *Transition from school to work: New challenges for youth with severe disabilities.* Baltimore, MD: Paul H. Brookes.

Wilkinson, D. (1993). Family ethnicity in America. In H.P. McAdoo (Ed.), *Family ethnicity.* London: Sage.

Wilmore, J.P., & Costill, D.L. (1994). *Physiology of sport and exercise.* Champaign, IL: Human Kinetics.

Wortham, A. (1992, September). Afrocentrism isn't the answer for black students in American society. *Executive Educator, 14*, 23–25

Wright, M.H. (1999). *Sounds like home: Growing up black and deaf in the south.* Washington, DC: Gallaudet University.

Yore, L.D. (2000). Enhancing science literacy for all students with embedded reading instruction and writing-to-learn activities. *Journal of Deaf Studies and Deaf Education, 5*(1), 105–122

INDEX